Textbook for Dental Nurses

Textbook for Dental Nurses

H. LEVISON
BDS ULond; FDS, DOrthRCSEng.
Emeritus Examiner,
National Examining Board for
Dental Nurses

EIGHTH EDITION

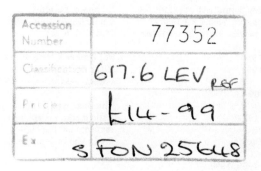

b

Blackwell
Science

© 1960, 1963, 1969, 1971, 1978, 1985, 1991,
1997
Blackwell Science Ltd
Editorial Offices:
Osney Mead, Oxford OX2 0EL
25 John Street, London WC1N 2BL
23 Ainslie Place, Edinburgh EH3 6AJ
350 Main Street, Malden
  MA 02148 5018, USA
54 University Street, Carlton
  Victoria 3053, Australia
10, rue Casimir Delavigne
  75006 Paris, France

Other Editorial Offices:
Blackwell Wissenschafts-Verlag GmbH
Kurfürstendamm 57
10707 Berlin, Germany

Blackwell Science KK
MG Kodenmacho Building
7–10 Kodenmacho Nihombashi
Chuo-ku, Tokyo 104, Japan

The right of the Author to be
identified as the Author of this Work
has been asserted in accordance
with the Copyright, Designs and
Patents Act 1988.

First published 1960
Second edition 1963
Reprinted 1966
Third edition 1969
Fourth edition 1971
Reprinted 1973, 1977
Fifth edition 1978
Reprinted 1982 (twice)
Sixth edition 1985
Reprinted 1988, 1989, 1990
Seventh edition 1991
Reprinted 1992, 1993, 1994, 1995, 1996
Eighth edition 1997
Reprinted 1998, 1999 (twice)

Set in 10 on 12 pt Melior
by DP Photosetting, Aylesbury, Bucks
Printed and bound in the United Kingdom
at the University Press, Cambridge

DISTRIBUTORS
Marston Book Services Ltd
PO Box 269
Abingdon, Oxon OX14 4YN
(Orders: Tel: 01235 465500
       Fax: 01235 465555)

USA
Blackwell Science, Inc.
Commerce Place
350 Main Street
Malden, MA 02148 5018
(Orders: Tel: 800 759 6102
              781 388 8250
       Fax: 781 388 8255)

Canada
Login Brothers Book Company
324 Saulteaux Crescent
Winnipeg, Manitoba R3J 3T2
(Orders: Tel: 204 837 2987
       Fax: 204 837 3116)

Australia
Blackwell Science Pty Ltd
54 University Street
Carlton, Victoria 3053
(Orders: Tel: 03 9347 0300
       Fax: 03 9347 5001)

A catalogue record for this title
is available from the British Library

ISBN 0–632–04031-9

Library of Congress
Cataloging-in-Publication Data
is available

For further information on
Blackwell Science, visit our website:
www.blackwell-science.com

The Blackwell Science logo is a
trade mark of Blackwell Science Ltd,
registered at the United Kingdom
Trade Marks Registry

Contents

Introduction

To the Eighth Edition

The seventh edition was written in 1990 and significant changes of importance to the dental team since then are likely to lead to implementation of even greater changes by the opening years of the next millennium.

This edition maintains the intentions mentioned in the introduction to the first edition; and also acts as an introduction to post-qualification certificates, none of which existed at that time. The text has accordingly been updated to cover the latest changes. They include more health and safety legislation; additional advice to dentists from the General Dental Council; the recommendations of the Poswillo Report and its effect on provision of general anaesthesia and sedation in dental practice; some simplification of the administrative structure of the National Health Service; and advances in dental materials technology.

For their help in the provision of new diagrams, information and material for this edition I am indebted to the National Examining Board for Dental Nurses; Dentsply Ltd, Portex Ltd, Kodak Ltd, Nobel Biocare; David Craig, Associate Specialist in Dental Sedation, Guy's Hospital; my sister, Mrs B. Tobias BDS, MSc; and Blackwell Science.

To the First Edition

This book is designed to cover the syllabus for the British Dental Nurses and Assistants Examination. Although written primarily for nurses preparing for this examination, it also provides an outline of dental surgery for those embarking on a career of dental nursing; thus helping them gain a greater understanding of the nature and aims of their duties. For examination purposes, the subject matter is deliberately presented in a dogmatic fashion and, to aid final revision, there is a summary after each chapter.

The text was prepared during a winter spent in the North Isles of Shetland with the School Health Service mobile dental unit; and for helpful advice and encouragement throughout, I am indebted to my former dental nurse, Miss M.E. Isbister. I wish to thank my wife for typing the manuscript; my sister, Miss B. Levison, for the drawings; the Amalgamated Dental Trade Distributors Ltd for providing some new blocks; and Mr P. Saugman of Blackwell Science for his guidance.

H. Levison

Abbreviations

ABC	airway, breathing, circulation
AIDS	acquired immune deficiency syndrome
ANUG	acute necrotizing ulcerative gingivitis
APF	acidulated phosphate fluoride
BADN	British Association of Dental Nurses
BDA	British Dental Association
BDJ	British Dental Journal
BDS	Bachelor of Dental Surgery
BNF	British National Formulary
COSHH	control of substances hazardous to health
CPITN	community periodontal index of treatment needs
CPR	cardiopulmonary resuscitation
DDPH	Diploma in Dental Public Health
DDR	Diploma in Dental Radiology
DGDP	Diploma in General Dental Practice
DMF	decayed, missing, filled
DNSTAB	Dental Nurses Standards and Training Advisory Board
do	distal occlusal
DPB	Dental Practice Board
DPF	Dental Practitioners' Formulary
DPT	dental panoramic tomograph
DRO	dental reference officer
EAR	expired air respiration
ECC	external cardiac compression
ECG	electrocardiogram
EDH	Enrolled Dental Hygienist
EDT	Enrolled Dental Therapist
EOT	extra-oral traction
F/	full upper denture
F/F	full upper and lower dentures
/F	lower full denture
FDI	International Dental Federation
FDS	Fellow in Dental Surgery
FGC	full gold crown
GA	general anaesthesia
GDC	General Dental Council
GI	gold inlay
GIC	glass ionomer cement
GP	gutta-percha
HA	health authority

HBV	hepatitis B virus
HIV	human immunodeficiency virus
IV	intravenous
LA	local anaesthesia (analgesia)
LDS	Licentiate in Dental Surgery
MCCD	Member in Clinical Community Dentistry
MDS	Master of Dental Surgery
MGDS	Member in General Dental Surgery
MIMS	Monthly Index of Medical Specialities
mo	mesial occlusal
mod	mesial occlusal distal
MOrth	Member in Orthodontics
MRD	Member in Restorative Dentistry
MSc	Master of Science
NEBDN	National Examining Board for Dental Nurses
NHS	National Health Service
NRPB	National Radiological Protection Board
NSAID	non-steroidal anti-inflammatory drug
OPG	dental panoramic tomograph (orthopantomograph)
P/	partial upper denture
P/P	partial upper and lower dentures
/P	partial lower denture
PBC	porcelain bonded crown
PE	partially erupted
PJC	porcelain jacket crown
PoM	prescription-only medicine
ppm	parts per million
PV	porcelain veneer
RA	relative analgesia
RDN	Registered Dental Nurse
RPA	radiation protection advisor
RPS	radiation protection supervisor
UE	unerupted
ZOE	zinc oxide and eugenol cement

1 Structure of the Dental Profession

The dentist

Dentists undergo a period of training at a University Dental School which lasts five years. On passing their final examinations students are awarded the degree of Bachelor of Dental Surgery (BDS) or the Licence in Dental Surgery (LDS). But they cannot use the title of dentist or practise the profession until their names have been entered in **The Dentists Register**.

The register is kept by the **General Dental Council** and contains the name, address and qualification of every person legally entitled to practise dentistry in the United Kingdom. Such persons may describe themselves as dentist, dental surgeon or dental practitioner. There is no difference between these titles. Dentists may also use the courtesy title of Doctor but must not imply that they are anything other than dentists. Following qualification all dentists are ethically obliged to continue their professional education for the duration of practice, in order to maintain and update their skills.

Registered dentists have a wide choice of opportunities within the profession: general practice, community dental service, hospital service, university teaching and research, industrial dental service and the armed forces. They may also take additional higher qualifications and become specialists in a particular branch of dentistry. Some examples of higher dental qualifications are the degree of Master of Dental Surgery (MDS) and the Fellowship in Dental Surgery (FDS). It is also possible to obtain extra qualifications in many dental specialities, for example:

- Master of Science (MSc) in a speciality
- Membership in Orthodontics (MOrth)
- Membership in General Dental Surgery (MGDS)
- Membership in Clinical Community Dentistry (MCCD)
- Membership in Restorative Dentistry (MRD)
- Diploma in Dental Public Health (DDPH)
- Diploma in Dental Radiology (DDR)
- Diploma in General Dental Practice (DGDP)

General Dental Council

The General Dental Council (GDC) is the governing body of the dental profession and its duties are set out in the **Dentists Act**. These duties

are to promote high standards of professional education and professional conduct among dentists. It thereby ensures that the status of the
profession in the community is upheld and that a proper code of
conduct is maintained for the protection of the public.

In performance of these duties the GDC must be satisfied that
courses of study at dental schools and the qualifying examinations are
adequate, and the same applies to postgraduate education.

It is the policy of the GDC for all dentists, after qualification, to
serve a period of vocational training before starting independent
practice. Such training schemes are already in force in National
Health Service general practice, the community and hospital services;
and also on a voluntary basis in private practice. As soon as adequate
resources and facilities are available, it will be mandatory for all
dentists to undergo vocational training after qualification.

The GDC is empowered to remove or suspend from the register any
dentist who has been convicted of a criminal offence or is guilty of
serious professional misconduct. It may also suspend any dentist
whose fitness to practise is seriously impaired because of physical or
mental condition.

Apart from registered dentists, the only other persons permitted to
undertake dental treatment are **dental hygienists** and **dental therapists**. The GDC is responsible for these auxiliary workers in much the
same way as for dentists. After qualification they must be enrolled by
the GDC and the strictly limited range of dental treatment which they
are permitted to undertake is laid down in the Dental Auxiliaries
Regulations.

The dental team

Dentists' training enables them to undertake, without assistance, all
treatment necessary for patients, including construction of their
dentures, crowns and bridges, etc. Except for the actual treatment
performed within the mouth, however, much of the work which a
dentist is qualified to do can be performed by others. For example, a
chairside **dental nurse** provides an extra pair of hands for preparing
and mixing filling and impression materials, and for helping with
suction, retraction and illumination to keep the operative field clear
and dry for the dentist and comfortable for the patient. A **dental
technician** can make dentures, crowns and bridges ready for the
dentist to fit; while dental hygienists and therapists are permitted to
undertake limited forms of dental treatment.

By utilizing all this assistance, a dentist becomes the captain of a
team which can practise in the most efficient way. Dentists carry out
all the treatment which they alone can perform, while the other
members of the team – hygienist, therapist, nurses and technician –

perform all the work which a dentist can delegate. Compared with a single-handed dentist, the dental team can provide far more treatment each day with less effort and fatigue for all concerned, and thereby give a better total service to the patient and the community.

Dental hygienist

After two years training at a dental hospital, or in the armed forces, hygienists are awarded a Diploma in Dental Hygiene. They may be employed in general practice and in the public health service, and are permitted to carry out the following dental work, prescribed in writing and directed by a dentist:

1   Cleaning and polishing teeth
2   Scaling teeth
3   Application of fluorides and fissure sealants

Hygienists may administer local infiltration analgesia for scaling but this is only permitted under direct personal supervision by a dentist on the premises. Apart from their treatment role, hygienists are also trained to be proficient dental health educators.

Dental therapist

Dental therapists are auxiliary dental workers who have completed a two-year course at a dental hospital. They are awarded a Diploma in Dental Therapy and are permitted to carry out the following treatment on patients attending community dental service or hospital clinics.

1   Cleaning and polishing teeth
2   Scaling teeth
3   Application of fluorides and fissure sealants
4   Simple fillings
5   Extraction of deciduous teeth

Therapists may administer local infiltration analgesia for extractions, fillings and scaling. All treatment must be prescribed in writing by a dentist and carried out under the dentist's direction.

Prior experience as dental nurses and possession of their National Certificate (see page 17) is the preferred requirement for admission to dental hospital training courses for hygienists and therapists. All dental hospitals provide the two-year course for hygienists but only two offer courses for therapists: the University of Wales has a two-year course; the Royal London Hospital has a slightly longer course for dual qualification as hygienist and therapist. As with hygienists, an important part of their role is dental health education.

Dental technician

Dental technicians are highly skilled craftsmen who construct dentures, crowns, bridges, inlays, orthodontic appliances, splints and replacements for fractured or diseased parts of the face and jaws. They work to the dentist's prescription in a dental laboratory. Training consists of a full-time course in a dental hospital or technical college; or by an apprenticeship with part-time attendance at a technical college. Technicians are not allowed to undertake any form of dental treatment.

Dental nurse

The role of dental nurses, their duties and training facilities are covered in the next chapter.

The National Health Service

Dental treatment in the United Kingdom is either provided privately or through the National Health Service (NHS). Private patients obtain treatment from a practitioner of their choice; and pay a fee to the practitioner for professional services given. NHS dental treatment differs from private practice in the range of treatment provided and the method of payment for such treatment. Certain types of treatment available in private practice are restricted in the NHS; while payments to the dentist are controlled by the State, with patients' contributions ranging from nil to a set maximum.

The cost of the NHS is borne by the State, and the government department responsible for it is the Department of Health. This delegates operational management of the Service to the NHS Executive. For administrative purposes the country is divided into a large number of health districts. Each district is called a **health authority** (HA) and contains hospitals, community clinics and general practitioner services. These services are grouped locally into NHS trusts funded by the HA.

Hospital and community service staff are employees of their NHS trust, but NHS general medical and dental practitioners are self-employed independent contractors.

Community dental service

This was formerly called the school dental service, providing examination and treatment for children and expectant and nursing mothers. It still meets the same needs but has acquired additional responsibilities. These vary according to local demand but can include treatment for handicapped patients of all ages; treatment of the elderly; provision of general anaesthetic facilities and orthodontic treatment for patients of general practitioners; and dental health programmes for the community at large.

The community dental service is administered by the NHS trust and co-operates with hospital staff and general practitioners in planning and co-ordinating all dental services in the district. Salaried community dental officers provide treatment in clinics with equipment and materials supplied by the trust.

Hospital dental service

Hospitals are administered by an NHS trust. Dental services are provided by the consultant oral surgeon and consultant orthodontist. They give specialist advice and treatment for patients referred by practitioners outside the hospital; and for patients referred from other departments of the hospital. They are also in overall charge of dental care for long-stay in-patients. In addition, most consultants provide postgraduate courses and part-time training posts for general practitioners.

General dental service

This is the general practitioner service which provides much of the dental treatment in this country. It is administered by the local HA which holds dentists' contracts and is responsible for NHS disciplinary procedures.

The **Dental Practice Board** (DPB) authorizes payment of treatment fees to practitioners. It can also arrange for patients to be examined by its dental reference officers (DROs).

General practitioners set up and equip their practices at their own expense and are entitled to have private patients as well as NHS patients.

British Dental Association

The British Dental Association (BDA) is the professional body representing the majority of dentists in the United Kingdom. It publishes the British Dental Journal (BDJ) and negotiates for the profession with the government and other bodies where dental interests are concerned. Membership of the BDA is voluntary and open to all dentists.

Summary

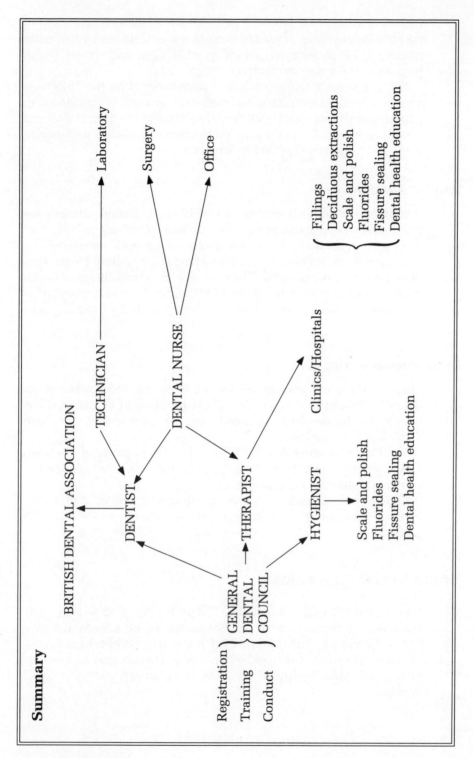

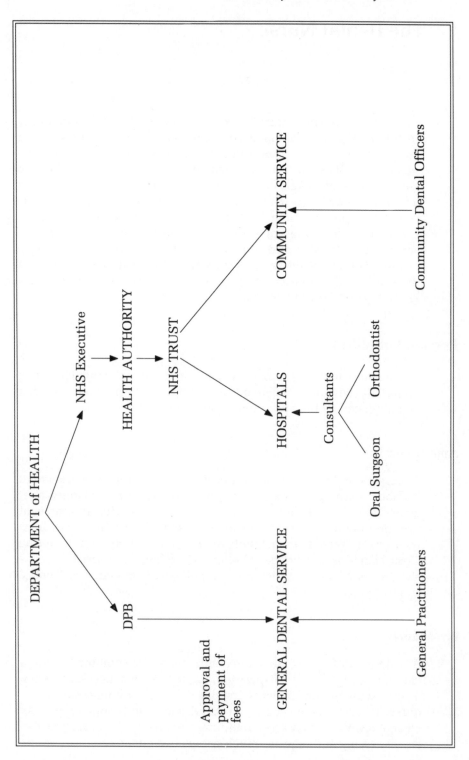

2   The Dental Nurse

Employers requiring a nurse look for the following attributes: ability to communicate; common sense; friendliness; sense of loyalty and responsibility; and awareness that the first priority in a practice is the patient. Of these attributes, common sense and the ability to communicate are likely to be regarded as far more important than academic knowledge. However, a command of written English is essential as poor grammar and spelling reflect badly on a practice.

Although the duties of a nurse vary from practice to practice, according to its size and number of staff employed, they may be classified under the headings of surgery and office duties. To perform these efficiently, nurses must possess certain personal qualities and a knowledge of the law and dental ethics.

Personal qualities

The nurse is usually the first person to receive a patient. This is an important occasion as a patient's confidence in the practice may well be influenced by the appearance and manner of the nurse.

Appearance

A nurse should be smartly dressed without going to extremes of fashion. Attention to personal hygiene is essential, not only as it affects appearance, but also to ensure good results and prevent infection in the surgery. Hair should be short, or secured away from the face, to prevent contact with working areas or equipment during close chairside assistance. Similarly, jewellery and wrist watches should not be worn as they can be unhygienic or liable to damage surgical gloves.

Personality

A calm, courteous and sympathetic manner, combined with a cheerful and friendly disposition, is an obvious necessity when dealing with anxious patients. It will gain their confidence; allow the nurse to keep cool under all conditions, and cope with any emergency which may arise. Handling patients in a busy practice can be very trying and requires much patience and tact.

Speech

The voice must be calm to inspire confidence; and clear enough to be understood on the telephone. Instructions to patients should be given in simple language to avoid misunderstanding.

Concentration

This requires an alert mind and attention to detail. Mistakes must not be made in patients' records, appointments, telephone messages, assisting with treatment or dealing with emergencies.

Punctuality

The smooth running of a busy practice depends on the staff and patients keeping appointments on time. Nurses must set an example by strict punctuality on duty.

The law

All nurses are affected directly or indirectly by two enactments: the Dentists Act, referred to in the previous chapter, and the *Health and Safety at Work Act*, which is covered in Chapter 31.

Dentists Act

Under the Act, the General Dental Council is given the important function of maintaining high standards of professional conduct among dentists, hygienists and therapists, with responsibility to their patients as the first priority. Anyone found guilty of a criminal offence or serious professional misconduct is liable to be removed or suspended from the register kept by the GDC, and is thereby legally forbidden to practise. This does not, of course, apply to nurses; but dentists may be held responsible for any acts or omissions of their staff. It is therefore necessary for nurses to know of the legal and ethical obligations in dental practice.

A dentist found guilty by the GDC of the following types of unprofessional conduct is liable to be struck off the register.

Illegal practice

Dentists commit this offence if they enable unqualified people to give dental treatment. They must not allow nurses to do dental work which is not permitted by law. The only people entitled to provide dental treatment are those registered with the GDC: which means dentists, dental hygienists and dental therapists only. It is illegal for dental nurses and technicians to carry out any work in a patient's mouth.

Nurses are not allowed to take X-rays unless they have been specially trained for this purpose. Further details are given in this chapter and in Chapter 29.

A dentist may delegate to a nurse the responsibility for giving patients instruction in oral hygiene, provided:

1 the dentist is satisfied that the nurse is fully competent to do so
2 it is understood that the dentist is personally responsible for whatever instruction is given

Alcohol and drugs

This includes drunkenness and abuse of drugs. There are strict legal rules for dentists relating to the purchase, storage, prescription and use of dangerous drugs (Chapter 11). Dentists must not abuse the privileges conferred upon them under the law. Nurses must strictly obey the dentist's instructions on the care and use of drugs.

False certification

A dentist must never sign, or allow a nurse to sign, or induce a patient to sign, any untrue or improper document or certificate. This includes false certification and improperly seeking fees under the NHS Acts. Special care is necessary in practices where both NHS and private treatment are provided. Patients must not be induced to accept private treatment by a false suggestion that similar treatment could not be carried out under the NHS.

Nurses should know that the dentist is held responsible for ensuring that a patient clearly understands whether treatment is being provided under the NHS or privately. All patients should be given an estimate of the cost of treatment, preferably in writing. If a patient indicates to the nurse any uncertainty or confusion about costs or whether treatment is being provided under the NHS or privately, the dentist must always be informed.

Advertising

The GDC stipulates that practice publicity and advertising material must be legal, decent, truthful and devoid of any unprofessional descriptions. No claims may be made which suggest superiority over any other dentist or practice; or that a dentist has specialist expertise, but may indicate that a practice is devoted to particular types of treatment: for example, confined to orthodontics.

Canvassing

Dentists must not make unsolicited telephone calls to promote their practice. Neither this rule nor any other advertising restrictions may be broken by a nurse or other person on behalf of the dentist.

General anaesthesia, sedation and resuscitation

Deaths have occurred under general anaesthesia and dentists are accordingly required to fulfil certain conditions laid down by the GDC. These are covered in Chapter 14 and are intended to safeguard the patient. They place upon dentists the responsibility of ensuring that general anaesthesia or sedation is administered safely by properly experienced and trained staff with adequate equipment and facilities for resuscitation of the patient.

Any failure to meet these requirements would be regarded as serious professional misconduct.

Cross-infection

Dentists must take proper precautions to protect their staff and patients from the risk of cross-infection. Failure to comply with this requirement is punishable not only by the GDC, but also under the provisions of the Health and Safety at Work Act. Nurses as well as dentists are covered by this Act, which means that a nurse is legally obliged to co-operate fully in carrying out instructions on sterilization and the prevention of cross-infection. Details are given in Chapters 10 and 31.

Dental radiography

Dentists using X-rays are legally obliged to comply with the Ionizing Radiation Regulations described in Chapter 29. They require dentists to ensure that nurses involved in the taking and processing of radiographs are adequately trained for their duties. These obligations applying to dentists and nurses are also covered by the Health and Safety at Work Act.

Complaints

All practices are expected to establish a procedure for dealing with complaints from patients. This is to ensure that complaints are not ignored or dismissed, but treated seriously, sympathetically and rapidly. They should be discussed with the patient, and appropriate action taken to resolve the matter and prevent the recurrence of avoidable incidents. Full records should be kept of complaints, investigations and action taken; and all such records should be kept in a separate complaints file.

Ethics

In addition to these obligations upon dentists, there is a code of ethics which all nurses should obey.

1   They must be honest and loyal; and serve their employers and patients to the best of their ability.
2   They must hold in strict confidence all details of professional services rendered by their employers. This is not only an ethical obligation but a legal one too. Confidentiality of patients' records is compulsory. This is covered in more detail in Chapter 30. Nurses must realize that breach of confidentiality constitutes grounds for dismissal.
3   They should strive to improve their own professional ability and that of their team colleagues; and inform their employer of any duties they feel unable to undertake satisfactorily.
4   They should disclose to an appropriate person any circumstances adversely affecting proper patient care or staff health and safety.

Duties of a dental nurse

It is of the utmost importance for nurses to realize the extent of patients' perception of the efficiency of a practice. The livelihood of a nurse, as well as that of a dentist, depends on meticulous attention by the entire practice staff to the following requirements:

1   Maintenance of a high standard of cleanliness throughout.
2   Adequate heating and ventilation.
3   Careful planning of appointments and an efficient recall system. Patients' time is just as important as that of dentists, and appointment times should accurately cater for varying lengths of visit. Some visits are unavoidably longer than planned and any patients kept waiting should be informed of delays and offered help if inconvenienced.
4   Strict confidentiality at all times. This includes preventing medical histories, conversations, financial transactions and reactions to treatment being overheard.
5   No delays in communicating information to patients or dentist. This entails the rapid retrieval of filed records, radiographs, models and correspondence; legible handwriting, proper typing format, good English and correct spelling; keeping written

records of telephone messages; and adequate back-up copies of computerized records.

6 Ready availability of addresses and telephone numbers of emergency, building and equipment maintenance services, taxis, public transport and welfare facilities.

7 Updated stock and maintenance records, to ensure that materials are never out of stock, equipment is always working properly, and a full range of spares is immediately available.

8 Orders for materials are precise, unambiguous and give correct catalogue descriptions.

9 Efficient liaison with the dental laboratory to prevent delays in despatch and receipt of work, and to ensure that work prescriptions for the technician include all required details.

10 Staff know how to maintain and service their equipment.

11 All practice staff are trained and regularly practised in the safety policies concerning infection control, X-rays, mercury hygiene, resuscitation, emergency procedures and fire drill (Chapter 31).

Office duties

The reception, clerical and administrative duties of a nurse may be summarized as follows:

1 Responsibility for, and supervision of general cleanliness
2 Reception of patients and dental company representatives
3 Arranging current and recall appointments
4 Completion and filing of patients' records
5 Recording all attendances and treatment
6 Ordering and storage of supplies
7 Management of financial records
8 Correspondence
9 Knowledge of NHS regulations and organization

Much of the secretarial work can be handled far more quickly and efficiently with a computer. This has not only taken over the role of typewriter, but also that of accounts ledger and filing cabinet; and has revolutionized the keeping, filing, storage, retrieval, display, printing and security of all types of practice records.

Surgery duties

Specific surgery duties are covered in the appropriate chapter but general preparation of the surgery is common to all procedures. Thorough preparation of the surgery is essential before the day starts, between patients, and at the end of a treatment session.

Beginning of day

1   Nurses should be well groomed with clean nails, clean uniform and without jewellery.
2   Switch on power, water and air supply to all equipment. Check temperature, ventilation and lighting throughout premises.
3   Check that domestic staff have cleaned the premises thoroughly.
4   Disinfect all working surfaces.
5   Discharge water for two minutes through air/water syringes and handpieces with water spray. Refill ultrasonic cleaner with fresh fluid.
6   Set out clean uniforms and linen as appropriate.
7   Check equipment is working satisfactorily.
8   Ensure that appointment book, day book, patients' notes, radiographs, laboratory work, emergency kit and all materials for the day are ready.
9   Prepare surgery for first patient. Fit new disposable covers where necessary; provide protective spectacles and supply of disposable masks and gloves. Lay out mirror, probe and tweezers.

Reception and treatment of patient

Before a patient enters the surgery, ensure that both you and the dentist know the patient's name, title, purpose of visit and length of appointment. Check that the dentist has the patient's notes and relevant records such as radiographs and models. Remind the dentist of any particular aspects of the patient, such as anxiety about treatment, nausea during impressions, fainting tendency, special medical history, time of patient's transport home, etc.

All unnecessary instruments should be out of view with no sign of a previous patient's visit. The surgery should always appear to patients as if their appointment is the first of the day. Adjust the dental chair and move any mobile equipment so that the patient will have no difficulty in access and getting seated.

Greet the patient by name, and with a smile, and introduce them to the dentist by name. Relieve the patient of any outer clothing or bags and hang them in the office section of the surgery. Seat the patient comfortably, fit a new disposable bib, supply a new disposable beaker of warm mouthwash, a receptacle for the patient's denture, and give the patient a new disposable napkin for the removal of lipstick or drying the lips after rinsing. Protective spectacles are provided for patients treated in the supine position. Always remember that what is all in a day's work for a nurse may well be a very worrying experience for a patient. The surgery atmosphere must be one of friendly communication, appreciation of the patient's feelings, and relaxed efficiency.

If the appointment is for examination only, the nurse records and charts the examination findings. For treatment, the nurse provides the dentist with a clear, dry operative field by attending to illumination, suction, and retraction of cheeks, lips and tongue. Instruments and materials are passed to the dentist, materials are mixed and assistance given in all procedures throughout the visit. In addition the nurse closely observes the patient so as to anticipate and forewarn the dentist of any impending complications such as fainting or sickness.

At the end of the visit the nurse ensures that no sign of the treatment is left on the patient's face or clothing. The next appointment is arranged and given in writing to the patient. Any post-operative instructions given by the dentist are repeated by the nurse, and given in writing when appropriate, before the patient leaves. Any work for the dental laboratory is disinfected, carefully packed and documented ready for despatch; treatment is entered in the day book, and used notes and records set aside ready for filing.

The surgery is then prepared for the next patient so that no traces of the previous visit remain. Used instruments are cleaned and sterilized; waste is placed in a waterproof disposable bag, except for sharp waste which requires a special safe container. Spittoon and work surfaces are cleaned with disinfectant; water discharged for 30 seconds through air/water syringe and handpiece; and new disposables provided. Instruments and records are then set out ready for the next patient.

End of the day

Instruments used on the last patient are cleaned and sterilized. Handpieces are cleaned and lubricated and appropriate sterilization procedures undertaken. The aspirator bottle is emptied and the whole system flushed with disinfectant. The spittoon, unit and work surfaces are also cleaned with disinfectant. All instruments and materials are returned to their proper place.

Laboratory work is checked for proper documentation and carefully prepared for despatch to the technician. Exposed X-ray films are checked for proper documentation and taken to the darkroom for processing. Treatment of the last patient is entered in the day book; all patients' notes and records filed; and back-up copies of computer records are made.

The appointment book is used for making out the next day's page in the day book and getting notes and records ready. A check is made of security arrangements, such as locking drug and filing cabinets, store cupboards, drawers, doors and windows. Finally all electric, gas, water and air services to surgery equipment are switched off.

These duties may be summarized as follows:

1   Care and maintenance of equipment and instruments
2   Care of drugs
3   Preparation of surgery and setting out instruments
4   Sterilization and prevention of cross-infection
5   Recording and charting
6   Chairside assistance during all operative procedures
7   Pre- and post-operative care of patients
8   Processing and mounting radiographs
9   Oral hygiene instruction (*see* page 10)

Legal aspects

In addition to the chairside duties mentioned, a nurse also performs the indispensable roles of chaperone and witness. Dentists are sometimes accused of improper or negligent conduct and, for this reason, a nurse must always be present in the surgery when the dentist is attending a patient. The presence of a third party has great legal value and protects both dentist and patient. If temporary absence is unavoidable, the door should be left open until the nurse returns or another member of staff stands in.

Consent to treatment

Any form of dental examination or treatment without appropriate consent is an assault which could lead to legal proceedings. Consent to treatment from any person of 16 years of age and over (unless mentally incapacitated) is legally valid; but only if the necessity, nature, complications, alternative options and treatment costs have been personally explained by the dentist, and are understood by the patient.

Consent may be verbal or written, but whenever possible it should be written. This is essential for general anaesthesia, sedation, and other procedures with significant side-effects or involving high fees. Written consent must be signed and dated by the patient and dentist. For patients under 16 (or mentally incapacitated), parental consent is required.

British Association of Dental Nurses

The British Association of Dental Nurses (BADN) aims to assist, protect and represent its members; improve education, training and career opportunities; promote and defend their professional status; and liaise with all appropriate bodies in pursuit of these aims.

It is in the best interests of all nurses to join their Association and take an active part therein. Full details of membership and the facilities it can provide for you are obtainable from:

The Secretary
BADN
11 Pharos Street
Fleetwood
Lancs FY7 6BG

National Examining Board for Dental Nurses

This Board (NEBDN) is the body solely responsible for the examination for the National Certificate for Dental Nurses. It consists of examiners from all branches of practice, and nurses representing the BADN. All the examiners are either dentists or nurses and they are elected to the Panel of Examiners by the NEBDN, again ensuring that all branches of dentistry are represented. All examiners must have been qualified for at least seven years.

The National Certificate Examination

The examination for the National Certificate is held twice a year, in May and November, at many centres throughout the country. It may be taken at any age, with any amount of experience and without any educational qualifications; but the certificate cannot be awarded until a nurse has two years' full-time (or equivalent part-time) chairside experience. Although the NEBDN may, at any time, alter the syllabus or vary the form of the examination, it consists at present of written, spotter, practical and oral sections.

Candidates for the examination may obtain copies of the syllabus and regulations, entry form, past examination papers and any further details from:

The Secretary
NEBDN
110 London Street
Fleetwood
Lancs FY7 6EU

Written examination

The written paper is in two parts, A and B. Part A has four sections:

1   Multiple choice questions
   e.g. Indicate the best answer:
   An extra tooth is called a:

    (a)   wisdom tooth
    (b)   supernumerary tooth
    (c)   retained tooth
    (d)   dilacerated tooth

2   A diagram with features to be identified and labelled. Types of diagram used are shown on pages 33, 42, 50, 111, 124, 125, 144.
3   Short-answer questions
e.g. Complete the sentence:
The abbreviation HBV stands for...
4   A charting exercise
An empty chart has to be filled in from the written information provided. An example of this type of exercise is shown in Figure 12.8.

Part B consists of five questions, of which only four have to be answered. Answers may be written in essay or note form, but must be clear and well ordered.

Examples of part B questions are given on page 22 and at the end of most other chapters. Each chapter concludes with a summary and their purpose is to aid final revision for the examination. They may also indicate how to answer written examination questions in note form for candidates who prefer that to essay-type answers.

Use of abbreviations can save time in written answers. Show the examiner that you know their meaning by using the full name first, followed by the abbreviation in brackets. Thereafter just use the abbreviation. A list of abbreviations is given at the beginning of the book.

Spotter test

This is a ten-minute test requiring rapid identification of a series of instruments, materials and other items which nurses are expected to know. They are set out in sequence on a table and the nurse writes the answer as each item is reached. Illustrations in this book show some examples of items used.

In both the spotter test and part A of the written examination, there are many questions to be answered, each carrying only a small mark. To achieve a total pass mark it is *very* important not to waste time on any individual item you are uncertain of, but proceed immediately to the next one that you can answer.

Practical examination

This consists of two tests:

1 Mixing a filling or impression material, e.g. alginate; or preparing an instrument ready for use, e.g. matrix outfit.
2 Selecting the correct instruments or materials for a specified procedure from the choice displayed.

Up to five minutes are allowed and two examiners are present. They understand how nervous you may be and make allowances accordingly. In test 1 they can provide manufacturers' instructions, or an alternative instrument of the same type and purpose, if you are unfamiliar with what is provided. Do not hesitate to tell the examiner if you are uncertain of what you are required to do, or have not used the particular brand of material or type of instrument.

If you are dissatisfied with your mix, e.g. too thick or too thin, or not enough prepared, tell the examiner what is wrong with it. You are not necessarily expected to produce a perfect result under the stress of examination with a brand you have never used before; but you are expected to know how a mix should appear when prepared with a familiar brand in a normal working situation; and the consequences for the patient of an unsatisfactory mix.

Inability to perform a test because your practice is restricted to specific procedures or patients is unacceptable. Examination candidates are expected to be familiar with all procedures covered by the syllabus. The same applies to the oral examination. Examples of test 1 are given at the end of the appropriate chapter.

Oral examination

This takes no longer than ten minutes and the same two examiners are present. You sit at a table covered with a selection of instruments, materials and other items you should know; but it is not a repetition of the spotter test. The table contents are only there for the promotion of questions and discussion. Remember that silence earns no marks. If you do not know the answer to a question, tell the examiner immediately.

Training facilities

Full-time courses, for one or two years, are held at some dental hospitals and technical colleges. Conditions of entry and duration of these courses vary from place to place but full details may be obtained on application to the hospital or college.

Evening courses are also available in many parts of the country, organized by local education authorities. A list of these courses is included with the examination syllabus and regulations obtainable from the NEBDN.

In addition to the courses mentioned, extra lectures are given at branch meetings of the BADN. It issues a quarterly journal and newsletters and has a library from which members may borrow dental books and periodicals.

Although you can enter and pass the examination without attending a course, you are strongly advised to attend one. If this is impossible, however, it is essential to find out for yourself what is required and to practise the various sections of the examination. To do this you will need the examination syllabus and regulations and a set of past examination papers. With these you will be able to test your knowledge of the syllabus by answering past questions. You can seek help from your employer, to mark your answers and also help you with the spotter, practical and oral sections, which consist mainly of mixing impression and filling materials, and identifying instruments.

Guidelines are available to help dentists and course organizers train their nurses to the full extent and depth of the examination syllabus. A special body called the *Dental Nurses Standards and Training Advisory Board* (DNSTAB) is responsible for this information. The Board includes representatives from the NEBDN, BADN, GDC and BDA.

Extra qualifications

After obtaining their National Certificate, nurses can take further courses of study to qualify them for work in specialized fields such as general anaesthesia, sedation, radiography and oral health education. These courses lead to a special certificate and are arranged by the NEBDN in conjunction with the DNSTAB and other interested bodies. Full details are obtainable from the NEBDN or BADN.

Although it is not necessary to attend a course for entry to these post-qualification examinations, all candidates must be on the dental nurses register described on page 21.

Nurses with the National Certificate are also eligible to train as hospital dental nurse tutors, hygienists and therapists. Those wishing to become tutors may need a Further Education Teachers' Certificate. Courses for this are held at local colleges of further education.

Details of hygienist and therapist training are mentioned in Chapter 1 and further information is obtainable from:

General Dental Council
37 Wimpole Street
London W1M 8DQ

Certificate in oral health education

As mentioned on page 10, dental nurses are permitted to give patients instruction in oral hygiene, provided a dentist is satisfied that they are competent to do so.

Although it is not necessary for nurses to have passed any examination for a dentist to be satisfied of their competence, they can prove it by obtaining the NEBDN Certificate in Oral Health Education. It covers the knowledge and experience necessary to comply with GDC requirements for dentists wishing to delegate this important function to their nurses.

Sedation

The full name of this qualification is: Certificate in Assisting in the Care of the Patient Relating to Treatment under Conscious Sedation. The examination covers the basic principles of sedation and patient care, and the knowledge and skills necessary to comply with GDC requirements for dentists to have fully trained and experienced nurses for these procedures.

General anaesthesia

The Certificate in Dental Sedation Nursing covers the practical role and knowledge required by dental nurses to satisfy GDC requirements for dentists to use adequately trained staff to assist the anaesthetist and dentist. The syllabus for this certificate has much in common with that for conscious sedation.

Dental radiography certificate

The College of Radiographers and DNSTAB have arranged courses and an examination for dental nurses which satisfy the legal requirements for dentists who train their nurses to take and process radiographs. Details of courses are obtainable from:

The College of Radiographers
2 Carriage Row
183 Eversholt Street
London NW1 1BU

Registration

There is a scheme of voluntary registration for dental nurses. The register is known as the Voluntary National Register of Dental Nurses. Its purpose is to encourage training and qualification of dental nurses; and to encourage the employment of qualified and registered dental nurses. Everybody on the Register is entitled to use the designation

Registered Dental Nurse (RDN). Only registered dental nurses can become examiners for the National Certificate or enter for the extra qualifications just described.

For admission to the Register, a nurse must have passed the NEBDN National Certificate examination; an examination recognized by the dental hospitals; any other dental nursing examination approved by the NEBDN; or have served an adequate period of training. Full details of the requirements for registration are obtainable from:

The Registrar
Voluntary National Register for Dental Nurses
110 London Street
Fleetwood
Lancs FY7 6EU

Past examination questions

Some typical questions set in part B of the National Certificate written examination are included at the end of their appropriate chapter, under the heading of Written examination.

Describe the non-clinical role of the DSA [Dental nurse] in organizing and running an efficient practice system (November 1989)

Summary

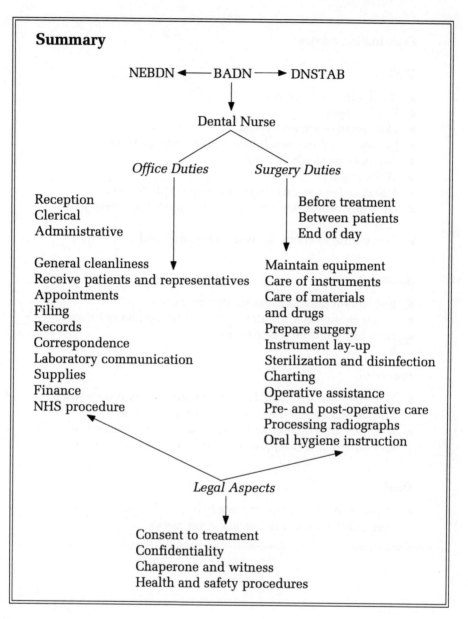

NEBDN ◄——— BADN ———► DNSTAB

↓

Dental Nurse

Office Duties   *Surgery Duties*

Reception
Clerical   Before treatment
Administrative   Between patients
                                              End of day

General cleanliness   Maintain equipment
Receive patients and representatives   Care of instruments
Appointments   Care of materials
Filing   and drugs
Records   Prepare surgery
Correspondence   Instrument lay-up
Laboratory communication   Sterilization and disinfection
Supplies   Charting
Finance   Operative assistance
NHS procedure   Pre- and post-operative care
                                       Processing radiographs
                                       Oral hygiene instruction

Legal Aspects

Consent to treatment
Confidentiality
Chaperone and witness
Health and safety procedures

Examination advice

Written

- Read question carefully
- Read it again
- Only answer what is asked
- Do not spend too much time on any one question
- Use note form where possible
- Write legibly
- Use simple coloured diagrams where appropriate
- Give answers in logical order – the most important points first
- Leave time to check answers when finished

Spotter

- Instrument may have name stamped on it.
- If you cannot identify item, proceed immediately to next.
- Give full but brief description.

Practical

- You may ask for manufacturer's instructions if unfamiliar with brand of material, or instrument supplied.
- If you are dissatisfied with your mix, tell the examiner why, and what the consequences would be for the patient.

Oral

- If you don't know the answer to a question, tell the examiner immediately. Silence earns no marks.

3 Outline of Anatomy and Physiology

The next few chapters deal with human **anatomy** and **physiology**, which are the study, respectively, of the normal structure and functioning of the body. Just as houses are built of individual bricks, so is the body made up of millions of microscopic individual units called **cells**. Each cell has a job to do and must be supplied with fuel and **oxygen** before it can do it. In this respect the body is no different from any other working engine or machine. A motor-car engine, for example, needs fuel in the form of petrol. This is burnt inside the engine cylinder to produce the energy which drives the car. But petrol, gas, coal, wood or any other form of fuel can only burn in the presence of oxygen. Thus all engines, machines and body cells are alike in requiring oxygen to burn their fuel and thereby produce the energy needed to perform their functions.

The *fuel* needed by the body comes from our food, while oxygen is present in the air we breathe. Fuel and oxygen are conveyed in the **blood** to all parts of the body by the **heart** and **circulation**.

The food we eat is turned into usable fuel by a process known as **digestion**. The digestive system contains the stomach and intestines.

Oxygen is obtained from the air we breathe. The process by which it enters the blood to reach the body cells is called **respiration**. The respiratory system consists of the air passages and lungs.

Just as engine and domestic fuels produce waste products, such as smoke, water and ash, so too do body cells. Cell waste is eliminated from the body by a process known as **excretion**.

Overall control and co-ordination of body functions is effected by the **nervous system**, which consists of the **brain** and **nerves**. The brain may be likened to a computerized telephone exchange with the nerves serving as telephone lines.

There are many different types of cell in the body, depending on their particular function, but they all contain a central **nucleus** and are bounded by a cell wall. The nucleus is responsible for growth by cell division; and contains **chromosomes** and **genes** which transmit the hereditary factors which make every person a unique individual. The cell wall is sufficiently thin to allow oxygen and nutrients from the blood to enter the cell and waste products to leave.

Summary

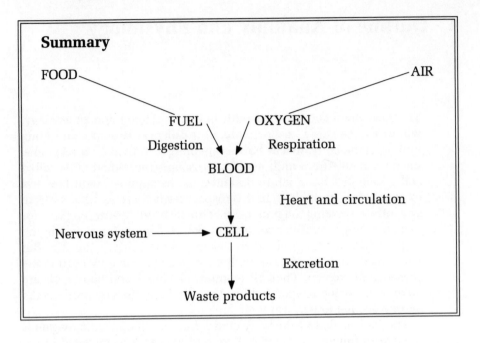

4 Blood

The body contains about five litres of blood, kept at a constant temperature of 37°C. Blood consists of three different types of cell floating in a liquid called **plasma**. The blood cells are known as **red cells**, **white cells** and **platelets**. Red cells and platelets are unique among body cells in having no nucleus. Blood cells are so small that one cubic millimetre of blood (the size of a pin head) contains about five million red cells, 7,000 white cells and 250,000 platelets.

Red cells

The red blood cells contain a pigment called **haemoglobin** which gives the blood its red colour. The main function of red cells is to carry oxygen (O_2) to the body cells.

For its journey from the lungs to the body cells, oxygen combines with the haemoglobin of the red cells. It is then released from the haemoglobin when the body cells are reached. Some people do not have enough haemoglobin in their red cells and are consequently short of oxygen. This condition is called **anaemia** and such people tire easily, become breathless on exertion and have a pale complexion. They need special care during general anaesthesia.

White cells

The white blood cells defend the body against disease. They do this by attacking germs and repairing damage.

Platelets

The function of blood platelets is to stop bleeding. They do this in two ways: by blocking the cut blood vessels; and by producing substances which help the blood to clot.

Plasma

Plasma is a straw-coloured liquid which consists mainly of water (90%) and the plasma proteins. It has many different functions:

1 It carries digested food (*fuel*) to the body cells.
2 It carries away waste products from body cells to the **kidneys**. In the kidneys, waste products filter out of the plasma to form a

liquid called **urine**. This is stored in the **bladder** until it is discharged from the body.

3 The waste gas **carbon dioxide** (CO_2) from body cells is carried in the plasma to the lungs, where it is expelled by breathing out.

4 Special glands in various parts of the body control certain important processes such as growth, reproduction, etc. They do this by producing chemicals called **hormones**. These are carried in the plasma to the part of the body concerned.

5 Plasma contains **antibodies** and **antitoxins** which give resistance to disease. They are formed from plasma proteins called globulins.

6 Plasma, together with the platelets, takes part in the blood-clotting process by which bleeding is stopped. It is a complex process involving a plasma protein called fibrinogen and many other factors found in the plasma and platelets.

Clotting

Heavy bleeding is dangerous to life as blood has so many vital functions. The natural response is clotting which seals off the severed blood vessels. Treatment of bleeding is aimed to assist this natural process, and is covered in Chapter 16.

Written examination

Describe briefly the main constituents of blood and their functions

What is the role of the dental nurse in the treatment of post-extraction haemorrhage? (November 1995)

Summary

Functions of blood

1 Carriage of oxygen to body cells
2 Carriage of digested food to body cells
3 Carriage of carbon dioxide and other waste products away from body cells
4 Carriage of hormones
5 Defence against disease and repair of injury
6 Maintenance of body temperature at 37°C
7 Clotting to seal off cut blood vessels and prevent loss of blood

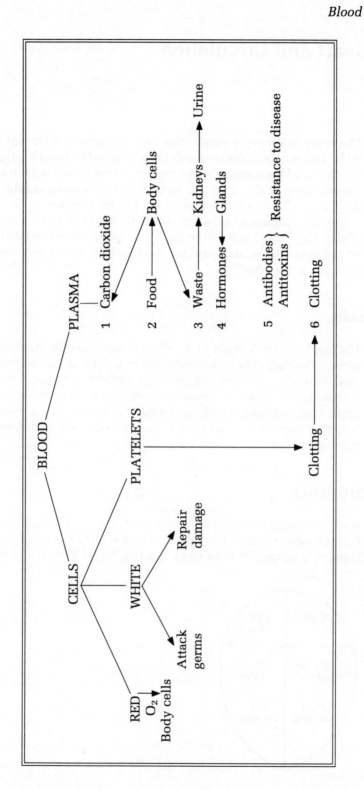

5   Heart and Circulation

The **heart** is simply a pump which circulates blood throughout the body. Tubes called blood vessels carry it from the heart to all parts of the body and back again. This round trip is known as the **circulation**. Vessels carrying blood *away* from the heart are known as **arteries** and those returning blood *to* the heart are known as **veins**.

The heart pumps blood round the body about 70 times a minute in adults. The heart beats can be felt as the **pulse** where certain arteries lie just beneath the skin, and the most well-known place where this occurs is at the wrist.

The heart

The heart (Figure 5.1) lies in the chest immediately behind the breast bone. It consists of two chambers, left and right, separated from each other by a wall. Each chamber is further divided into upper and lower compartments which communicate with each other by valves. Each upper compartment is called an **atrium** and each lower a **ventricle**. Note that there is no communication at all between the left and right sides of the heart.

The circulation

Blood returning from all parts of the body, *except* the lungs, enters the **right atrium**. All this blood enters the right atrium through two great veins – the **superior vena cava** bringing blood from the head, neck

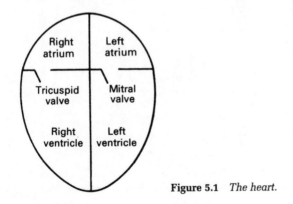

Figure 5.1   *The heart.*

and arms, and the **inferior vena cava** bringing it back from the rest of the body (Figure 5.2). Of course the heart is really much more complicated in shape than these diagrams suggest, but for examination purposes they will suffice. Figure 5.5 shows the real appearance.

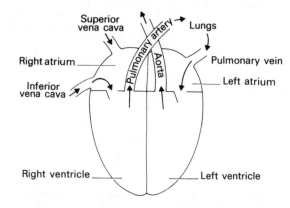

Figure 5.2 *Heart and great vessels.*

From the right atrium, blood passes through the **tricuspid valve** into the **right ventricle**. It then passes out of the right ventricle through the **pulmonary artery** to the lungs.

Here the blood gives up the waste carbon dioxide it is carrying and takes in fresh oxygen, which is part of the fuel necessary for the working of the body. This **oxygenated blood** is carried from the lungs in the **pulmonary vein** to the **left atrium** of the heart. From here it passes through the **mitral valve** into the **left ventricle**. Then it is pumped out of the left ventricle into the **aorta**. This great artery divides into many smaller arteries which convey oxygenated blood all round the body.

When these smaller arteries reach their destination they divide again into very thin-walled vessels called **capillaries**. Oxygen from the blood passes through the walls of these capillaries to the body cells. Carbon dioxide, which is a waste product formed in the body cells, also passes through the capillary walls, but in the reverse direction, from the body cells to the blood (Figure 5.3). The capillaries then unite to form veins which carry the blood and waste carbon dioxide back to the right atrium of the heart via the superior and inferior vena cava. As already described, the blood then passes on again via the tricuspid valve, right ventricle and pulmonary artery to the lungs.

In the lungs a similar but reverse process occurs (Figure 5.4). The pulmonary artery, carrying blood from the right ventricle, divides up into a capillary network in the lungs. These capillaries give up waste carbon dioxide from the blood into the air spaces of the lungs. At the same time oxygen from the air in the lungs passes into the capillaries

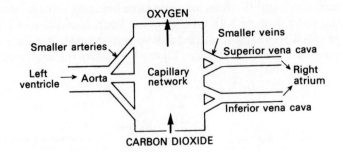

Figure 5.3 *Body capillaries.*

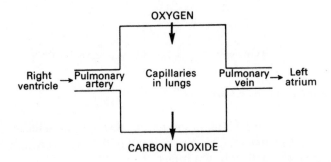

Figure 5.4 *Lung capillaries.*

to refill the blood with oxygen again. The capillaries then unite to form the pulmonary vein which carries the oxygenated blood to the left atrium of the heart. From here it passes through the mitral valve to the left ventricle and aorta to start another journey round the body.

It should now be clear that the function of the left side of the heart is solely to pump oxygenated blood from the lungs to the rest of the body; while the right side returns deoxygenated blood from the rest of the body back to the lungs (Figure 5.5). Oxygenated blood is bright red in colour, but when it has given up its oxygen to the body cells and received waste carbon dioxide instead, the deoxygenated blood appears much darker in colour.

Systemic circulation

The journey made by blood from the left ventricle through arteries, body capillaries and veins back to the right atrium is known as the **systemic circulation**. These arteries carry only oxygenated blood, while the veins carry only deoxygenated blood.

The systemic circulation has two important subdivisions: the coronary circulation and portal circulation. The former is described in this chapter and the latter in Chapter 7.

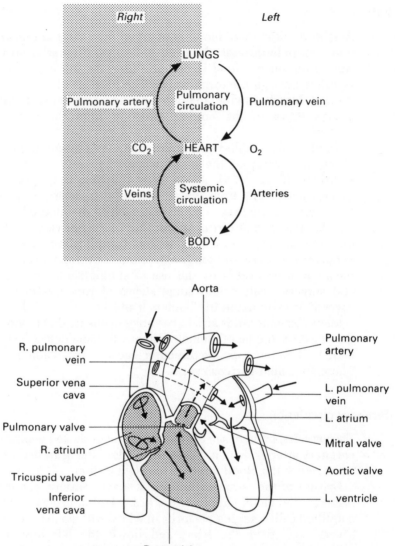

Figure 5.5 *Heart and circulation* (Deoxygenated blood shaded).
Source: *Emergency Procedures and First Aid for Nurses*, M. Skeet, Blackwell Science Ltd, Oxford.

Pulmonary circulation

The passage of blood from the right ventricle through the pulmonary artery, lungs and pulmonary vein back to the left atrium is called the **pulmonary circulation**. It is unique in being the only part of the circulation where an artery carries deoxygenated blood (pulmonary artery) and a vein carries oxygenated blood (pulmonary vein).

Valves

As already described, blood is pumped from the right atrium to the right ventricle through the tricuspid valve. Similarly, on the other side of the heart, blood is pumped from the left atrium to the left ventricle through the mitral valve. The purpose of these valves is to prevent blood flowing the wrong way. They ensure that blood always flows in the correct direction from the atrium to the ventricle.

Similar valves called **semilunar valves** are present in the aorta and pulmonary artery at the point where they leave their respective ventricles (Figure 5.5). Again their function is to prevent blood flowing backwards from the arteries into the heart. Sometimes the heart valves are damaged by disease such as **rheumatic fever** or they may be defective at birth. Any of these forms of valvular heart disease present a risk of a very serious complication called **infective endocarditis** following tooth extraction. Development of this complication is prevented by the use of antibiotics before extractions, oral surgery, scaling and some stages of root treatment. This is covered in more detail in Chapters 9 and 11.

Many systemic veins also have valves to ensure that blood will only flow towards the heart. Sometimes they become defective and blood leaks back in the opposite direction, causing distension of the veins. These are called **varicose veins**.

Coronary circulation

The very first branches of the aorta as it leaves the left ventricle are the **coronary** arteries, which supply the walls of the heart itself. Coronary veins return the blood direct to the right atrium.

Disease of the coronary arteries is a very serious condition as it obstructs the blood supply of the heart. Partial obstruction causes a condition called **angina pectoris**, in which sudden exertion produces severe pain over the heart and down the left arm. Complete obstruction may be caused by a clot of blood. This condition is even more painful and is known as **coronary thrombosis**. It is a common cause of collapse and sudden death. Patients with disease of the heart and circulation need special care during dental treatment, and surgery staff must know how to deal with heart attacks.

The aorta

After giving off the coronary arteries the aorta ascends inside the chest where it supplies branches to the head, neck and arms. It then arches downwards through the chest and abdomen giving off branches which supply all the rest of the body.

Heart failure

Heart failure, or cardiac arrest, means that the heart has stopped beating. This, of course, means that no blood is being pumped round the body and death occurs in a few minutes. But as the heart is just a simple pump, it can be made to beat artificially by rhythmically applying pressure to the chest. This squeezes the heart between the breast bone and spine and forces blood out of the heart into the circulation. When pressure on the chest is relaxed, blood returns to the heart again (Figure 5.6).

This simple first-aid procedure is repeated 80 times a minute and is called **external cardiac compression** (ECC). Combined with artificial respiration it can keep a patient alive until expert medical help is available. Treatment of cardiac arrest in the dental surgery is covered in Chapters 14 and 15 (Figures 5.6, 14.7).

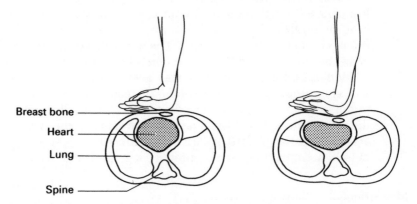

Breast bone
Heart
Lung
Spine

Figure 5.6 *External cardiac compression.*
Source: *Emergency Procedures and First Aid for Nurses*, (2nd edn). M. Skeet, Blackwell Science Ltd, Oxford.

Body temperature

Apart from supplying body cells with fuel and oxygen, another function of the circulation is the maintenance of body temperature. As mentioned in the previous chapter, blood is kept at a constant temperature of 37°C, which is essential for the normal functioning of the body. Indeed, a change of only 5°C either way can be fatal.

The **skin** is mainly responsible for controlling body temperature, by acting as a radiator when it gets too hot, or as a layer of insulation against heat loss when it gets too cold. It does this in the following ways.

High body temperature

Muscular exercise and a high air temperature make the body too hot. When this happens the blood vessels of the skin dilate and allow an increased volume of blood to circulate through the skin. This diversion of extra blood to the skin raises its surface temperature and the excess heat radiates away into the air.

At the same time the skin produces a layer of sweat on its surface. This evaporates by absorbing excess heat from the skin. When the body is trying to lose heat in these ways the skin appears pink, warm and moist.

Low body temperature

When the body gets too cold a reverse process occurs. Skin vessels contract and the circulation of blood through the skin is greatly reduced. This is tantamount to switching off a radiator. The layer of fat beneath the skin then acts as a natural insulator which prevents loss of heat through the skin. Sweating also ceases in order to preserve heat. Blood flow through the skin may become so reduced that very little oxygenated blood is present. The remaining deoxygenated blood gives the skin a bluish tinge and it feels cold and dry.

Sudden chilling of the body may also give rise to *goose-pimples* and shivering which are involuntary reactions to cold. A goose-pimple appearance is caused by the erection of tiny hairs which cover the skin surface. This traps a layer of warm air on the surface which acts as a barrier to further heat loss. Shivering is caused by strong muscular contractions which produce a great deal of heat.

Measurement of body temperature

A healthy body functions at a constant temperature of 37°C. But this may change during illness as the body's reaction can cause a rise in temperature. In feverish conditions, for example, the skin becomes hot and flushed and profuse sweating occurs as the body attempts to restore normal temperature.

Measurement of body temperature therefore provides a useful indication of the state of health. It was formerly done with a clinical thermometer, but nowadays a disposable heat-sensitive strip (Tempa-Dot) is used instead. It is placed under the tongue, and changes colour to accurately indicate body temperature. Every practice should have some as a raised temperature may occur with an acute abscess or acute gingivitis and necessitate use of antibiotics; and some dental procedures should not be undertaken if a patient is unwell.

Summary

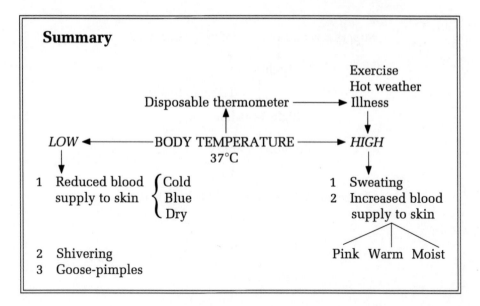

Superior vena cava   Inferior vena cava

↓   ↓

Right atrium

Tricuspid valve

↓

Right ventricle

↓

Pulmonary artery

CO_2

↓

O_2 breathed in → Lungs → CO_2 breathed out

↓ O_2

Pulmonary vein

↓

Left atrium

Mitral valve

↓

Left ventricle

↓

Aorta

↓

Small arteries

↓ O_2

CO_2 → Body capillaries → O_2

↓ CO_2

Small veins

↓   ↓

Superior vena cava   Inferior vena cava

6   Respiration

Respiration means breathing. Its function is to provide the means whereby oxygen enters the blood and carbon dioxide leaves. This interchange of gases occurs in the **lungs** which are situated in the chest, one on each side of the heart (Figure 6.1).

The chest forms a protective cage for the heart and lungs. The bars of the cage are formed by the ribs – which are joined to the breast bone in front and spine behind. The spaces between the ribs are filled by the rib muscles. The floor of the cage is formed by the **diaphragm** which is a sheet of muscle separating the chest from the abdomen.

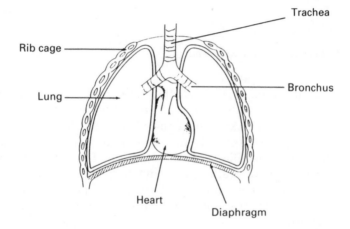

Figure 6.1   *The chest.*
Source: *Lecture Notes on Human Physiology*, (3rd edn). J.J. Bray *et al.*, Blackwell Science Ltd, Oxford.

In order to reach the lungs, the air we breathe enters the throat through the nose or mouth and passes into the **larynx** or voice box. (This is the *Adam's apple* in men.) Below the larynx the air passes along a tube called the **trachea**, or windpipe, which runs down the neck to the chest where it divides into two. These two branches are known as the right and left **bronchi** and they enter their respective lungs (Fig. 6.2). Just as arteries divide up into smaller arteries and finally into thin-walled capillaries, so do the bronchi divide inside the lungs. Each bronchus divides into many smaller and smaller tubes until it eventually ends up as a huge number of tiny **air sacs** which comprise each lung. A network of capillaries originating from the pulmonary artery passes round each air sac.

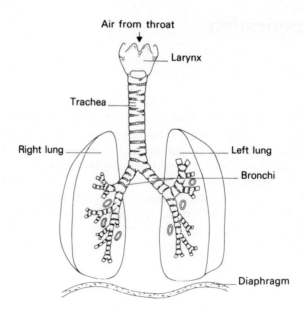

Figure 6.2   *Respiratory system.*

Air breathed in through the nose passes via the throat, larynx, trachea and bronchi to the air sacs of the lungs. This passage from nose to lungs is known as the **airway**. In the lungs, oxygen from the air passes through the thin walls of each air sac and its surrounding capillary to reach the blood. In the same way carbon dioxide passes simultaneously out of the blood into the air sacs. This gaseous exchange for replenishing the blood with oxygen and eliminating the waste product, carbon dioxide, is the sole purpose of respiration.

Oxygen enters the blood by combining with haemoglobin in the red cells; whereas carbon dioxide is carried by the plasma.

External and internal respiration

The exchange of gases just described is sometimes referred to as **external respiration**. It occurs between the pulmonary circulation and lungs, with oxygen entering the blood and carbon dioxide leaving (Figures 5.4 and 5.5). The reverse process between capillaries of the systemic circulation and body cells was described in Chapter 5. It is known as **internal respiration**, with carbon dioxide entering the blood and oxygen leaving it (Figures 5.3 and 5.5).

Importance of the airway

The airway is the only route available for air to enter the lungs. For life to continue, it must stay open at all times and has accordingly been specially constructed.

The nostrils form the entrance to the airway and are guarded by hairs which filter out dust. Inside the nose a very rich blood supply warms and moistens the air as it passes into the throat. Here it shares the same passage as food *en route* for the stomach; and to ensure that food goes the right way, and does not obstruct the airway, special protective mechanisms operate:

1 *Swallowing* is a complex act which not only propels food towards the stomach but specifically prevents it entering the nose or larynx.
2 *Sneezing* forcibly expels foreign bodies from the nose.
3 *Coughing* does the same for the larynx, trachea and bronchi.

Some of these protective mechanisms may be put out of action during general anaesthesia, and the maintenance of an open airway and freedom from obstruction become matters of paramount importance.

The larynx, trachea and bronchi are reinforced by a rigid gristly material called **cartilage**. This keeps them open and prevents them being squashed during swallowing or other activities. The larynx is made almost entirely of cartilage while the trachea and bronchi are protected by rings of cartilage throughout their length (Figure 6.2). The rigidity of the larynx and upper part of the trachea can be felt with your fingers on the front of the neck. The nose, too, is largely made of cartilage which ensures that the entrance to the airway is always open.

The entrance to the larynx is protected by a flap of cartilage called the **epiglottis** (Figure 6.3) which prevents food entering the larynx during swallowing. The larynx itself has the special function of voice production. It contains two fibrous folds called **vocal cords** which adjust themselves to vibrate at different rates and thereby produce speech.

The trachea terminates inside the chest by dividing into right and left bronchi which enter their respective lungs. The right bronchus is almost vertically in line with the trachea so that a small foreign body entering the larynx may drop straight through into the right lung (Figure 6.2). This could happen during dental treatment, even on a conscious patient, and give rise to grave consequences. It is of the utmost importance for nurses to realize this danger while assisting at the chairside and be constantly on their guard to prevent extracted teeth, loose milk teeth, small instruments or other foreign bodies getting lost in the mouth.

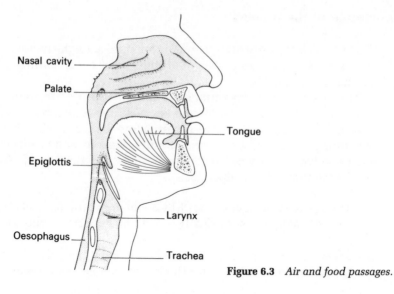

Nasal cavity

Palate

Tongue

Epiglottis

Larynx

Oesophagus

Trachea

Figure 6.3 *Air and food passages.*

The entire airway is covered with a fine layer of sticky fluid, called **mucus**, which collects dust and dirt particles from the air. Contaminated mucus is propelled upwards, away from the lungs, by special cells containing minute whip-like hairs. These hairs lash the mucus along towards the entrance of the airway, whence it can be removed by blowing the nose or coughing.

Breathing

Breathing is the means whereby air is sucked into and expelled from the lungs. It is brought about by movements of the chest which have the same effect as bellows. When the chest expands air is sucked into the lungs, and when it contracts air is expelled. Fresh air reaches the lungs when we breathe in. This is called **inspiration** and occurs about 15 times a minute. Breathing out, or **expiration**, rids the lungs of carbon dioxide.

For inspiration to take place, the chest cavity must expand, and this is brought about by the action of the respiratory muscles. These are the diaphragm and rib muscles (Figures 6.1, 6.2). As already described, the diaphragm is a sheet of muscle separating the chest from the abdomen. It moves up and down like a piston, enlarging the chest cavity each time it descends. The rib muscles expand the chest by pulling the ribs upwards and outwards. This combined action of diaphragm and rib muscles sucks air into the lungs during inspiration, while their passive recoil during expiration expels air from the lungs.

Inspired air contains 20% oxygen and a negligible amount of

carbon dioxide. Expired air contains about 16% oxygen and 4% carbon dioxide.

Artificial respiration

If natural breathing stops it can often be restored by artificially inflating the lungs with air and then allowing the chest to contract. This is repeated at the natural breathing rate of 15 times a minute. In this way a person whose heart is still beating, and whose airway is clear, can be kept alive until natural breathing recommences.

Artificial respiration makes use of the fact that expired air contains 16% oxygen. Expired air is blown directly into the patient's mouth and this provides the lungs with a fresh supply of oxygen. This is called **expired air respiration** (EAR). It is commonly known as mouth to mouth respiration and is a most effective first-aid measure (Figure 6.4). The subject of artificial respiration is covered more fully in Chapter 14.

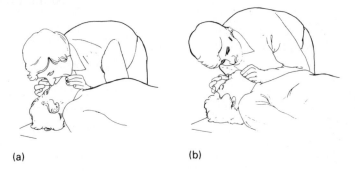

(a)   (b)

Figure 6.4   *Expired air respiration* (a) Inflation (b) Expiration.
Source: *Lecture Notes on Anaesthetics.* Lunn, Blackwell Science Ltd, Oxford.

Summary

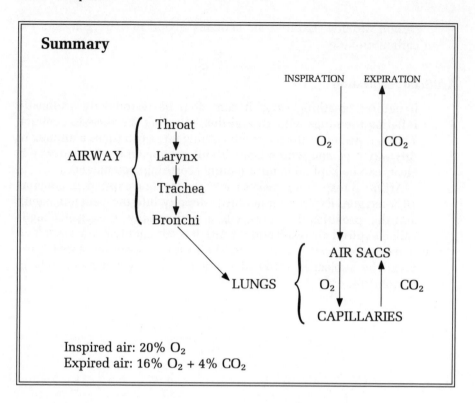

Inspired air: 20% O_2
Expired air: 16% O_2 + 4% CO_2

7 Digestion

For life to continue, the body requires fuel in the form of oxygen and food. Respiration provides the oxygen. Our food, however, cannot be utilized by the body in the form in which it is eaten. It must be specially processed by the body before it can be of any use. This special processing is known as **digestion**. It is brought about by the action on the food of certain substances called **enzymes** which are made by the body and mixed with the food during its passage through the body.

Food

The food we eat consists of protein, carbohydrate and fat. It also contains small quantities of vitamins and minerals.

Protein

Proteins are found in meat, fish, eggs, milk and cheese. They are broken down into **amino-acids** during digestion. Protein is necessary for cell growth and repair.

Carbohydrate

Carbohydrates are found in sweet and starchy foods such as sugar, flour and potatoes. They are broken down into **glucose** during digestion. Carbohydrates provide body cells with the energy required to perform their functions.

Fat

Fats are found in meat, fish, dairy products and vegetable oils. The digestive process breaks them down into **fatty acids**. Fats provide energy and body fat, which is stored in a layer beneath the skin. It acts as a reserve source of energy when needed, and also as insulation which helps maintain body temperature in cold weather.

Vitamins

Vitamins are essential ingredients of food but are only needed in minute quantities. There are many different vitamins but the most important for examination purposes are vitamins B, C and D.

Vitamin B is really a complex of related vitamins found in cereals and liver. They take part in the production of energy from digested food, and in the formation of red blood cells. Deficiency may cause anaemia (page 27) and is often associated with a sore tongue.

Vitamin C, found in fresh fruit and vegetables, is necessary for the formation of capillary blood vessels. Deficiency leads to bleeding and gum disorders.

Vitamin D is present in meat fat, fish and dairy products. It is necessary for bone and tooth formation, and deficiency may affect their structure.

Minerals

Minerals, like vitamins, are needed in comparatively small amounts but are nevertheless essential food constituents. For examination purposes the most important ones are calcium, phosphorus and iron.

Calcium and phosphorus, together with vitamin D, are necessary for bone and tooth formation. Deficiency has the same effect as for vitamin D.

Iron is necessary for the production of haemoglobin. Deficiency causes anaemia.

Water

The body requires water for the production of blood, digestive juices, urine and sweat. Many foods contain a large quantity of water but it is still necessary to drink more than a litre of fluid daily.

Diet

The food we eat is called our diet. All the constituents of food – protein, fat, carbohydrates, vitamins and minerals – are present in adequate quantities in a normal balanced diet. There is no need to eat excessive quantities of one or the other. Over-eating is dangerous to health as the body only requires a certain amount of energy. Food eaten in excess of the body's energy requirements is stored in the form of surplus fat and thus increases body weight. This is potentially dangerous to health as it puts an extra strain on the heart and circulation and may lead to disease of the heart and arteries, resulting in high blood pressure and heart failure.

Thus all the food we eat undergoes digestion by enzymes, which turn it into amino-acids, fatty acids, glucose, vitamins and minerals. Only when it is in this form can it be absorbed into the blood and utilized by the body cells.

Mastication

The first stage of digestion occurs in the mouth. The food is chewed, which breaks it up and mixes it with **saliva**. Chewing, or **mastication**, is very important as it is the means whereby food is thoroughly mixed with saliva. The tongue helps to roll this mixture of food and saliva into a slippery ball which is easily swallowed. A set of teeth capable of chewing food properly is accordingly important. False teeth are not a perfect substitute for one's own teeth as mastication cannot be carried out so efficiently with them.

Saliva

The functions of saliva are:

1   Lubrication
2   Cleansing
3   Digestion
4   Antacid
5   Antibacterial

The main constituent of saliva is water (99%). Thus saliva moistens and lubricates all parts of the mouth. This facilitates the movements of the tongue, lips and cheeks which are essential for eating, swallowing and speech; and which also help to keep the teeth clean.

The digestive action of saliva is caused by an enzyme it contains called **ptyalin**. This initiates digestion of carbohydrates.

Saliva contains substances which help to neutralize the acid responsible for tooth decay. This antacid function of saliva is called **buffer action** and is described in Chapter 17.

Chapter 8 mentions that the mouth is full of germs. Most of them are normal residents of the mouth and quite harmless. Antibacterial constituents of saliva help maintain this natural balance by preventing the growth of harmful germs.

The importance of these functions of saliva is dramatically shown in conditions where there is a deficiency of saliva. Radiotherapy for oral cancer, AIDS, disease of the salivary glands, and certain drugs can all cause a severe deficiency of saliva. This results in a dry mouth, difficulties with speech, eating and swallowing, bad breath, gum disease and extensive tooth decay. The medical term for dry mouth is **xerostomia**.

Saliva is produced by three pairs of glands situated close to the lower jaw. They are the **parotid**, **submandibular** and **sublingual** salivary glands (Figure 12.21). Saliva reaches the mouth through tubes, called *ducts*, which pass from each gland into the mouth.

Saliva is always present in the mouth but is needed in much larger amounts when eating. Hunger and the thought, smell, sight and taste of food all stimulate an increased flow of saliva from the glands. Salivary glands only produce saliva. They must not be confused with the glands mentioned in Chapter 4 which produce hormones.

Swallowing

After being thoroughly chewed and mixed with saliva, food is swallowed. This is a complex muscular act which prevents the ball of food entering the nasal cavity or larynx, where it could obstruct the airway. It is propelled by the tongue from the mouth to the back of the throat. From there it goes down a long tube, called the **oesophagus**, which passes through the neck (behind the trachea) and chest (behind the heart and lungs) into the **abdomen** where it enters the **stomach**.

To understand how the swallowing mechanism works it is necessary to realize that the throat is a cavity open to the nose and mouth. The upper part of the throat behind the nose is called the **naso-pharynx**; while the lower part, at the back of the mouth, is called the **oro-pharynx** (Figures 6.3 and 7.1). The sequence of events in swallowing is as follows:

1 The slippery ball of food is propelled backwards into the oro-pharynx by the tongue.
2 To prevent food entering the naso-pharynx, the soft palate rises up and seals itself like a trapdoor against the back of the throat. This completely seals off the naso-pharynx from the oro-pharynx and food cannot enter the nasal cavity.
3 At the same time the larynx rises bodily and seals itself off against the epiglottis, thereby preventing ingress of food into the airway (Figure 7.1). By placing your fingers on the front of the neck, over the larynx, and then swallowing, you can feel it rise as it seeks the shelter of the epiglottis.
4 The food is now propelled downwards from the oro-pharynx into the oesophagus by the muscles of the throat. Oesophageal muscles then take over to propel it into the stomach.

The abdomen

The abdomen is a cavity containing the main organs of digestion (Figure 7.2). It is immediately below the chest but separated from it by the diaphragm (Figure 6.1).

The stomach lies just below the diaphragm and receives all the food which has passed down the oesophagus after being swallowed. Food

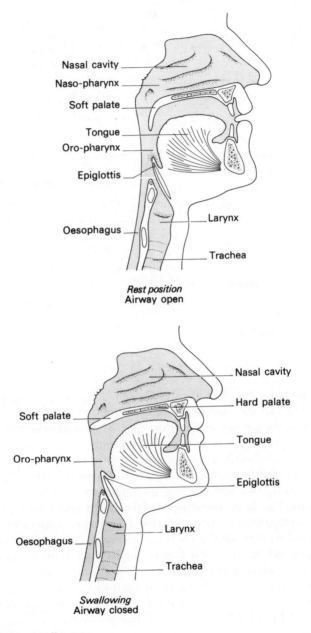

Figure 7.1 *Swallowing.*

stays in the stomach for a few hours while the stomach enzymes begin the first stages of digestion.

After leaving the stomach, the partially digested food enters the **small intestine**. This is a long coiled tube about six metres long in which digestion is completed. It manufactures its own enzymes for

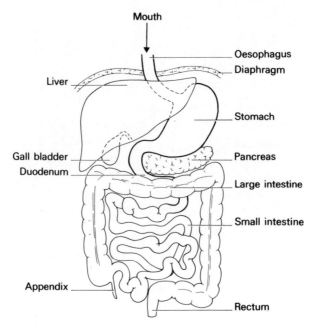

Figure 7.2 *Digestive system.*

this purpose but also receives some help from the **pancreas**. This gland lies in the loop of the **duodenum**, which is the first part of the small intestine after the stomach. The pancreas produces some enzymes which pass into the duodenum.

When the food has been completely digested in the small intestine, the indigestible residue passes into the **large intestine**. This is a wider tube, nearly two metres long, leading from the small intestine to the **rectum**. The large intestine absorbs water and minerals from waste food remnants. The rectum carries this waste to the external orifice or **anus** where it is eliminated from the body. The whole system of tubes through which the food passes on its way from mouth to anus is called the **alimentary canal**.

After digestion has been completed in the intestines, the digested food, which is now in a state the body can use, passes through the walls of the intestines into capillaries where the blood carries it to the **liver**.

The liver lies just below the diaphragm to the right of the stomach. It is a storehouse for digested food and distributes it to those parts of the body requiring it. It also produces a digestive juice known as **bile**. This is stored in the **gall bladder**, which lies underneath the liver. Bile passes into the duodenum at the same point as the digestive juice from the pancreas.

Digestion

The first stage of digestion takes place in the mouth where the salivary enzyme pytalin initiates digestion of carbohydrates. This occurs during mastication which mixes food and saliva together. The ball of food is then swallowed and passes down the oesophagus into the stomach.

Food is propelled down the oesophagus by a muscular action called **peristalsis**. But this form of muscular propulsion is not confined to the oesophagus. It occurs progressively, along the entire alimentary canal, and consists of alternating waves of muscular contraction and relaxation. Peristalsis thus produces a milking effect which squeezes food through the whole system of tubes from oesophagus to rectum.

Stomach

The next stage of digestion occurs in the stomach, which produces a mixture of acid and enzymes called *gastric juice*. The acid kills germs and extracts any iron from the food – for haemoglobin formation. The enzymes initiate digestion of proteins and fat.

Food is churned up in the gastric juice for up to five hours before being released into the duodenum. That is why patients must not eat for at least four hours before receiving a general anaesthetic. If such precautions were not taken, the stomach might still contain food which could be vomited during anaesthesia and cause blockage of the airway. It must be remembered that the protective mechanism of swallowing, which prevents food entering the airway, may be paralysed during general anaesthesia.

Small intestine

Partially digested food leaves the stomach and enters the duodenum, which is the first loop of the small intestine. Also entering the duodenum are the duct from the gall bladder, carrying bile from the liver, and the duct from the pancreas, carrying *pancreatic juice*.

Bile is the digestive juice produced by the liver. It neutralizes the acid from the gastric juice, aids the digestion of fat and carries waste products away from the liver.

Pancreatic juice contains enzymes which digest fat, protein and carbohydrate.

Digestion is then completed by other enzymes produced by the rest of the small intestine.

Absorption

Food has now been digested into a form the body can use – broken down by enzymes into amino-acids, fatty acids, glucose, vitamins and minerals. These are absorbed into the blood by passing through the intestinal walls into capillaries. These capillaries join up to form the **portal vein** which carries digested food to the liver. Here the portal vein divides up into a second set of capillaries through which the digested food leaves the blood and enters the liver cells. The portal vein is therefore unique in being the only blood vessel which begins and ends as capillaries.

This passage of blood carrying digested food from intestines to liver is called the **portal circulation**. It is quite separate from the systemic circulation through the liver which brings in oxygen and carries away carbon dioxide. Oxygenated blood reaches the liver through a branch of the aorta, while deoxygenated blood leaves by another vein which joins the inferior vena cava. The portal circulation also carries minerals and drugs absorbed from the stomach and large intestine. Iron, for example, is extracted from food in the stomach and goes direct to the liver.

The final stage of absorption takes place in the large intestine where any remaining minerals enter the portal circulation. The undigested food remnants still contain a large quantity of water and most of this is absorbed through the walls of the large intestine into the blood stream.

Liver

The liver is a large complex organ which acts as the body's chemical factory. Its functions include:

1 Storage and distribution of carbohydrate
2 Storage of vitamins
3 Manufacture of bile
4 Manufacture of plasma proteins
5 Disposal of waste products

Excretion

Excretion means the removal of waste products from the body. Many different products are involved and their disposal occurs as follows:

1 Unusable food remnants in the large intestine pass into the rectum and are discharged from the body through the anus. This form of waste is called **faeces**. Bile contains some waste products from the liver and these are eliminated in the faeces.

2 Carbon dioxide is breathed out through the lungs.
3 Other waste products from the body cells are carried by the blood to the liver. Here they are specially processed and returned to the blood for carriage to the kidneys. As described in Chapter 4, the kidneys filter out these waste products and excess water to form urine, which is then stored in the bladder until ready for discharge.
4 Excess water is excreted mainly in the urine. The remainder is eliminated by the skin, as sweat; and by the lungs, as moisture in expired air.

Written examination

Write notes on:

(a) the main functions of saliva
(b) the principal salivary glands
(c) the results of reduced salivary flow (November 1992)

Summary

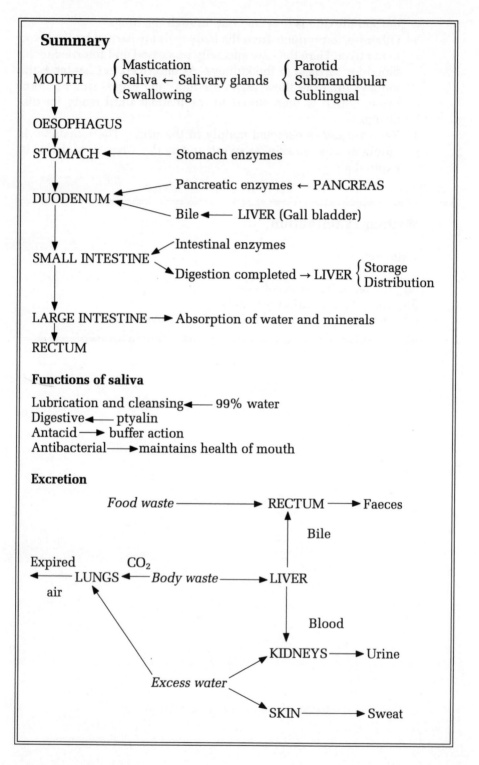

MOUTH $\left\{\begin{array}{l}\text{Mastication}\\ \text{Saliva} \leftarrow \text{Salivary glands}\\ \text{Swallowing}\end{array}\right.$ $\left\{\begin{array}{l}\text{Parotid}\\ \text{Submandibular}\\ \text{Sublingual}\end{array}\right.$

OESOPHAGUS

STOMACH ◄——— Stomach enzymes

DUODENUM ◄——— Pancreatic enzymes ← PANCREAS
◄——— Bile ◄——— LIVER (Gall bladder)

SMALL INTESTINE ⟋ Intestinal enzymes
⟍ Digestion completed → LIVER $\left\{\begin{array}{l}\text{Storage}\\ \text{Distribution}\end{array}\right.$

LARGE INTESTINE ——► Absorption of water and minerals

RECTUM

Functions of saliva

Lubrication and cleansing ◄—— 99% water
Digestive ◄—— ptyalin
Antacid ——► buffer action
Antibacterial ——► maintains health of mouth

Excretion

Food waste ————————► RECTUM ——► Faeces

Bile

Expired
air ◄—— LUNGS ◄— CO_2 *Body waste* ——► LIVER

Blood

KIDNEYS ——► Urine

Excess water

SKIN ————► Sweat

8 Microbiology

Chapters 3 to 7 have covered the structure and functions of the normal healthy body. The following chapters are concerned with the causes, effects and treatment of the changes produced by disease. Many diseases are caused by microscopic organisms, commonly called germs, but more correctly known as **micro-organisms**.

The mouth provides a warm sheltered home for countless numbers of micro-organisms. Most are quite harmless but some take part in dental diseases such as decay and gum disorders. Other micro-organisms, which are not normally present in healthy people, can be transmitted from persons affected by certain diseases. In such cases transmission of the disease to a healthy person can occur. There are three different groups of micro-organisms: fungi, bacteria and viruses. They are all of microscopic size and each group contains many different kinds, both harmless and dangerous.

Fungi

Fungi are larger than bacteria and the most important one found in the mouth is **candida albicans**. The most common oral condition associated with this organism is **denture stomatitis** (denture sore mouth), which appears as a conspicuous red area under dentures and orthodontic appliances.

A less common condition is called **thrush**. This appears as a white film or sore patches on the tongue and other parts of the mouth. Thrush can occur in babies, debilitated elderly people, and in any condition where resistance to infection is poor, such as AIDS (Chapter 10).

Bacteria

Bacteria are subdivided into groups according to their shape (Figure 8.1).

Bacilli

Bacilli (singular, *bacillus*) are rod-shaped bacteria. Examples are the **lactobacillus** found in decayed teeth; and **bacillus fusiformis** found in acute necrotizing ulcerative gingivitis (ANUG).

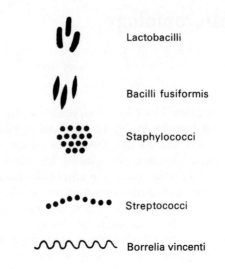

Lactobacilli

Bacilli fusiformis

Staphylococci

Streptococci

Figure 8.1 *Bacteria found in the mouth.*

Borrelia vincenti

Cocci

Cocci (singular, *coccus*) are round bacteria; for example, **staphylo-cocci** and **streptococci**. They are distinguished by their growth patterns: staphylococci grow in clumps like a bunch of grapes; streptococci in single lines like a string of beads. Each of these two groups is subdivided into different strains which are associated with different diseases. For example, one strain of staphylococcus causes skin boils, but a different strain may be found in gum boils. Similarly with streptococci, one particular strain, **streptococcus mutans**, initiates tooth decay (caries); while another causes sore throats.

Spirochaetes

These are spiral bacteria; for example, **borrelia vincenti** found in ANUG.

Spores

If conditions are unfavourable for their growth, some bacteria can exist in the form of **spores**. They do this by forming a tough protec-tive coating around themselves, rather like a nutshell. Spores can survive extremes of temperature and drought and may live in this dormant state for years until conditions become favourable again, whereupon they regain their normal shape and activities. The prac-tical importance of bacterial spores is that they are highly resistant to destruction and special methods of sterilization are necessary to deal with them.

Viruses

Viruses are far smaller than bacteria and cannot be seen with an ordinary microscope. They are responsible for a very wide range of diseases such as colds, German measles, mumps, herpes, hepatitis B (serum hepatitis) and AIDS.

Unlike fungal and bacterial diseases, which can be cured by drugs that kill micro-organisms, most viruses are unaffected by such drugs. Viral diseases are accordingly difficult to cure and some, such as **AIDS**, are incurable and fatal; while **hepatitis B** is dangerous and highly infective. Fortunately, however, many viral diseases, such as hepatitis B and German measles, can be prevented by vaccination. Chapter 10 covers AIDS and hepatitis B.

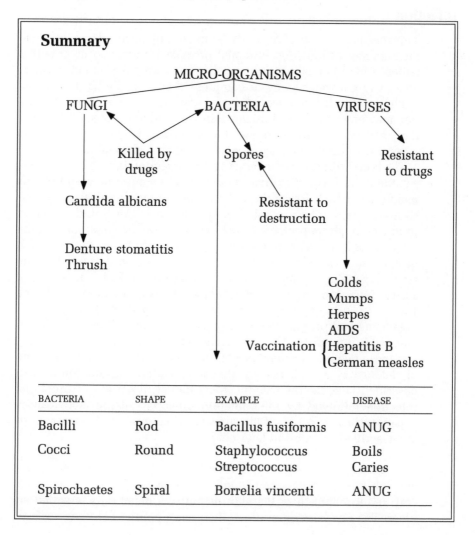

Summary

MICRO-ORGANISMS

FUNGI · BACTERIA · VIRUSES

Killed by drugs · Spores · Resistant to drugs

Candida albicans · Resistant to destruction

Denture stomatitis
Thrush

Colds
Mumps
Herpes
AIDS
Vaccination {Hepatitis B
{German measles

BACTERIA	SHAPE	EXAMPLE	DISEASE
Bacilli	Rod	Bacillus fusiformis	ANUG
Cocci	Round	Staphylococcus	Boils
		Streptococcus	Caries
Spirochaetes	Spiral	Borrelia vincenti	ANUG

9 Pathology

Pathology is the study of disease. It covers the changes in normal anatomy and physiology brought about by disease and the body's reaction to it. This chapter begins with the general effects of disease and continues with a consideration of diseases which are of importance in dental practice. Some common pathological terms are explained first.

Infection

This means invasion of the body by micro-organisms. The most common sources of infection in dental practice are direct contact with a patient's blood or saliva; airborne droplets containing blood or saliva when using a water spray or compressed air; and flying particles of tooth, tartar or filling released during drilling. These sources of infection may enter the body through skin cuts and abrasions, or the eyes; they may also be inhaled or swallowed. That is why it is necessary to wear gloves, mask and glasses when working at the chairside.

The body's first line of defence against infection is an intact surface, e.g. the outer layer of skin; and the protective outer layer of **mucous membrane** which forms the red *skin* of the mouth, airway and alimentary canal. The second line of defence is the liquid secretion produced by these protective surfaces. The mucous membrane of the mouth, together with the salivary glands, produces saliva which dilutes and neutralizes some bacterial poisons and can kill some micro-organisms. Tears and sweat have a similar effect. The acidity of gastric juice kills many of the micro-organisms in food; while the sticky film of mucus which covers the airway helps to trap micro-organisms and propels them away from the lungs. The third line of defence is immunity. This is covered later in the chapter.

If these defence mechanisms fail to prevent infection, the last line of defence is a response by the body called **inflammation**, also described later in this chapter. Most dental disease is of this type: infection followed by inflammation. Infection of the teeth causes decay (caries); infection of the gums causes periodontal disease. Both are described in detail in later chapters.

Ulcer

Any shallow breach of the skin or mucous membrane is called an ulcer. The raw base of an ulcer often has a painful bleeding surface.

The *herpes* virus can cause a severe and painful ulceration of the gums called herpetic gingivitis. Another type of painful gum ulceration is acute necrotizing ulcerative gingivitis, mentioned in Chapter 8.

Cyst

A cyst is an abnormal sac of fluid. Cysts are usually small and localized and can occur in soft tissues or bone anywhere in the body. Cysts of the jaws are described in Chapter 16.

Tumour

A tumour is a swelling caused by an abnormal and uncontrolled growth of body cells. It serves no useful purpose and may cause displacement or destruction of adjacent structures. Some types of tumour can spread throughout the body causing severe, and often fatal, destructive effects. This condition is commonly known as **cancer**.

Oral cancer

About 3,000 people a year get cancer of the mouth (oral cancer) and about half of them die from it. But this high mortality rate is mainly due to the late detection of the disease; and that is because its early stages are painless. If it is detected and treated early enough, about 80% can be cured.

Early signs of oral cancer, or conditions which may become cancerous, are any ulcer, lump, white or red patch which persists for more than two or three weeks. They usually occur on the side or undersurface of the tongue, the floor of the mouth, inside the cheeks, on the lower lip and the throat.

Heavy smokers and drinkers are most at risk, and 85% of cases occur in people over 50. Oral cancer may therefore be prevented by giving up smoking, cutting down on alcohol, and by having a dental check-up every year. If the dentist detects any suspicious signs, referral for hospital tests will tell whether or not it is cancerous and enable early treatment to be undertaken.

Congenital defects

This means defects which are present at birth, such as heart and valvular defects, cleft palate or other deformities.

Biopsy

The cause or nature of an ulcer or tumour cannot always be determined by physical or X-ray examination. Confirmation of the diagnosis often necessitates surgical removal of some diseased tissue for examination under a microscope. This minor operation is called a **biopsy**. The biopsy specimen is sent to a hospital pathology department in a bottle of formol-saline preservative.

The diagnosis of infections often requires bacteriological examination of a swab or smear from an infected surface. Other types of disease are commonly diagnosed by blood and urine tests.

Inflammation

Inflammation may be defined as the reaction of the body to irritation. It is a defence reaction, *not* a disease. The irritant may be infective, chemical or physical, e.g. bacteria, burns or wounds, but whatever the cause, the reaction is basically the same. Inflammation arising suddenly and lasting only a short time is called **acute inflammation**. If it lasts for a long time it is known as **chronic inflammation**, e.g. chronic alveolar abscess. The suffix *itis* means inflammation. Thus inflammation of the bronchi is bronchitis; of the gum is gingivitis; of the mouth is stomatitis.

The white cells of the blood are the body's main defence against infection. Inflammation is, therefore, characterized by a tremendous increase of blood flow to the infected part, in order to bring as many white blood cells as possible into battle against the invading bacteria or other micro-organisms. To obtain this extra supply of blood, all the blood vessels in the area dilate and this causes what are known as the cardinal signs of inflammation:

1   Swelling
2   Redness
3   Heat
4   Pain
5   Loss of function

Swelling, redness and heat result from the extra volume of blood in the inflamed area. Pain is caused by the increased pressure of blood on the nerves. Because of the pain and swelling, the affected part is unable to function properly. For example, an inflamed tooth is too tender to bite on and cannot be used for its normal function of chewing. There may also be a rise in body temperature, caused by the effect of poisons produced by the micro-organisms concerned. This can be checked with a clinical thermometer or as described on page 36. Normal body temperature is 37°C.

The inflamed area is now engorged with blood, caused by dilation of the blood vessels. White cells then wriggle through the capillary walls to reach the bacteria. At the same time an exudate of plasma, containing antibodies and antitoxins, seeps out of the capillaries to help the white cells. The exudate dilutes bacterial poisons, while antitoxins neutralize them; antibodies and white cells can then overcome the bacteria. During the battle between invading bacteria and white cells in the inflamed area, many casualties occur. These dead white cells and bacteria form the creamy liquid known as **pus**. A localized collection of pus is called an **abscess**. Abscesses involving the teeth are called *alveolar abscesses*, and abscesses of the skin are called boils. Sometimes pus formation spreads diffusely instead of forming an abscess. This is called **cellulitis** and may occur around an infected lower wisdom tooth.

This description of the inflammatory process is typical of acute inflammation following infection. In chronic inflammation the process is less obvious, as it is spread over a much longer period of time. Generally there is little or no pain in chronic inflammation; the main feature is usually swelling. Acute and chronic inflammatory processes affecting the teeth and gums are described in Chapters 17 and 25.

In the absence of infection, pus formation does not occur and any damage done by the causal irritant is repaired. But if an infection is too virulent, or the body resistance too weak, the white cells are unable to contain the infection and it can spread throughout the body. Before the discovery of antibiotics, such spread was usually fatal. If the balance between infection and body resistance is equal, a condition of stalemate may supervene, often leading to a persistent state of chronic infection. This usually occurs with alveolar abscesses and in gum disease.

Repair

Following inflammation, any damage is repaired by white cells which rebuild the area by filling the breach with a temporary repair tissue called **granulation tissue**. This consists of rapidly growing white cells and new capillaries which form a fibrous scaffolding in which damaged parts are removed and reconstruction takes place. But repair cannot take place in the presence of pus. Thus an abscessed tooth requires extraction or root treatment to drain off the pus before the destroyed area of bone can be repaired.

When a tooth is extracted an inflammatory reaction is set up as a wound has been inflicted. The increased blood supply brings white cells to the area and they repair the socket by replacing the blood clot with granulation tissue. No infection is present in the socket so there is no 'battle' or pus formation in the normal course of events. The granulation tissue is later replaced by the formation of new bone.

Immunity

Immunity means resistance to disease. It is provided by certain white blood cells which release antibodies and antitoxins into the blood plasma. Many causative factors can stimulate white cells to produce antibodies and antitoxins; for example, micro-organisms; bacterial, plant and animal toxins; foreign bodies; transplants; transfusion of incompatible blood cells. All such factors are called **antigens**.

When infection occurs, inflammation results, and part of this defensive reaction involves antibodies and antitoxins. They are present in the blood and help overcome the micro-organisms concerned. Some of these antibodies and antitoxins can remain in the blood for life and prevent any repetition of the same infection. Such life-long protection is called **acquired immunity**; but unfortunately it does not occur for every type of micro-organism. However, where immunity is possible it can be reproduced artificially in people who have never been infected by a particular micro-organism. It may be done by giving a non-immune person a dose of dead micro-organisms. This is called **vaccination**. Dead micro-organisms cannot produce disease but they do stimulate the host's body to produce antibodies and antitoxins against the particular micro-organisms concerned. Thus any subsequent infection with these organisms is immediately overcome by the antibodies and antitoxins already present.

Vaccination can give life-long immunity against many very serious diseases, such as hepatitis B, poliomyelitis, tuberculosis, German measles (rubella), whooping cough and tetanus. All nurses should be vaccinated against these as some are virus infections which are resistant to any other form of treatment. Much research has been done to create vaccines against tooth decay and gum disease, but without practicable results so far.

If there has been no vaccination or prior exposure to disease, acquired immunity is not present. However, all individuals inherit some degree of **natural immunity** and this helps explain why some people are more resistant to disease than others.

Where immunity to a particular disease is not present, it can be provided by vaccination to prevent that disease; but it can also be introduced by injecting antibodies or antitoxins to treat or temporarily prevent the disease concerned. Such protection is called **passive immunity** and is commonly used against tetanus. During pregnancy a mother passes on her own antibodies and antitoxins to her unborn baby and this provides passive immunity for the first few months after birth.

Some people have a defective immune system and are accordingly much more susceptible to infection. Such individuals are said to be **immuno-compromised** and one of the most important examples is the destruction of the body's defence mechanism by the AIDS virus, resulting in death from an inability to resist infection. AIDS is described in detail in Chapter 10.

Other immuno-compromised patients may be those suffering from leukaemia, kidney failure and diabetes; and those taking drugs which suppress immunity; for example, cytotoxics, used for the treatment of cancer, and drugs used to prevent rejection of transplants.

Allergy

Sometimes a normal immune response does not occur. Instead, a violent reaction called allergy is produced. This can cause sudden death but usually involves consequences of varying degrees of ser-iousness, ranging from skin rashes or mouth ulcers to partial obstruction of the airway. Sensitivity to certain types of pollen, food, stings, latex products and drugs can produce an allergic response.

This can happen to both dental staff and patients. For example; some brands of latex gloves, or materials and drugs used in routine treatment, can produce skin reactions. These are usually mild and can be easily overcome by changing to a different brand of glove or material.

A much more serious type of allergy which could happen in dental practice is that affecting patients sensitive to penicillin and its deri-vatives (e.g. amoxycillin). If one of these drugs were given to such patients, the above-mentioned reactions could occur – the worst effect of all being the rapid onset of a severe state of collapse which may be fatal. This is called **anaphylactic shock** and is covered in Chapter 15. The patients most at risk of allergic responses are those with a history of asthma, eczema and hay fever.

Diseases affecting dental practice

Many dental patients suffer from diseases which may lead to serious complications during certain forms of dental treatment. It is accord-ingly necessary for nurses to know of these conditions and realize how important it is to be aware of patients' medical histories.

Disorders of the blood

These may affect its oxygen-carrying function, clotting, or the white cells which resist infection. Diagnosis is confirmed by blood tests.

Anaemia

Anaemia is a disease in which the capacity of red blood cells to carry oxygen is diminished. Anaemic patients tire easily, become breathless on exertion, may have a pale complexion, or suffer from a sore tongue and mouth. They need special care during general anaesthesia.

Anaemia may be caused by iron deficiency or liver malfunction. A hereditary form of anaemia called **sickle cell disease** often affects patients of African or Caribbean origin. All patients of this ethnic group requiring general anaesthesia should have a blood test to check their fitness for it.

Excessive bleeding

Any disorders of the blood-clotting mechanism result in excessive bleeding which may be difficult to stop. This is of obvious importance in dental practice when tooth extraction is necessary. It may be caused by a deficiency of platelets, liver disease, anticoagulant drugs, or a hereditary condition such as **haemophilia** in which certain plasma factors are missing. Even the injection of a local anaesthetic can cause dangerous bleeding in a haemophiliac.

Leukaemia

This is a form of blood cancer affecting the white cells. Instead of normal white cells, enormous numbers of immature cells are produced which cannot perform their normal functions. This results in loss of resistance to disease, anaemia and excessive bleeding. Such patients often have enlarged bleeding gums.

Cardiovascular disease

This means disorders of the heart and circulation, some of which were mentioned in Chapter 5. They can affect the heart's ability to pump oxygenated blood round the body, or lead to the blockage or leakage of blood vessels. Special care of such patients is necessary during general anaesthesia to ensure adequate oxygenation of the blood. Local anaesthesia is used instead of general anaesthesia in most cases.

Valvular heart disease

This condition may be congenital or result from **rheumatic fever** in childhood.

Infective endocarditis

This is a serious, and sometimes fatal, complication of congenital or rheumatic valvular heart disease. Whenever teeth are extracted, or scaled, or root treatment performed, bacteria enter the blood. This is called **bacteraemia**. Normally, such bacteria would soon be killed by white blood cells, but damaged heart valves are able to harbour bacteria circulating in the blood and afford them protection from white cells. Infected clots of blood from these valves may spread throughout the body, causing infections or blocking blood vessels. Fortunately infective endocarditis can be prevented by giving antibiotic cover (Chapter 11) before extractions, surgery, scaling and some root treatments in patients with a history of valvular disease.

Patients at risk are those with congenital heart defects, a history of rheumatic fever, previous infective endocarditis, and those with artificial heart valves. They should be warned to see their doctor or dentist if any minor illness develops after dental treatment, whether or not antibiotic cover was given. If infective endocarditis occurs it is usually within a month of treatment, but the symptoms may be of such gradual onset that their significance is not realized by the patient. This can lead to late diagnosis and the possible failure of medical treatment.

Arterial disease

The internal surfaces of arteries may be damaged by fatty deposits on their walls. These produce a rough surface which encourages blood clots to form and create blockage of an artery. If this occurs in the coronary arteries which supply the heart itself, blood flow may be so restricted that chest pain called **angina pectoris** occurs on exertion. An even worse complication is complete blockage of a coronary artery by clotted blood. This is **coronary thrombosis** and is characterized by severe chest pain and collapse. It is a common cause of sudden death, as it produces **myocardial infarction** which means the death of an area of heart muscle supplied by the blocked artery. Emergency treatment of heart attacks is covered in Chapter 15.

Hypertension

This means high blood pressure. It is a complication of arterial disease, and may be caused by a generalized constriction of the arteries. Hypertension is treated with drugs which can cause adverse effects during general anaesthesia. Local anaesthesia is accordingly preferred.

Stroke

A stroke is a very serious, and often fatal, form of collapse caused by sudden brain damage. It may occur in arterial disease: from blockage of a brain artery by a blood clot; or because of hypertension bursting a blood vessel in the brain. Whatever the cause it may leave the patient with varying degrees of paralysis.

Respiratory disease

Disease of the airway or lungs can seriously impair oxygenation of the blood, and this in turn makes general anaesthesia hazardous. Again, local anaesthesia is preferred. Chronic bronchitis and asthma cause partial obstruction of the bronchi.

Asthma

This condition causes spasmodic constriction of the bronchi resulting in wheezing and difficulty in breathing. Attacks may be triggered by the stress of dental treatment and are accordingly covered in Chapter 15. Asthma is a type of allergy and can result from environmental allergens such as pollen, dust, traffic fumes and animal hair. Any patient with a history of asthma is at risk of allergic reactions to the drugs, materials and equipment (e.g. latex gloves) used in dentistry.

Liver disease

The liver has so many essential functions that many different effects can result from liver disease. They include excessive bleeding and altered response to drugs, including complications from some used in general anaesthesia. Drug treatment should be minimal or avoided altogether in severe forms of liver disease.

In many forms of liver disease bile is prevented from entering the duodenum and accumulates in the blood instead. This gives the skin and whites of the eyes a yellowish tinge known as **jaundice**.

Any inflammation of the liver is called **hepatitis**. The most important type is hepatitis B, already mentioned in chapter 8 and the section on immunity. Special care is necessary with jaundiced patients as this is a diagnostic sign of liver disease. Such patients may be highly infective (if suffering from hepatitis B) or liable to excessive bleeding.

Diabetes

Chapter 7 on the digestive system described the role of the pancreas in producing enzymes which are discharged into the duodenum. Another entirely different function of the pancreas is the production of a hormone called **insulin**. This enters the blood directly from the pancreas and is responsible for maintaining the correct level of glucose in the blood.

Diabetes is a disease in which the pancreas is unable to produce insulin. This results in a build-up of glucose in the blood and its excretion in urine. The effect of this accumulation of blood glucose is a serious range of complications ranging from collapse (**hypergly-caemic coma**) to arterial disease, blindness, gangrene and poor resistance to infection.

Fortunately insulin can be manufactured synthetically and is accordingly used for the treatment of diabetics. However, it requires careful dietary control to maintain the correct levels of blood glucose. This balance can be upset by starving a diabetic patient prior to general anaesthesia or keeping them waiting beyond normal meal-times if appointments are running late. In either case, if the blood glucose becomes too low they are liable to a different form of collapse called **hypoglycaemic coma**. This is remedied by giving some sugar and is covered in Chapter 15.

Medical history

This account of general disease and its effects in dental practice should make it clear that an adequate and up-to-date medical history must be kept for every patient attending a practice. Any failure to detect or be aware of such diseases can lead to serious complications, or even death, during the course of dental treatment. Complications may be caused by the disease itself, the dental treatment, or an interaction between drugs taken by the patient and those used in dental treatment. It is therefore essential for the medical history to include full details of drugs being taken as well as details of past and present illness.

Any dentist failing to keep regularly updated records of patients' medical histories is liable to a charge of serious professional mis-conduct if complications occur. History-taking is covered in more detail in Chapter 30.

Written examination

What precautions need to be taken when treating a dental patient who:

(a) is pregnant
(b) is a known hepatitis B carrier
(c) has suffered from rheumatic fever? (November 1994)

List the five signs of inflammation.
With these in mind, describe the sequence of events which may lead from healthy gingivae to deep periodontal pockets. (May 1996)

Summary

- *Infection:* invasion by micro-organisms
- *Ulcer:* raw area of skin or mucous membrane
- *Cyst:* localized collection of fluid
- *Tumour:* swelling due to uncontrolled cell growth
- *Congenital defect:* present at birth, e.g. heart defects, cleft palate
- *Immunity:* previous disease or vaccination → antibodies → life-long protection
- *Allergy:* abnormal immune response → rashes, ulceration, sometimes fatal. May be due to drug sensitivity, e.g. penicillin
- *Biopsy:* surgical removal of diseased tissue for diagnosis by microscopic examination

Inflammation

Defence mechanism – not disease

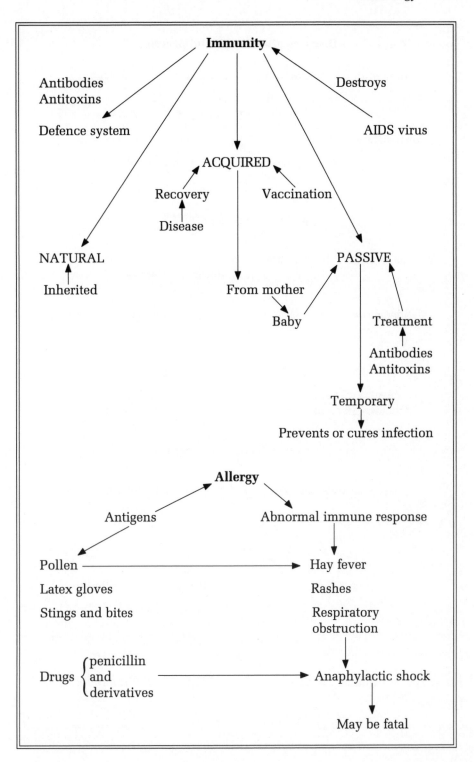

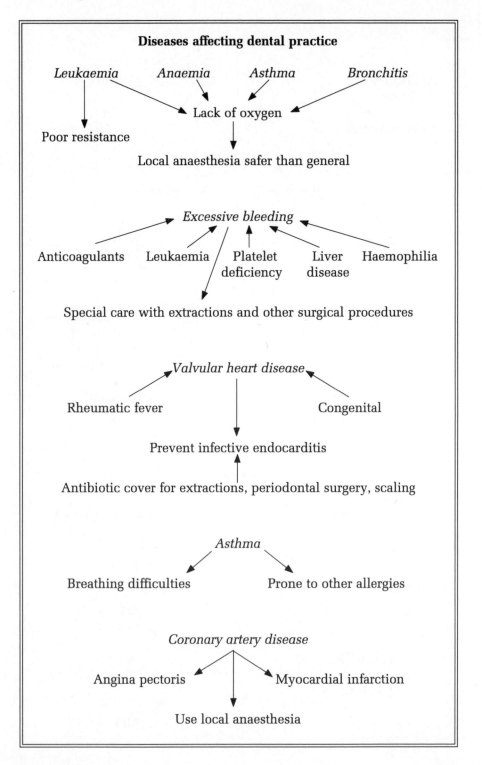

Diseases affecting dental practice

Leukaemia   *Anaemia*   *Asthma*   *Bronchitis*

Lack of oxygen

Poor resistance

Local anaesthesia safer than general

Excessive bleeding

Anticoagulants   Leukaemia   Platelet   Liver   Haemophilia
deficiency   disease

Special care with extractions and other surgical procedures

Valvular heart disease

Rheumatic fever   Congenital

Prevent infective endocarditis

Antibiotic cover for extractions, periodontal surgery, scaling

Asthma

Breathing difficulties   Prone to other allergies

Coronary artery disease

Angina pectoris   Myocardial infarction

Use local anaesthesia

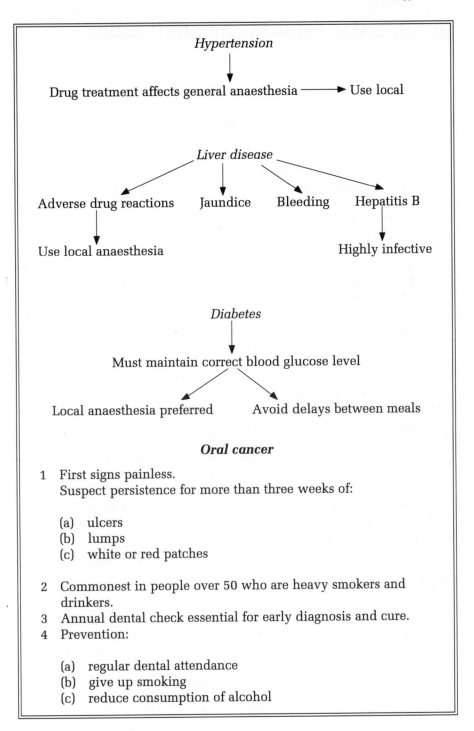

Hypertension

Drug treatment affects general anaesthesia ⟶ Use local

Liver disease

Adverse drug reactions   Jaundice   Bleeding   Hepatitis B

Use local anaesthesia   Highly infective

Diabetes

Must maintain correct blood glucose level

Local anaesthesia preferred   Avoid delays between meals

Oral cancer

1 First signs painless.
   Suspect persistence for more than three weeks of:

   (a) ulcers
   (b) lumps
   (c) white or red patches

2 Commonest in people over 50 who are heavy smokers and
   drinkers.
3 Annual dental check essential for early diagnosis and cure.
4 Prevention:

   (a) regular dental attendance
   (b) give up smoking
   (c) reduce consumption of alcohol

10 Infection Control and Sterilization

As shown in Chapter 8, the mouth is full of micro-organisms, some of which are harmful. Consequently instruments and equipment used in dental treatment become contaminated whenever they are used. If no action were taken, infection from this contamination would be passed on from patient to patient, from patient to dental staff, and from staff to patient. This involvement is called **cross-infection**. In order to prevent cross-infection it is essential to kill all the micro-organisms on infected instruments. This process is known as **sterilization** and means the killing of all micro-organisms: bacteria, spores, fungi and viruses. It is carried out immediately after completion of treatment so that all instruments are sterile again before use on the next patient.

Countless numbers of micro-organisms live on the skin and in the mouth, nose and throat. Normally they do no harm to their host as they are living on an external surface and not among delicate internal cells. However, they may become harmful if they are introduced inside the body tissues, or are transferred from one person's mouth to another. This can occur when the tissues are penetrated by a contaminated forceps blade, scaler or syringe needle, and may give rise to a harmful reaction. After each patient has left the surgery, it is the nurse's duty to see that all instruments are properly sterilized before being used again for another patient.

As already mentioned, sterilization means killing not only bacteria and fungi, but all other micro-organisms, including viruses and bacterial spores. Any method which kills bacteria and fungi but allows some spores or viruses to survive cannot be called sterilization. The term used for this restricted range of action is **disinfection**. In dental practice the goal is sterilization, not disinfection.

Sterilization

Instruments and dressings requiring sterilization are made of different materials: some cannot be heated; some go rusty; others must remain dry to be of any use. To meet these differences there are various methods of sterilization, each suitable for certain instruments or materials. Basically the methods used in a dental surgery are moist heat (steam), dry heat, and chemical sterilization.

Steam

Steam under pressure kills all bacteria, spores, fungi and viruses. It is the most effective method available for dental practice and is the most common method of sterilization in hospitals. Steam is produced in an **autoclave**, which resembles a pressure cooker in principle, and is kept at a temperature of 134°C for at least three minutes. In practice, however, it takes much longer as the instruments are inserted cold. Time must be allowed for the autoclave to reach its sterilizing temperature and cool down again afterwards. In fact, autoclaves are so made that once any instruments are inserted, they cannot be removed until the full cycle of up to 20 minutes has been completed.

Sterility can be checked by means of **TST strips**. These are paper strips which change colour from yellow to purple on exposure to steam at 134°C for three minutes. A strip is included with the instruments when they are placed in the autoclave.

Steam is suitable for metal instruments, diamond and tungsten carbide burs, rubber, most plastics, swabs, cotton wool and paper points, etc. Handpieces are autoclavable if they are lubricated beforehand in accordance with their manufacturers' instructions. Instruments and dressings must be placed in open containers to ensure full exposure to the steam.

Autoclaves are expensive but, overall, they are the most convenient and acceptable method in practice. Health and safety legislation (Chapter 31) requires autoclaves to be regularly inspected, tested and serviced in accordance with the manufacturers' instructions.

Hot air

Sterilization is effected by very hot air produced in an electrically heated oven called a **hot air sterilizer**. Its contents are kept at 160°C for two hours, but time must be allowed for warming up and cooling down; thus giving a cycle of well over two hours. Furthermore the sterilizer must not be opened during this time. However, it is convenient for sterilizing large batches of instruments overnight. Like an autoclave it will kill all micro-organisms but is generally regarded as of limited value in a dental surgery as its disadvantages outweigh its advantages.

It is used for all metal instruments and is particularly suitable for those which must be kept dry, such as root treatment kits; or liable to rust, such as steel burs. Although the cotton wool and paper points used in root treatment kits may become discoloured or brittle at this high temperature, their absorbent qualities are not seriously affected. Low-speed handpieces can also be sterilized in this way if suitable lubricants are used. Hot air ovens have the advantage of allowing kits of instruments for any particular procedure to be sterilized inside a closed metal container. Such kits may then be stored elsewhere and will remain sterile, ready for immediate use at any time.

Sterility can be checked by means of **Browne's tubes**. These are sealed glass tubes containing a liquid which changes colour on exposure to 160°C. One of these tubes is included with the instruments when they are placed in the sterilizer.

The most serious disadvantage of some hot air ovens is the absence of a fan for ensuring the correct temperature throughout the sterilizing chamber. Other disadvantages are the long time and high temperature involved, which is too hot for modern handpieces, rubber and plastics.

Hot oil

This is confined to instruments with moving parts which can go rusty, and are unsuitable for an autoclave or hot air sterilizer. Thus it is used primarily for old low-speed handpieces. The temperature and time vary according to the oil used; the handpiece being lubricated as well as sterilized.

Oil sterilizers specially made for low-speed handpieces, are used. Spores are destroyed if the oil is kept at 140°C for 15 minutes. However, most modern handpieces can be sterilized in an autoclave and this is the method of choice whenever possible.

Flaming

Flaming is simple and immediate but has only a limited application. It is particularly useful for sterilizing the caps of local anaesthetic cartridges.

Disinfectants

This method uses chemicals called disinfectants which kill or prevent the growth of bacteria. Many different disinfectants are available but some of the most useful in dental practice are **chlorhexidine** (*Hibitane*) and **sodium hypochlorite** (*Milton*, domestic bleaches). Their main use is for cleaning and disinfecting work surfaces.

The time required varies with each disinfectant and they are only used for items or equipment which cannot be sterilized by the previous high temperature methods. Most disinfectants do not kill spores and some are unreliable against viruses. For this reason, the use of disinfectants cannot be accepted as a satisfactory method of sterilization; they may only produce disinfection, have a limited shelf life and should be freshly made up before use. They are routinely used in surgical procedures, however, for the disinfection of body surfaces prior to incisions and injections; and for rinsing hands before treatment.

The disadvantage of most disinfectants is their poisonous nature and unpleasant taste. Instruments taken from a disinfectant must therefore be rinsed in sterile water or carefully wiped with a sterile towel before use.

Disinfectants must be used in strict accordance with manufacturers' instructions; prepared to the correct strength; used for the correct period of time; and not kept beyond their active life or expiry date.

Hypochlorite is effective against spores, hepatitis B and AIDS viruses. It is the best overall disinfectant for work surfaces, impressions, denture work, and items which cannot be heat sterilized. The disadvantages are that it can bleach clothing and corrode metal.

Glutaraldehyde has been used as an alternative to hypochlorite but has the disadvantage of being irritant if it contacts eyes or skin, and if its vapour is inhaled. Its use is therefore confined to items which are damaged by hypochlorite. It should be stored in covered containers, and used with eye protection, mask and gloves, and good ventilation. The same applies to any other irritant solutions used in a practice.

Industrial sterilization

Although steam and hot air kill all micro-organisms, they are not satisfactory for sterilizing syringe needles. Even the minutest trace of infected blood in the lumen of a used syringe needle can transmit the hepatitis B virus from one patient to another. As hepatitis B is a very serious disease which may result in death, used needles must never be used again on another patient. Normally a hot air sterilizer or autoclave will kill these viruses but in the case of contaminated syringe needles they cannot be relied upon; the space inside the needle is too small to allow complete penetration of hot air or steam into clotted blood remnants.

A new pre-sterilized disposable needle must be used for every patient. Each needle is supplied in a sealed plastic cover and is sterilized by the manufacturer, using modern industrial methods. After use it is discarded. Many other items such as scalpels, syringes, suture needles, intravenous injection kits and dressings are supplied in this way and are similarly disposable.

The manufacturers sterilize these articles by exposing them to **radiation**. This is done by exposure to gamma rays which are obtained from a radioactive source and are similar to X-rays.

This method is cold and dry, and destroys all bacteria, fungi, spores and viruses. Unfortunately it cannot be used in a dental surgery as it is an industrial process entailing the skilled operation of elaborate equipment.

Cross-infection

Infection control involves far more than the sterilization of instruments between patients. It is concerned with surgery hygiene as well as sterilization. Furthermore, it is not only the patients who must be protected from infection, but surgery staff themselves.

Occupational hazards

There are three major occupational hazards in dentistry: radiation, mercury poisoning and cross-infection. All three concern the dental nurse who must be aware of their dangers and know how to avoid them. The former two are described in later chapters; but cross-infection is covered here as its prevention is the purpose of infection control.

The most serious diseases which can be contracted from cross-infection are **hepatitis B** and **AIDS**, both of which are spread by contact with blood containing these viruses. Patients infected with hepatitis B or AIDS viruses are usually unaware of their condition until symptoms arise, but their blood contains the virus nonetheless.

Dental practice often involves the shedding of blood; and even the minutest blood-stained droplets may contain viruses. Furthermore, such blood-borne viruses can be sprayed over a wide area of the surgery when using high-speed handpieces, ultrasonic scalers and air/water syringes. Thus, not only instruments, but work surfaces, surgery equipment and surgery staff are exposed to contamination in this way.

Hepatitis B and AIDS are covered in detail later in the chapter but less serious viral infections are conveniently discussed here. Special care should be taken if child patients have been in contact with virus infections such as **mumps** and **rubella** (German measles). The virus is present in saliva before any signs of illness are apparent, and surgery staff may become infected in this way from an apparently fit child. If there is any evidence of contact, appropriate questioning of parents will allow the dentist to assess the risk of infection and decide whether to postpone treatment. Although such infections are usually trivial in children, they can cause serious complications in susceptible adults.

If rubella occurs in the first three months of pregnancy it can affect the unborn child – and this may happen before pregnancy is confirmed. Such a child is likely to have serious physical defects; and in such cases there are strong medical grounds for advising the termination of pregnancy.

Adult males are most at risk from mumps as it may cause sterility. All practice staff should, therefore, check their own medical history and vaccination records. They should be immune from common childhood infections previously contracted and are only at risk from any which are not included in these records.

Cold sores on the lips are another condition commonly met in the surgery. They are caused by a **herpes** virus and can transmit the infection to persons with no immunity to this virus. Dental staff should accordingly take great care to avoid direct skin contact with cold sores, as they can result in a very painful herpetic *whitlow* if operating gloves are not worn.

Even such a trivial viral infection as the common cold is infectious. If surgery staff or their patients have a cold, transmission to others can be prevented by wearing protective clothing. Although the effects of a cold are not serious, they often necessitate time off work with the resultant inconvenience caused by staff shortage.

Bearing in mind that it will rarely be known if a patient is infectious or carrying a dangerous virus, and very likely that the patient is unaware of it too, or unwilling to admit it, the safest approach to the problem of cross-infection is to assume that *every* patient is infectious. Fortunately, protection is available against hepatitis B, rubella, poliomyelitis, diphtheria, pertussis (whooping cough), tuberculosis and tetanus by vaccination. All practice staff should be protected in this way.

Protective clothing

Infected debris from a patient's mouth may be scattered in all directions when using a high-speed handpiece, ultrasonic scaler or air/water syringe. Good ventilation and an efficient aspirator (which exhausts externally) reduces, but cannot eliminate this source of infection. Chairside staff should protect their eyes by wearing glasses with full lenses and side shields; their airway with a mask; their hands by wearing gloves; and clothing by an operating gown or uniform coat. Any open skin wounds or cuts should be covered with a waterproof dressing. Wrist watches and jewellery should not be worn in the surgery as they can harbour infection and damage gloves.

Dentists are legally obliged to provide all necessary protective clothing for their staff.

Surgery hygiene and sterilization

After a patient's treatment is finished the instruments must be carefully scrubbed with detergent and warm water to remove all traces of saliva, blood, amalgam and other filling materials, etc. An ultrasonic cleaner is very useful and effective for this purpose. The cleaned instruments are then rinsed under running water and autoclaved. Heavy-duty gloves should be worn when cleaning instruments; and manufacturers' instructions must be followed when using ultrasonic cleaners and sterilizing handpieces.

All non-sharp contaminated waste material on the bracket table, such as napkins, cotton rolls, extracted teeth, etc., is placed in a disposable plastic bag and transferred to a yellow clinical waste sack kept away from the surgery. To prevent injury to refuse collectors or re-use by addicts, special puncture-proof rigid sharps containers are used for syringe needles, scalpel blades, steel burs, root canal broaches, matrix bands and other disposable sharp items.

To prevent accidental injury and cross-infection from non-disposable sharp instruments, nurses should use heavy-duty gloves, a long-handled brush, and hold sharp ends away from them when cleaning up.

The surgery is then prepared for the next patient by covering the bracket table with a new disposable waterproof cover or cleaning with a detergent, followed by a disinfectant. A new disposable headrest cover is fitted; water is discharged for 30 seconds from the air/water syringe and handpieces with water spray; the spittoon is flushed clean and a new disposable beaker of warm mouthwash is provided. Many other disposable products are available: saliva ejectors, aspirator and air/water syringe tips, impression trays, hand towels and refuse bags. Their use simplifies surgery procedure, saves time and should be used whenever possible.

Special arrangements must be made for items which cannot be sterilized by the methods described. Wherever possible, switches, handles and taps should be adapted to avoid hand contact. This may be done by electronic means, foot-operated switches or using your elbow. Alternatively, kitchen clingfilm can be used to cover the handles and switches of surgery equipment.

Special zone routines should be devised for minimizing the number and extent of potentially contaminated surfaces. Depending on the particular surgery layout, this may be achieved by allotting various functions, such as the preparation and mixing of surgery materials, hand washing and clerical work, to *clean* zones; while chairside units and work surfaces are regarded as contaminated zones.

Whichever type of sterilizer is used, instruments must be sterile when they come out. To ensure this, they must be kept in the sterilizer at the correct temperature for the correct time, and should not be added to a batch of instruments already being sterilized. It is of the utmost importance to ensure that no traces of amalgam or mercury get into a sterilizer as they emit poisonous mercury vapour when heated. Some types of handpiece cannot be placed in a hot air oven and some cannot be autoclaved. Manufacturers' instructions should always be obeyed; and in this respect it is fortunate that modern handpieces are specially designed to permit easy cleaning, autoclaving and lubrication.

After sterilization the instruments are removed from the autoclave in their tray containers. Individual instruments are handled with sterile Cheatle's forceps (Figure 10.1). The sterilized instruments must then remain sterile until used again. Sterile containers or trays with lids are used where practicable; but if instrument cabinets or drawers are used for storage, instruments should be placed on, and covered with, a new disposable waterproof lining.

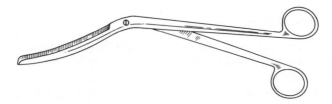

Figure 10.1 *Cheatle's forceps.*

The purpose of sterilization is to prevent the spread of infection from one source to another. It must, therefore, be constantly borne in mind that sterilization of instruments is a waste of time if they are immediately brought into contact with contaminated hands or gloves. Disinfectant liquid soaps (e.g. *Hibiscrub, Hibisol*) are best for washing hands, and paper towels for drying them. After hands are thoroughly washed and dry, any cuts or abrasions are covered with waterproof dressings, and a new pair of gloves worn. If gloves are torn or punctured during treatment, they should be discarded immediately, hands washed again and new gloves fitted before continuing treatment. A new mask is also worn for each patient.

At the end of the day, the spittoon and aspiration system should be flushed with disinfectant. Surgery waste is stored in heavy-duty yellow plastic sacks ready for incineration. Sharps containers are also incinerated but should be kept separate from other surgery waste. Domestic waste is kept separate from sharps containers and surgery waste, and is collected by the normal waste-disposal service.

The nurse's duty

Sterilization and the procedures just described for infection control are some of the dental nurses' most important duties. Dentists rely upon them to accept this responsibility conscientiously and to undertake their duties with the utmost care and diligence. Nurses are legally obliged to comply with employers' instructions in all aspects of health and safety at work. Short cuts, omissions and untidiness cannot be tolerated. Always remember that the object of treatment is to make patients better, not worse!

Prevention of cross-infection

In view of the increasing publicity and concern among the general public about the dangers of cross-infection, hepatitis B and AIDS, the following guidelines to good dental practice have been issued. As mentioned in Chapter 2, the GDC requires all dentists to ensure that they and their staff comply with such guidelines. Any failure to do so can result in disciplinary proceedings.

Infection control policy

Every practice must draft an appropriate policy describing its infection control procedure; who is responsible for it; and who to consult about any accidents, problems or doubts which may arise. A copy of the policy should be given to all practice staff; signed by the principal and staff member; and displayed in the surgery.

Vaccination

All practice staff should be vaccinated against rubella, poliomyelitis, pertussis, diphtheria, tuberculosis, tetanus and hepatitis B.

Medical history

A thorough and regularly updated medical history must be taken by the dentist for every patient. This subject is covered in Chapter 30.

Sterilization

Instruments must be thoroughly cleaned before sterilization. Use an ultrasonic cleaner where appropriate. Autoclaving is the method of choice for sterilization. Correct times and temperatures must be used without interruption.

Cold sterilizing in disinfectants should only be used for instruments and other items which cannot be exposed to heat.

Disposables

Use these whenever possible.
Never reuse disposable materials or equipment, especially syringes, needles and local anaesthetic cartridges.

Work surfaces

Avoid contamination by using instrument trays or disposable protective coverings wherever possible. Use rubber dam whenever possible to reduce contamination. Clean and disinfect surfaces and flush all water-spray equipment after each patient leaves.

Protective clothing

- Uniform coats, operating gowns or other surgery clothing should not be worn in eating areas or outside the practice. It should be washable at 65°C.
- Gloves, mask and eye protection should be worn routinely by all surgery staff.
- Protective glasses should have full lenses and side-shields and be provided for patients as well as surgery staff.
- Hands should be washed with disinfectant liquid soaps before and after donning gloves.
- Cuts and abrasions should be covered with waterproof dressings and gloves should be worn on top.
- Wear a new pair of gloves and mask for each patient.

Waste disposal

Health and safety legislation (Chapter 31) requires special arrangements for the collection and incineration of clinical waste by authorized personnel.

Rigid, puncture-proof, sealable sharps containers conforming to the British Standard must be used and should not be overfilled. All other surgery waste and infected material must be stored in heavy-duty yellow plastic sacks and sealed ready for collection. Sharps containers should be kept separate from other surgery waste while awaiting collection.

Ordinary domestic and office refuse is stored in black plastic sacks ready for collection by the normal domestic waste-disposal service.

To prevent contamination of public water supplies, the water supply to surgery equipment must incorporate an air gap to prevent backflow into the mains supply.

Laboratory work

- Impressions, appliances and other work for the laboratory should be thoroughly rinsed in cold running water and disinfected with hypochlorite before despatch.
- Technicians should wear gloves when handling impressions.
- Appliances and other work *from* the laboratory should be treated in the same way (Chapter 27).
- All disinfected material should be labelled as such and the same applies to instruments and equipment sent away for servicing or repair.

Pathology specimens

Biopsy and other specimens (Chapter 9) for pathology departments must be packaged and labelled in accordance with Post Office requirements.

Aspiration and ventilation

- Surgery and laboratory aspiration and ventilation systems should have their exhaust outlets vented externally.
- Ensure good ventilation.

Training

- All staff must be thoroughly trained to understand and comply with procedures for prevention of cross-infection.
- Such procedures must be reviewed to ensure their adequacy.

Inoculation injuries

Any incident where a contaminated object or substance breaches the skin or mucous membrane, or contacts the eyes, is called an inoculation injury. It is most likely to occur from:

(a) accidental stabbing with a used syringe or suture needle
(b) any other sharp instrument or equipment
(c) splashing of the eyes, skin cuts or abrasions, with blood, saliva or other contaminated substances
(d) bites or scratches from patients

It most commonly occurs when resheathing needles after local anaesthetic injections. This is called **needlestick injury** (Chapter 13) and can be avoided by the use of resheathing devices.

If an inoculation injury occurs, the following procedure should be followed:

1 Encourage bleeding by washing the wound in hot running water.
2 Apply a sterile dressing and inform the dentist.
3 If it occurs during treatment, or before the sterilization of contaminated instruments, the patient's medical history should be checked.
4 If there is a possibility of a serious infection, advice should be sought from the public health authority and appropriate arrangements made for tests and observation.
5 All such incidents should be recorded in the practice accident book.

6   The incident should be investigated by the practice principal and safety procedures reviewed to prevent recurrence.

Hepatitis B

Hepatitis B (serum hepatitis) is an inflammation of the liver caused by a virus. Its effect varies from a mild attack of jaundice to a severe or fatal illness. Over 50% of cases are undiagnosed as their symptoms are too mild to indicate the disease. On the other hand, 80% of primary liver cancers are a result of hepatitis B.

The hepatitis B virus (HBV) is always present in the blood of people suffering from the disease. It may also be present in people who have no symptoms of the disease. Such people are called **carriers**; they may or may not have had any symptoms before; and most of them are unaware that they are carriers. About one person in every thousand of the population is an HBV carrier. Thus all dentists are likely to treat patients who are carriers.

Infectivity

Hepatitis B is highly infective. As mentioned in Chapter 8, HBV is very resistant to destruction. It can survive boiling for up to half an hour, immersion in chlorhexidine (*Hibitane*), and can live outside the body for some weeks. Disinfectants capable of killing HBV are hypochlorites and glutaraldehyde.

HBV has been found in all body fluids, including blood, saliva and breast milk. It is transmitted by people suffering from the disease, and by carriers who have no symptoms at all and are unaware of their condition. Diagnosis is by blood test.

In dental practice the main source of infection is direct contact with blood containing HBV. This is most likely to occur from needlestick injury, i.e. accidentally pricking yourself with a syringe needle used on an HBV carrier; 40% of such accidents result in HBV infection.

Staff are also at risk from the use of high speed equipment, such as an air turbine handpiece with water spray, an ultrasonic scaler or an air/water syringe. These release a cloud of water and saliva particles into the air which, if contaminated with a carrier's blood, may infect the dentist or nurse via the nose, eyes or skin abrasions. Furthermore, adjacent working surfaces become infected too; while inadequate sterilization procedures may cause infection of other patients.

High risk groups

Among the general population the main modes of transmission of HBV are childbirth; the sharing of needles by drug addicts; sexual contact. Thus certain groups of people are much more likely to be carriers; they include:

1 Drug addicts
2 The sexually promiscuous
3 Those who have received long-term regular blood transfusions, such as haemophiliacs, dialysis and transplant patients
4 Mentally handicapped patients living in institutions, and staff in close contact with them
5 Those working or living in institutions such as prisons or reha- bilitation centres for drug addicts and alcoholics
6 Partners and close relatives of carriers, not necessarily with sexual contact.

Prevention

As the majority of HBV carriers are unaware of their condition, it has been estimated that 400 are treated daily in dental practice. But provided the sterilization and surgery hygiene procedures in this chapter are adopted, there need be no cause for alarm. However, the existence of high risk groups emphasizes the importance of obtaining an adequate medical history before treatment.

Fortunately all dental staff can obtain protection against hepatitis B by vaccination. This will also protect their patients against HBV infection from dental staff. Vaccination is freely available under the NHS. It involves a series of three injections, followed by a blood test to check its success. A booster injection may be needed three to five years later. As vaccination is a requirement for chairside employ- ment, documentary evidence of successful immunization must be kept.

Treatment of known carriers

The basic principle of preventing infection with HBV is to avoid contact with the patient's blood. In addition to the sterilization and surgery hygiene procedures already detailed, the following extra precautions have been recommended for general practice.

1 For operations involving extensive loss of blood, such as multiple extractions and minor oral surgery; or if the disease is in an active state, refer the patient to hospital – where full sterile surgical facilities are available.
2 Reserve the last appointment of the day for treatment of carriers. This allows full sterilization procedures to be undertaken before other patients are treated again.
3 Move all unnecessary equipment and materials away from the

chairside. Protect essential working surfaces and equipment controls, such as switches, operating light handle and air/water syringe, with plastic bags or clingfilm.

4 Take great care to avoid inoculation injuries. If they occur, or the eyes, mouth or skin are splashed with blood, proceed as described on page 82.

5 Regard steel burs and matrix bands as disposable. After treatment, flush aspirator with glutaraldehyde and leave the solution in a collection jar overnight.

6 Items which cannot be sterilized by heat or hypochlorite should be immersed in glutaraldehyde for three hours.

7 Launder linen and towelling in a hot wash – 90°C for ten minutes.

8 Pregnant staff or those who have not been vaccinated against HBV should not be involved in the treatment of known carriers.

AIDS

AIDS is an abbreviation for **acquired immune deficiency syndrome**. This means that the body's natural defence mechanism (Chapter 9) against infection is seriously impaired. Consequently AIDS patients succumb to infections which are not normally serious or which are not normally experienced. The outcome of AIDS is invariably fatal as there is no cure, no vaccination and no resistance to infection.

AIDS is caused by infection with a virus called the *human immuno-deficiency virus* which is abbreviated to HIV. There are no particular symptoms of AIDS as they depend solely upon whichever chance infection affects the sufferer. Like hepatitis B the AIDS virus has been found in most body fluids but is transmitted mainly by contact with blood containing the virus. HIV is present in the blood of all infected persons but it usually takes years before they suffer any effects. Furthermore, as there are no specific symptoms, many of those infected with HIV are unaware that they have AIDS. Diagnosis is by blood test.

Infectivity

Unlike HBV, the AIDS virus is not very infective and is not resistant to heat or disinfectants. Although every infected person is potentially infectious, repeated exposure to HIV in blood or body fluids is usually required for the transmission of AIDS. Among the general population the usual modes of transmission are sexual promiscuity, especially in homosexual men; the sharing of needles by drug addicts; childbirth; and repeated transfusions with contaminated blood.

In dental practice the main hazard is needlestick injury, but the infectivity of HIV is so low that a single such accident would rarely result in AIDS. However, no chances can be taken as AIDS is a fatal disease for which there is no cure and no vaccine.

High risk groups

From the modes of transmission of HIV just described, those most at risk of being carriers are:

1   The sexually promiscuous
2   Drug addicts
3   Haemophiliacs and other patients who have received long-term regular blood transfusions
4   Sexual partners of these groups
5   Infants born to infected mothers

Prevention

Although no preventive treatment by drugs or vaccination is possible, AIDS is easily avoided. All that is required as far as the general population is concerned is to avoid any form of sexual promiscuity, or the sharing of needles with drug addicts.

In dental practice, prevention is the same as for hepatitis B: by correct sterilization and surgery hygiene procedures.

Treatment of known carriers

This is the same as for HBV carriers. Fortunately HIV has a very low infectivity and is easily destroyed by routine sterilization procedures. Nevertheless, no chances can be taken as AIDS is fatal and no vaccination or cure is available.

Known carriers of HIV and HBV are those who are aware of their condition and have informed the dentist when their medical history is taken. The requirement of confidentiality mentioned in Chapter 2 is of paramount importance in such cases. Most carriers are either unaware of their condition; or unwilling to disclose it in case their affliction is revealed to unauthorized people. Some are also afraid of being denied dental treatment if they admit to being carriers. When any medical history is taken, it is ethically and legally essential to ensure that it cannot be overheard anywhere else in the practice; and under conditions that give patients the confidence to provide a complete relevant history.

As only a minority of carriers are known to be such, most are treated without the dentist being aware of their condition. This emphasizes the importance of strict adherence, by all practice staff, to correct procedures for the prevention of cross-infection.

Written examination

What is meant by the term 'cross-infection'?
What is the role of the dental nurse in minimizing the risk of cross-infection before, during and after treatment of a patient known to be a carrier of hepatitis B virus? (May 1992)

Define the term 'cross infection'.
Describe how the following should be handled after use to prevent cross infection.
(a) dental extraction forceps
(b) local anaesthetic needle, cartridge and syringe
(c) a recently taken alginate impression.
(November 1996).

Summary

Purposes of sterilization

- Kill all micro-organisms: bacteria, fungi, spores and viruses
- Prevent cross-infection: conveyance of bacteria, fungi, spores and viruses from one patient, or any other source, to another person

Methods of sterilization

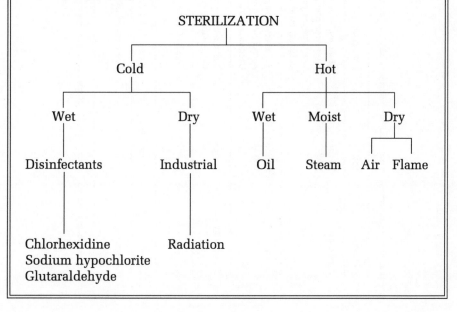

METHOD	TIME	USED FOR	ADVANTAGES	DISADVANTAGES
Autoclave	3 min. 134°C	Most metal instruments, swabs, towels, throat packs, cotton wool, paper points, rubber, plastics, modern handpieces	Kills all micro-organisms Best method of all	Equipment expensive
Hot air	2 hours 160°C	All metal instruments, old low-speed handpieces, root treatment kits	Kills all micro-organisms	Too hot, too long for rubber and plastics
Disinfectants	Varies	Items damaged by heat Work surfaces	Simple	Disinfection only
Oil	15 min. 140°C	Old low-speed handpieces	Lubricates Prevents rusting	Unsuitable for air turbine handpieces
Flaming	Immediate	Anaesthetic cartridge caps	Quick, simple	Very limited use
Radiation		Pre-packed disposable needles, etc.	Cold and dry Kills all micro-organisms	Not possible in dental surgery

Prevention of cross-infection

- Vaccination: hepatitis B, rubella, poliomyelitis, pertussis, diphtheria, tuberculosis, tetanus
- Medical history for all patients
- Good ventilation and efficient suction (exhausted externally)
- Protective clothing: mask, spectacles, gloves; waterproof dressings on all skin abrasions
- No jewellery or wrist watches
- Use disposable materials and equipment whenever possible. Never reuse
- New gloves and mask for each patient
- Wash hands in disinfectant liquid soap before gloving
- Use rubber dam whenever possible
- Clean work surfaces with detergent and disinfect with hypochlorite
- Confine glutaraldehyde to items unsuitable for hypochlorite
- Cover handles and switches in plastic bags or clingfilm
- Discharge water from handpieces, air/water syringes and other waterspray equipment before use
- Clean suction equipment by flushing with disinfectant
- Scrub used instruments with detergent and hot water, or use ultrasonic cleaner, before sterilization. Wear heavy-duty gloves
- Rinse laboratory work in water and disinfect with hypochlorite
- Seal clinical waste in yellow plastic sacks and sharps containers for incineration

Inoculation injuries

Causes

- Needlestick → use sheathing devices
- Sharp instruments → clean with long-handled brushes and point away from you
- Splashes → blood, saliva → skin or eyes
- Patient → bites or scratches

Treatment

- Make wound bleed → hot running water; waterproof dressing
- Inform dentist → check patient's medical history
- Advice from public health service → tests and observation
- Review surgery procedures

Hepatitis B

- Inflammation of liver due to hepatitis B virus (HBV)

- Sometimes fatal. Often so mild that patient unaware of infection
- All infected persons, with or without symptoms, are HBV carriers
- All carriers highly infective
- Vaccination is the best safeguard against hepatitis B
- HBV resistant to boiling and most disinfectants. Killed by autoclaving, hot air, glutaraldehyde and hypochlorites
- Transmitted in dental practice by blood or blood-stained saliva and spray
- Most prevalent in drug addicts; the sexually promiscuous; regularly transfused patients (haemophiliacs, dialysis and transplants); institutionalized mentally handicapped, prisoners, alcoholics, and staff; partners and close relatives of carriers.

AIDS

- Acquired immune deficiency syndrome caused by human immuno-deficiency virus (HIV)
- HIV destroys body's resistance to infection
- HIV easily killed by heat and disinfectants
- AIDS is fatal and incurable. No vaccine available
- Transmitted by blood or body fluids, mainly by sexual contact or drug addicts sharing needles
- All those infected with HIV, with or without symptoms, are carriers
- Most prevalent in the sexually promiscuous; drug addicts, patients receiving long-term regular blood transfusions; sexual partners of all these; children borne by infected mothers.

Treatment of HBV and HIV carriers

Apply same measures as for prevention of cross-infection.

Extra additional precautions

- Refer to hospital if disease in active state; and for multiple extractions and minor oral surgery
- Treat only as last appointment
- Use glutaraldehyde for items which cannot be sterilized by heat or hypochlorite
- Flush aspirator with glutaraldehyde after treatment and leave it in collection jar overnight
- Launder linen and towels in hot wash – 90°C for ten minutes
- Thoroughly wash needlestick injury or blood splashes on skin; notify public health authority.

11 Drugs

Dosage

The metric system is used exclusively when ordering and prescribing drugs. The metric unit of weight is the gram (g) and this is divided into thousandths called milligrams (mg).

The unit of volume is the litre (l) which is subdivided into thousandths called millilitres (ml). A litre is equivalent to just under two pints. The standard medicine teaspoon holds 5 ml.

Various reference books are available to help practitioners keep up to date with new drugs, the trade names of drugs, dosages and precautions with particular drugs. The most useful of these are the combined edition of the *Dental Practitioners' Formulary* and the *British National Formulary* (DPF/BNF), and the *Monthly Index of Medical Specialities* (MIMS). Manufacturers are also legally required to provide data sheets for all new drugs, giving full details of usage.

Administration

Drugs may be administered externally or internally.

External application

This is the commonest method used in dentistry. The drug may be applied in the form of a:

- Mouthwash, e.g. chlorhexidine
- Gel, e.g. miconazole
- Pastille, e.g. nystatin
- Lozenge, e.g. hydrocortisone
- Cement, e.g. zinc oxide and eugenol

Internal application

May be given by:

- Mouth, e.g. aspirin tablets
- Injection, e.g. local anaesthetics
- Inhalation, e.g. general anaesthetics

Classification

Drugs are classified into groups which have a specific action, such as antibacterial drugs which are used for the treatment of infections; or local anaesthetics which abolish pain. Some drugs belong to more than one group; for example, lignocaine, which is a local and surface anaesthetic. Groups used in dentistry are as follows:

Disinfectants

These are solutions used externally to kill or prevent the growth of bacteria. They are not administered internally as they are poisonous. Their main uses are:

1   Disinfecting work surfaces and instruments where heat sterilization methods are inapplicable
2   As a disinfectant liquid soap
3   Disinfecting a skin or mouth surface prior to injection
4   Disinfecting root canals
5   Temporary storage of sterile instruments

To ensure effective action they should be freshly made up to their manufacturers' recommended strength. Disinfectants applied to living tissue, such as the teeth, skin or mouth were formerly called **antiseptics**.

Sodium hypochlorite

A solution which forms the basis of some domestic bleaching agents and disinfectants, e.g. *Milton, Domestos*. It is effective against HBV and HIV and is used for disinfecting work surfaces, blood stains, impressions and other laboratory work. It is also used for irrigating root canals. Care should be taken to avoid contact with metal as it may cause corrosion.

Glutaraldehyde (Cidex)

A solution effective against HBV and HIV. It is only used for items which are unsuitable for sodium hypochlorite, as it is irritant to skin, eyes and lungs. It should be stored and used in a well-ventilated place and containers must be securely sealed. Gloves, mask and eye protection are necessary when working with glutaraldehyde.

Chlorhexidine (Hibitane)

A 0.5% solution in surgical spirit used to disinfect the surface prior to injections; and for the temporary storage of sterile instruments.

It is also available as a 0.2% antiseptic mouthwash or 1% gel to keep the mouth clean and inhibit plaque formation when oral ulceration makes toothbrushing too painful. These are also used to reduce gingival (gum) infection before treatment requiring antibiotic cover.

Chlorhexidine varnish (*Cervitec*) is a new product which is recommended for treatment of exposed sensitive roots; arrest of early root decay; and as a temporary fissure sealant (Chapters 21 and 26).

Hydrogen peroxide

Used as a 3% solution for irrigation of dry sockets; and, diluted to 0.5%, as a deodorant and cleansing mouthwash.

Tincture of iodine

A solution used to disinfect the surface prior to an injection of local anaesthetic; or the gingival crevice (Chapter 12) before tooth extraction.

Antibacterial drugs

These include antibiotics and metronidazole. They are administered internally to kill bacteria.

Antibiotics are drugs originally derived from micro-organisms; for example, penicillins, tetracyclines and erythromycin. Many people are allergic to penicillin and its derivatives. If such people are given any of these drugs they are liable to develop a dangerous reaction. Patients must always be asked beforehand if they are allergic to penicillin or any other drugs.

Penicillin

An antibiotic used to prevent the spread of infection in severe pericoronitis, cellulitis and jaw fractures; and to prevent secondary infection after minor oral surgery. It is given by mouth or injection.

Amoxycillin

A derivative of penicillin with a much wider range of antibacterial action. Taken by mouth for infections which do not respond to penicillin.

Its most important use in dentistry is for patients with valvular heart disease. In such cases it is given before extractions, surgery, scaling and some stages of root treatment, in order to prevent infective endocarditis.

Erythromycin

An antibiotic taken by mouth. It is used for patients who are allergic to penicillin and amoxycillin; or for infections resistant to them.

Clindamycin

An antibiotic given by mouth or injection. It is reserved for the prevention of infective endocarditis in patients allergic to amoxycillin and other penicillin derivatives.

Tetracycline

Sometimes used externally as a mouthwash to relieve discomfort from recurrent ulcers which do not respond to other drugs; and as a local application to gum pockets in periodontal disease.

If tetracycline, or one of its derivatives, is given internally for medical purposes while the teeth are still being formed, it may cause permanent discoloration of these teeth. It could affect the milk teeth of an unborn child if it is given in pregnancy; or the permanent teeth if given to children under twelve.

Metronidazole (Flagyl)

Taken by mouth for the treatment of acute necrotizing ulcerative gingivitis and pericoronitis (Chapters 8, 25); and as an alternative to the penicillins and erythromycin.

It should not be given during pregnancy and breast-feeding. Alcohol should be avoided by any patient taking metronidazole.

Antibiotic cover

As already described on page 65, bacteria are forced into the blood (bacteraemia) whenever any surgical manipulation of the gums occurs; for example, in extractions, minor oral surgery and scaling. Normally it causes no harm as the white blood cells rapidly overcome this mild invasion of bacteria. In some cases, however, the potentially fatal disease of infective endocarditis can follow. Patients at risk are those with congenital heart defects; diseased or replaced heart valves; a history of rheumatic fever or previous infective endocarditis.

Antibiotic cover is used to prevent infective endocarditis in these patients. An antibiotic is given as a short, high dose just before extractions, scaling, surgery and some endodontic procedures. The antibiotic of choice is amoxycillin; but for patients allergic to penicillin and its derivatives, clindamycin is used instead.

Antibiotic cover may also be necessary for some patients who are immuno-compromised (page 63). In such cases of poor resistance to infection, bacteraemia could permit the development of a very serious infection out of all proportion to what normally occurs.

Patients who would not normally require antibiotic cover are sometimes given it to prevent local complications from the surgical removal of impacted lower wisdom teeth. Amoxycillin or metronidazole are usually given in such cases.

Antifungal drugs

Used for treatment of *Candida albicans* infections such as denture stomatitis (denture sore mouth); and soreness at the angle of the mouth (*angular cheilitis*). Applied externally in the form of a gel to the fitting surface of a denture; as a gel to the angle of the mouth; or as pastilles or lozenges. For example:

- Nystatin pastilles
- Amphotericin (*Fungilin*) lozenges
- Miconazole (*Daktarin*). This gel should not be used during pregnancy and breast-feeding; or for patients taking anti-coagulants.

Antiviral drugs

Most viral infections are not susceptible to drug treatment. However, cold sores on the lips and mouth ulcers caused by the herpes virus can be treated with a new antiviral drug called **aciclovir**.

The ulcers and sores start off as tiny blisters, and treatment with aciclovir cream (*Zovirax*) is most effective if started just before this stage is reached.

Anti-inflammatory drugs

These are corticosteroids, used externally to relieve pain and promote healing of mouth ulcers. For example:

- Hydrocortisone lozenges
- Triamcinolone paste (*Adcortyl in Orabase*)

Corticosteroids combined with an antibacterial drug are sometimes used to suppress inflammation of the pulp or periapical tissues during cavity preparation or endodontic treatment. For example:

- *Ledermix*
- *Endomethasone*

Analgesics

Analgesics are drugs administered internally or externally for the relief of pain.

Most dental pain is caused by inflammation and the most effective drugs for relief of dental pain are accordingly those that combine analgesic and anti-inflammatory effects. However, the anti-inflammatory drugs mentioned in the preceding section are all corticosteroids, and these cannot be taken internally for dental treatment. Non-steroidal anti-inflammatory drugs (**NSAIDs**) are used instead and those that have analgesic properties may be taken internally for dental pain.

Aspirin

Taken by mouth to relieve toothache and post-operative pain. It forms the basis of many proprietary tablets obtainable without a prescription and is both analgesic and anti-inflammatory.

Aspirin is not given to children under 12 as it may cause a rare brain disease. It is also unsuitable during pregnancy and breast-feeding; and for any patients with bleeding disorders or peptic ulcers as it may cause bleeding from the stomach. It is also inadvisable for people with allergic conditions such as asthma. In all such cases, paracetamol is a suitable alternative.

Paracetamol

Taken by mouth as an alternative to aspirin. Commonly available in many proprietary brands without a prescription, e.g. *Panadol*. It has no anti-inflammatory effect.

Serious, and possibly fatal, liver damage may ensue if the recommended dose is exceeded.

Ibuprofen

Taken by mouth as an analgesic NSAID alternative to aspirin. It is safe for children and is obtainable without a prescription in many proprietary brands, such as *Nurofen*.

As in the case of aspirin, it should not be used for patients with peptic ulcers or asthma.

Regular use of NSAIDs should be avoided during pregnancy.

Eugenol

Eugenol (*oil of cloves*) is applied externally to painful dry sockets. Mixed with zinc oxide it makes an analgesic cement – applied to the gums following gingivectomy, and to cavities in aching teeth.

Tranquillizers

Tranquillizers are administered internally by *mouth* to relieve anxiety prior to dental treatment. They do not relieve pain or produce sleep. For example:

- Diazepam (*Valium*): started the night before treatment
- Temazepam
- Only obtainable on prescription as they are addictive.

Patients given tranquillizers must be warned against alcohol. This increases the effect of the drug and could result in overdosage. They are also forbidden to drive or operate machinery for up to 24 hours.

Tranquillizers are also used by *injection* immediately before treatment to sedate nervous patients sufficiently to accept local anaesthesia. This technique, called **conscious sedation**, is covered in Chapter 14. Drugs used are diazepam (*Diazemuls*) and midazolam (*Hypnovel*). They should not be given during pregnancy or breast-feeding.

General anaesthetics

General anaesthetics (Chapter 14) are drugs administered internally by inhalation or injection to produce unconsciousness with abolition of pain and reflexes. For example:

- Nitrous oxide
- Halothane (*Fluothane*)
- Methohexitone (*Brietal*)

Patients who are given general anaesthetics are forbidden to drive a vehicle or operate machinery until they are fully recovered from the effects of the drug.

Local anaesthetics

Local anaesthetics are drugs given internally by injection for the abolition of pain locally. For example:

- Lignocaine (lidocaine)
- Prilocaine (*Citanest*)

Surface anaesthetics

Surface anaesthetics are applied externally to numb the gum prior to injections, scaling, application of matrices, etc; or to numb the mouth and throat to prevent sickness during impressions. For example:

- Lignocaine paste or mouthwash

Haemostatics (*Styptics*)

Haemostatics, or styptics, are drugs applied externally to arrest hae-morrhage.

Adrenaline (epinephrine)

Applied externally as a 0.1% solution. Acts by constricting the bleeding capillaries.

This **vasoconstrictor** action of adrenaline is also used (in a strength of 1:80,000) as a constituent of local anaesthetics to prolong their action.

Absorbable packs

These act by coagulating the blood. Various types are available; for example, gelatine sponge, oxidized cellulose (*Surgicel*). They protect the bleeding surface and allow the blood to clot.

Care of drugs

There are strict legal requirements for the purchase, storage, use, identification, dispensing and prescription of drugs used in dental practice.

Storage

Many drugs are poisonous if taken accidentally or in excess; others are caustic and may cause painful burns. Some common sense pre-cautions in storing drugs are to keep them well away from food and drinks; keep poisons locked up in a special poisons cabinet; and to keep caustics on the lowest shelf where accidental spillage cannot affect the eyes or burn the face.

Stocks of drugs in the practice must be stored in accordance with manufacturers' instructions and not kept beyond their expiry date. Records of their purchase, supply and expiry date must be kept for at least 11 years. Any drugs which have passed their expiry date should be discarded, together with any solutions which have become dis-coloured or cloudy.

Certain drugs, such as adrenaline, halothane and hydrogen per-oxide must be stored in dark bottles to prevent premature deteriora-tion, while poisons bottles are ribbed to indicate by touch that their contents are dangerous.

Identification

All drug containers and bottles *must* be clearly labelled with the name of the drug and, where necessary, its strength. Very serious accidents have occurred through the wrong drug being given from an inadequately labelled bottle. Similarly, labels not indicating the strength are a potential source of danger. For example, a 3% solution of hydrogen peroxide may be used for irrigating root canals and dry sockets, but a 30% solution is a dangerous caustic which produces a chemical burn if it contacts the soft tissues of the mouth.

When nurses are asked for a drug it is their duty to read the label carefully in order to provide the dentist with the right drug. If they have to fill a small medicament bottle from a stock bottle, or a syringe from an ampoule, they must correctly label the new bottle or syringe with the name and strength of the drug, and ask the dentist or senior nurse to check it.

Dispensing

If drugs are given to patients to take home they must include manufacturers' instructions; be in childproof containers; and labelled with the date, name and dosage of the drug, directions and precautions for use, name of patient and name and address of the dentist.

Security

The rapid increase in drug addiction makes it imperative for dental staff to take careful precautions to prevent theft of drugs from the surgery. Not only must drugs be securely locked in a cupboard or cabinet where they are not exposed to view; but similar precautions must apply to syringes, needles and prescription pads. The latter must not be signed or stamped until given to the patient.

Disposal of drugs

In order to prevent harm to refuse collectors, or recovery by addicts, domestic refuse-collection services must not be used for the disposal of old drugs, syringes and needles.

Patients prescribed or given drugs for use at home are told to return unused drugs to a pharmacy for disposal, and not to use sinks or toilets for that purpose.

Controlled drugs

Controlled drugs are those which may be used by addicts or are otherwise liable to misuse. They cannot be obtained by the public without a prescription; and their supply is rigidly controlled by law under the Misuse of Drugs Regulations.

Misuse of drugs regulations

These regulations control the use of drugs of addiction such as cocaine, morphine and pethidine, but in general dental practice they are rarely used. Cocaine was the first local anaesthetic used in dentistry but has long been superseded by lignocaine and prilocaine. Morphine and pethidine are used to control very severe pain but conditions causing such pain are usually treated in hospital or by the patient's doctor.

The only controlled drugs likely to be used in dental practice are some of the general anaesthetic and sedation agents covered in Chapter 14. They must be kept in a locked cupboard and the key kept by the dentist.

Medicines (prescriptions only) order

This order specifies all the drugs which cannot be supplied without a prescription. These are indicated in the DPF/BNF by the symbol PoM. They include antibiotics, tranquillizers, local and general anaesthetics, adrenaline and stimulants.

Prescriptions must be written in ink or typewritten and give the date, name and address of the patient (including age, if a child); signature, title and address of the dentist; total quantity of the drug prescribed, and the dosage. Form FP14 is used for NHS prescriptions.

Adverse reactions to drugs

When drugs are administered to some patients a severe adverse reaction, such as collapse, may occur. This may be caused by an allergy to the drug administered, e.g. penicillin, or interaction with another drug which the patient is already taking for medical reasons.

To prevent these untoward effects a careful history must always be taken before any drugs are used. If it is found that a drug allergy exists, or a patient is taking drugs prescribed by a doctor; or taking non-prescription drugs for self-medication; this information must be recorded on the patient's chart, regularly up-dated and appropriate precautions taken. Particular drugs which may cause collapse are mentioned in Chapter 15.

As already stated, special care must also be taken when administering tranquillizers and general anaesthetics. Patients given tranquillizers are warned of the danger of taking alcohol; and patients given tranquillizers or general anaesthetics are forbidden to drive a vehicle until they are fully recovered.

Allergy

As already mentioned, allergy may cause collapse. Less serious but nonetheless unpleasant reactions can also occur. Severe ulceration of the mouth may result from cytotoxic drugs used for the treatment of cancer, and from many other drugs in susceptible patients.

Bleeding

Anticoagulant drugs are used for patients who have experienced or are at risk of blood clots (thrombosis) after operations or heart disease. These drugs naturally suppress the capacity of the blood to clot and may result in excessive bleeding after extractions and other dental procedures.

Some drugs used for medical or dental treatment can enhance the effect of anticoagulants and could give rise to more serious bleeding. Drugs which can interact with anticoagulants in this way include aspirin and other NSAIDs; miconazole, metronidazole and many antibiotics.

Elderly patients

Special care is necessary for elderly patients. They may have some degree of kidney or liver impairment and usually need a lower dosage of drugs. They may also find it difficult to read, remember or comply with the instructions on dose and frequency, especially if they are already taking many other drugs for medical treatment.

Pregnancy and breast-feeding

Drugs are best avoided altogether during pregnancy and breast-feeding as they may harm the baby. They include tetracyclines, general anaesthetics, tranquillizers, metronidazole, miconazole, aspirin and other NSAIDs. The DPF/BNF lists all drugs that may affect pregnancy and breast-feeding.

Children

As for elderly patients, children require lower doses of drugs. They are usually given by mouth to avoid the discomfort of injection; but they must be palatable enough to ensure a child's co-operation, and are accordingly prepared in the form of a sweet syrup to mask any unpleasant taste. An unfortunate side-effect of syrups sweetened with sugar has been extensive tooth decay when the drug is administered frequently over a long period of time. This danger can be overcome by using preparations made with artificial sweeteners instead of sugar;

and these should be used whenever possible. The DPF/BNF indicates preparations which are sugar-free.

Further advice

So many patients are taking drugs nowadays and so many different brands are used that it may be difficult for the dentist to know if an adverse reaction is likely. The reference books mentioned at the beginning of this chapter are an invaluable aid in such cases, but if any doubt remains the patient's doctor is consulted. If these sources are not available or applicable, advice is obtainable from local pharmacy services or telephone helplines listed in the DPF/BNF.

Drugs for emergency use

Chapters 14 and 15 cover equipment and drugs used for the treatment of collapse and other possible emergencies in a dental surgery. Some drugs recommended for inclusion in emergency kits are listed alphabetically here and mentioned in more detail in Chapters 14 and 15.

- Adrenaline: anaphylactic shock; cardiac arrest
- Aspirin: heart attack
- Chlorpheniramine (*Piriton*): anaphylactic shock
- Midazolam (*Hypnovel*): epileptic fits
- Flumazenil (*Anexate*): antidote to sedation agent
- Glucagon: diabetic hypoglycaemia
- Glyceryl trinitrate: angina pectoris
- Hydrocortisone: corticosteroid and anaphylactic shock; asthma
- Salbutamol (*Ventolin*): asthma; anaphylactic shock.

Written examination

What do you understand by 'antibiotic cover' and under what circumstances may it be indicated?
How should drugs be handled and stored in the dental practice? (May 1992)

Summary

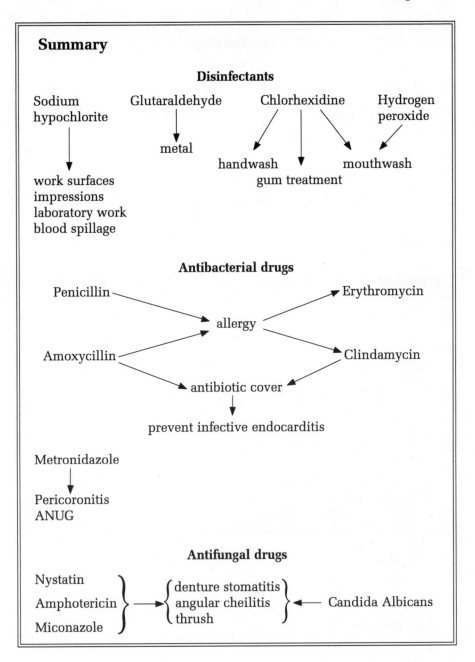

Disinfectants

Sodium hypochlorite   Glutaraldehyde   Chlorhexidine   Hydrogen peroxide

↓ metal

work surfaces
impressions
laboratory work
blood spillage

handwash   gum treatment   mouthwash

Antibacterial drugs

Penicillin → allergy → Erythromycin

Amoxycillin → allergy → Clindamycin

Amoxycillin → antibiotic cover ← Clindamycin

↓

prevent infective endocarditis

Metronidazole
↓
Pericoronitis
ANUG

Antifungal drugs

Nystatin
Amphotericin   } → { denture stomatitis, angular cheilitis, thrush } ← Candida Albicans
Miconazole

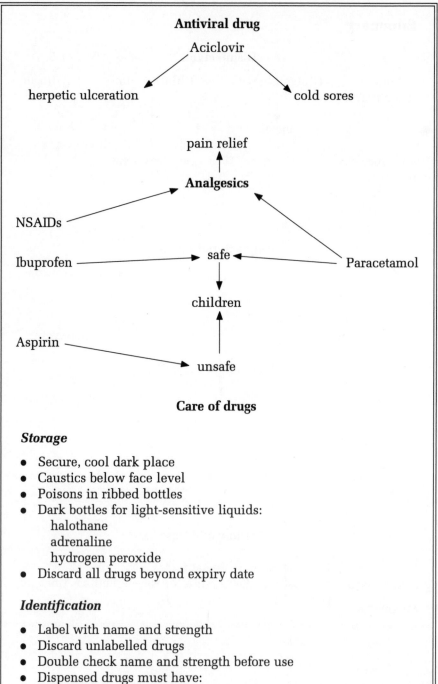

Antiviral drug

Aciclovir

herpetic ulceration   cold sores

pain relief

Analgesics

NSAIDs

Ibuprofen → safe ← Paracetamol

children

Aspirin → unsafe

Care of drugs

Storage

- Secure, cool dark place
- Caustics below face level
- Poisons in ribbed bottles
- Dark bottles for light-sensitive liquids:
    halothane
    adrenaline
    hydrogen peroxide
- Discard all drugs beyond expiry date

Identification

- Label with name and strength
- Discard unlabelled drugs
- Double check name and strength before use
- Dispensed drugs must have:
    childproof container
    date, name and address of patient and dentist
    full instructions on dose, frequency and precautions

Security

- Lock up syringes, needles, prescription pads (unstamped, unsigned)
- Lock up tranquillizers, general anaesthetics, sedation agents and other drugs liable to misuse or addiction

Disposal

- Do not use domestic refuse-collection service
- Return old and surplus drugs to pharmacy

Adverse reactions to drugs

Interaction between drugs used for treatment and those taken by patients.

Allergy

For example, penicillin and derivatives; effects mild to serious:

- itching, skin rashes
- mouth ulceration
- swelling
- breathing difficulties
- collapse

Overdosage

Overdosage effects from enhancement of normal dose by alcohol:

- tranquillizers and general anaesthetics
- metronidazole.

Bleeding

Interaction with anticoagulants and:

- aspirin and NSAIDs
- miconazole
- metronidazole
- many antibiotics

Pregnancy and breast-feeding

Avoid *all* drugs if possible, especially:

- tetracyclines
- general anaesthetics and tranquillizers
- metronidazole
- miconazole
- aspirin and NSAIDs

Children

- Low dosage
- Use paracetamol or ibuprofen instead of aspirin
- No tetracyclines

Elderly

- Low dosage
- Precise written and verbal instructions

Drugs for emergency use

- Adrenaline: anaphylactic shock; cardiac arrest
- Aspirin: heart attack
- Chlorpheniramine (*Piriton*): anaphylactic shock
- Midazolam (*Hypnovel*): epileptic fits
- Flumazenil (*Anexate*): antidote to sedation agent
- Glucagon: diabetic hypoglycaemia
- Glyceryl trinitrate: angina pectoris
- Hydrocortisone: corticosteroid and anaphylactic shock; asthma
- Salbutamol (*Ventolin*): asthma; anaphylactic shock

DRUG	STRENGTH	CLASSIFICATION	APPLICATION	USE
Aciclovir (*Zovirax*)	—	Antiviral	External	Cold sores
Adrenaline	0.1% 1:80,000	Haemostatic Vasoconstrictor	" Internal	Haemorrhage Added to local anaesthetics
		Emergency drug	"	Collapse
Amoxycillin	—	Antibiotic	"	Prevention of infective endocarditis
Amphotericin (*Fungilin*)	—	Antifungal	External	Denture stomatitis
Aspirin	—	Analgesic NSAID	Internal	Toothache; after-pain
Chlorhexidine (*Hibitane*)	0.5% 0.2%	Disinfectant "	External "	Disinfection Mouthwash
Clindamycin		Antibiotic	Internal	Prevention of infective endocarditis
Diazepam (*Valium*) (*Diazemuls*)	—	Tranquillizer	"	Sedation
Erythromycin	—	Antibiotic	"	Patients allergic to penicillin
Eugenol (*oil of cloves*)	—	Analgesic	External	Zinc oxide cement Dry sockets
Glutaraldehyde (*Cidex*)	2%	Disinfectant	"	Disinfection
Halothane (*Fluothane*)	—	General anaesthetic	Internal	General anaesthesia
Hydrocortisone	—	Emergency drug	"	Collapse
		Anti- inflammatory	External	Mouth ulcers
Hydrogen peroxide	3%	Disinfectant	"	Dry sockets
	0.5%	"	"	Deodorant mouthwash
Ibuprofen (*Nurofen*)		Analgesic NSAID	Internal	Alternative to aspirin
Iodine	—	Disinfectant	External	Skin and mucous membrane disinfection

DRUG	STRENGTH	CLASSIFICATION	APPLICATION	USE
Lignocaine (*Xylocaine*)	2%	Local anaesthetic	Internal	Local anaesthesia
	5%	Surface anaesthetic	External	Surface anaesthesia
Methohexitone (*Brietal*)	—	General anaesthetic	Internal	General anaesthesia
Miconazole (*Daktarin*)	—	Antifungal	External	Denture stomatitis
Midazolam (*Hypnovel*)	—	Tranquillizer	Internal	Sedation
Nitrous oxide	—	General anaesthetic	"	General anaesthesia
Nystatin	—	Antifungal	External	Denture stomatitis
Paracetamol	—	Analgesic	Internal	Alternative to aspirin
Penicillin	—	Antibiotic	"	Treatment of infection
Prilocaine (*Citanest*)	3%	Local anaesthetic	"	Local anaesthesia
Sodium hypochlorite (*Milton*)	—	Disinfectant	External	Disinfection; root treatment
Temazepam		Tranquillizer	Internal	Sedation

12 Dental Anatomy

Structure of the teeth

Every tooth consists of a **crown** and one or more **roots**. The crown is the part visible in the mouth and the root is the part hidden inside the jaw. The junction of crown and root is called the **neck** and the end of the root is called the **apex**. Every tooth is composed of enamel, dentine, cementum and pulp (Figure 12.1).

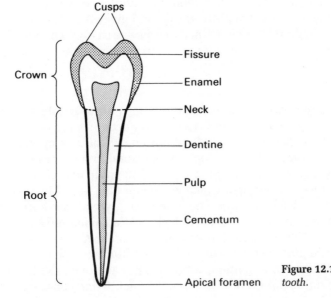

Figure 12.1 *Structure of a tooth.*

Enamel

This is the protective outer covering of the crown and is the hardest substance in the body. It does not contain any nerves or blood vessels and is insensitive to pain. Unlike most other body tissues it cannot undergo repair as described on page 61; damage caused by progressive decay or injury is permanent.

A microscope shows that enamel consists of long solid rods, called enamel prisms, cemented together by the interprismatic substance. The prisms run roughly at right angles to the surface.

Cementum

This is the protective outer covering of the root and is similar in structure to bone. Cementum meets enamel at the neck of the tooth. The thickness of cementum may vary at different parts of the root, and changes throughout life, depending on the forces exerted on individual teeth.

Dentine

This forms the main bulk of a tooth and occupies the interior of the crown and root. It is very sensitive to pain but is normally sheltered from painful stimuli – such as extremes of temperature or chemical irritation – by its outer coating of enamel which acts as a protective layer of insulation.

Dentine is harder than bone, but less solid than enamel as it is full of microscopic tubes called **dentinal tubules** which contain soft tissue. This renders it slightly elastic and gives it a shock-absorbing capacity. Dentine from elephants' tusks is commonly known as ivory but is the same dentine as that found in human teeth.

Pulp

Unlike enamel, dentine and cementum, the pulp is purely soft tissue. It contains blood vessels and nerves, and occupies the centre of the dentine. Vessels and nerves of the pulp enter the root apex through the **apical foramen** and pass up the **root canal** into the crown, where the space occupied by the pulp is called the **pulp chamber**.

The nerves of the pulp are responsible for pain felt when dentine is drilled or toothache occurs. The outermost layer of the pulp, next to the dentine, consists of special cells, called **odontoblasts**, which actually form the dentine. Under a microscope, odontoblasts are seen to have fine prolongations called **dentinal fibrils** which pass into the dentine through the dentinal tubules. They perforate the full thickness of dentine but do not penetrate enamel. Being continuous with the pulp they act as a vital link whereby irritation of the dentine, or any damage to it, can provoke a response by the pulp. The usual response to irritation is pain; but damage (such as tooth decay) is repaired by the odontoblasts which form a new inner layer of **secondary dentine**. Even in the absence of damage, secondary dentine slowly forms throughout life as part of the ageing process, and results in gradual obliteration of the pulp chamber and narrowing of the root canal.

Supporting structures

Every tooth fits into a socket (*alveolus*) in the jaw. The part of the jaw containing the teeth is a ridge of bone called the **alveolar process**. It contains all the tooth sockets and is covered with a soft tissue called **gum**. The jaw bones consist of a dense outer layer known as **compact bone** and a softer interior called **spongy bone**.

The compact bone lining the tooth socket (Figure 12.2) is called the **lamina dura**. It shows up very well in X-ray films (Figure 29.1), where any loss in its continuity is a good indicator of dental disease.

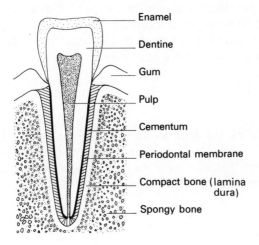

- Enamel
- Dentine
- Gum
- Pulp
- Cementum
- Periodontal membrane
- Compact bone (lamina dura)
- Spongy bone

Figure 12.2 *Supporting structure of a tooth.*

Gum

The anatomical term for gum is **gingiva**. It is firmly attached to the underlying alveolar bone and fits round the neck of each tooth like a tight cuff. A shallow crevice is present between the tooth surface and gum margin. It is called the **gingival crevice** (Figure 25.1). The triangular mound of gum between each tooth is called the **interdental papilla**. Healthy gums are firm and pink with a stippled surface and the gingival crevice is less than 3 mm deep.

Periodontal membrane

A tooth is attached to its socket in the jaw by a soft fibrous tissue called the **periodontal membrane**; but many authorities prefer to call it the **periodontal ligament**. It acts as a shock absorber and is attached to the cementum of the root and the compact bone lining the socket (Figure 12.2).

The periodontal membrane contains nerves and blood vessels, but consists mainly of bundles of fibres which pass obliquely from bone to cementum. They run in an apical direction and form a fibrous sling which attaches the tooth to its socket. Other bundles of fibres at the neck of the tooth firmly attach the gum margin to its adjoining cementum and crest of the alveolar bone; and also join the necks of adjacent teeth to each other.

Thus the periodontal membrane attaches the tooth to its socket; the gum margin to the tooth and alveolar bone; and each tooth to its neighbour. In this way the teeth are kept firmly in position but are still mobile enough to absorb the enormous forces exerted on them when biting and chewing.

The nerves of the periodontal membrane are particularly sensitive to excess pressure. This causes discomfort or pain and warns of abnormal forces acting on the tooth, such as food packing, high spots on fillings, attempting to chew extra hard substances, etc.

Deciduous teeth

The deciduous teeth are the first set and are also known as milk, temporary or primary teeth. There are twenty of them; ten in each jaw with five on each side. The five teeth on each side of both jaws are named as follows from the front backwards (Figure 12.3).

A   CENTRAL INCISOR
B   LATERAL INCISOR
C   CANINE
D   1ST MOLAR
E   2ND MOLAR

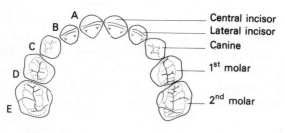

Figure 12.3   *Deciduous teeth.*

Eruption

All teeth start developing inside the jaws and their arrival in the mouth is known as **eruption**. Deciduous teeth start developing *before* birth and erupt after birth. Eruption starts at six months and is completed at two years. Individual variation is common but the average ages are as follows:

A   Central incisor   6 months
B   Lateral incisor   8 months
C   Canine   18 months

D 1st molar   12 months
E 2nd molar   24 months

Lower teeth usually erupt before their corresponding upper.

Permanent teeth

Permanent teeth are the second and final set. There are 32 of them; 16 in each jaw, eight on each side. Like deciduous teeth, the eight on each side of both jaws have the same names (Figure 12.4):

1   CENTRAL INCISOR
2   LATERAL INCISOR
3   CANINE
4   1ST PREMOLAR
5   2ND PREMOLAR
6   1ST MOLAR
7   2ND MOLAR
8   3RD MOLAR (wisdom tooth)

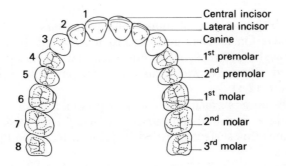

Figure 12.4 *Permanent teeth.*

Eruption

Permanent teeth start developing at birth. Eruption commences at six years of age and is completed at 18 to 25 years. Eruption times are subject to considerable individual variation but the average ages are:

1   Central incisor   7 years
2   Lateral incisor   8 years
3   Canine   9 years (lower); 11 years (upper)
4   1st premolar   10 years (lower); 9 years (upper)
5   2nd premolar   11 years (lower); 10 years (upper)
6   1st molar   6 years
7   2nd molar   12 years
8   3rd molar   18–25 years

After the deciduous teeth loosen, they are shed and replaced by the eruption of their permanent successors. Deciduous incisors and canines are replaced by permanent teeth of the same name. Deciduous molars, however, are replaced by premolars. Thus the permanent molars erupt without having any deciduous predecessors.

Deciduous teeth become loose by **resorption** of their roots which deprives them of their attachment to the jaws. This gradual process begins about three years before the eruption of their successors. The unerupted permanent successors lie adjacent to the absorbing deciduous roots and are thus able to erupt into their places when the deciduous teeth are finally shed (Figure 12.12).

Permanent teeth erupt before their roots are fully grown. About two-thirds of their root length has formed when permanent teeth erupt and the apex is still wide open. It takes another three years before root growth is complete and the apex closes. The only exceptions are canines and third molars which do not erupt until root growth is complete.

Surfaces of the teeth

The biting surface of molars and premolars is called the **occlusal surface**. On incisors and canines it is called the **incisal edge**. The occlusal surface of molars and premolars is raised up into mounds called **cusps**. Between the cusps are crevices known as **fissures** (Figure 12.1).

The outer surface of molars and premolars – the surface facing the cheeks – is called the **buccal** surface. In the case of incisors and canines this surface is called **labial** as it faces the lips instead of the cheeks.

The inner surface of every lower tooth faces the tongue so it is called the **lingual** surface. This surface in all upper teeth is known as the **palatal** surface (Figure 12.5).

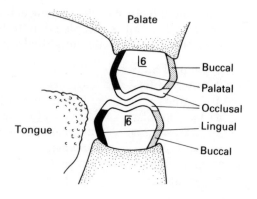

Figure 12.5 *Surfaces of the teeth – mesial aspect.*

The remaining surfaces are those between adjoining teeth. These are called **proximal** surfaces; the one facing towards the front of the mouth is called **mesial** and that facing backwards is called **distal** (Figure 12.6). The point where the proximal surface of a tooth touches its neighbour is called the **contact point**.

The adjective **cervical** is used for the neck of a tooth.

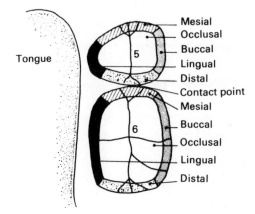

Figure 12.6 *Surfaces of the teeth – occlusal aspect.*

Charting

A chart is a diagrammatic representation of the teeth showing all their surfaces. It is used to show which teeth are present or missing, and the surfaces with cavities and fillings. Teeth can be divided into four groups: upper right, upper left, lower right and lower left. By drawing an imaginary cross over the mouth each group fits into a corner of the cross (Figure 12.7). Thus the patient's upper right teeth are repre-sented as ⌋, upper left as⌊ , lower right as ⌐, and lower left as ⌐.

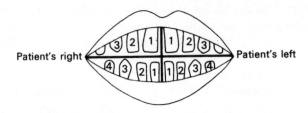

Figure 12.7 *Grouping of the teeth for charting.*

Permanent upper and lower teeth of each side are numbered from the centre backwards as follows:

Deciduous teeth are similarly represented by capital letters:

Central incisor	1
Lateral incisor	2
Canine	3
1st premolar	4
2nd premolar	5
1st molar	6
2nd molar	7
3rd molar	8

Central incisor	A
Lateral incisor	B
Canine	C
1st molar	D
2nd molar	E

Some examples of this representation are as follows:

Permanent upper right 2nd molar	7⌋
upper left	⌊7
lower left	⌈7
lower right	7⌉
Permanent upper left central incisor	⌊1
upper right	1⌋
lower right	1⌉
lower left	⌈1
Deciduous lower left 1st molar	⌈D
lower right	D⌉
upper right	D⌋
upper left	⌊D

There are various kinds of dental chart but perhaps the best known is the National Health Service Chart (Form FP25). Various symbols and abbreviations are used to denote missing or filled teeth, and the treatment required (Figure 12.8).

Part A of the National Certificate written examination includes a charting exercise similar to that in Figure 12.8. Some additional symbols and abbreviations used in charting are as follows:

+	retained root	FGC	full gold crown
#	fracture	FS	fissure sealant
A	artificial tooth	GIC	glass ionomer filling
Am	amalgam filling	PBC	porcelain bonded crown
BA	bridge abutment	PC	post crown
BP	bridge pontic	PV	porcelain veneer
Cm	composite filling	Tm	temporary filling

The system of tooth notation just described is used by the vast majority of practitioners in the United Kingdom. However, the

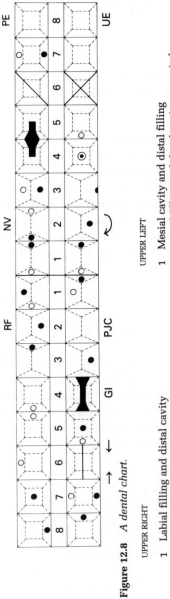

Figure 12.8   *A dental chart.*

UPPER RIGHT

1 Labial filling and distal cavity
2 Palatal filling; root filling
3 Mesial filling
4 Distal cavity
5 Mesial cavity
6 Buccal cavity
7 Occlusal filling
8 Palatal filling

LOWER RIGHT

1 Mesial filling and lingual cavity
2 Porcelain jacket crown
3 Labial filling
4 Mesial-occlusal-distal gold inlay
5 Occlusal filling and distal cavity; drifted distally
6 Missing
7 Buccal filling and lingual cavity; drifted mesially
8 Mesial filling

UPPER LEFT

1 Mesial cavity and distal filling
2 Mesial filling and distal cavity; non-vital
3 Labial cavity and palatal filling
4 Distal-occlusal filling
5 Mesial-occlusal filling
6 To be extracted
7 Buccal cavity and palatal filling
8 Partially erupted

LOWER LEFT

1 Mesial cavity and distal filling
2 Labial filling; rotated
3 Labial cervical filling
4 Occlusal filling to be replaced
5 Mesial cavity
6 Recently extracted
7 Sound tooth
8 Unerupted

quadrant symbols are inconvenient for reproduction by typewriters or word processors; while the quadrants must be quoted fully in spoken communications, e.g. 'upper left 8, lower right 4'.

This has led to a recommendation by the International Dental Federation (FDI) that a new two-digit system be adopted to overcome these difficulties and allow the easy transmission of dental information in a form which can be used irrespective of the language spoken.

FDI two-digit system

This system replaces the quadrant symbol by a number: 1 for upper right; 2 for upper left; 3 for lower left and 4 for lower right. Thus the quadrants are represented as:

quadrant 1	quadrant 2
quadrant 4	quadrant 3

The quadrant number forms the first digit while the second identifies an individual tooth as 1 to 8 in the same way as the existing system. Reading clockwise from the upper right third molar, all 32 teeth have their own two-digit number indicating their quadrant (first digit) and identity (second digit) as shown:

18 17 16 15 14 13 12 11	21 22 23 24 25 26 27 28
48 47 46 45 44 43 42 41	31 32 33 34 35 36 37 38

The lower left second premolar, for example, is written as 35 and pronounced 'three five', *not* thirty-five. If all dentists get into the habit of starting their charting from the back of the upper right quadrant the FDI system could soon become universally accepted.

Deciduous teeth are similarly treated by using quadrant numbers 5 to 8, and tooth numbers 1 to 5 as shown.

quadrant 5	quadrant 6
quadrant 8	quadrant 7

55 54 53 52 51	61 62 63 64 65
85 84 83 82 81	71 72 73 74 75

Thus the upper right deciduous first molar would be written as 54 and pronounced 'five four'.

The following example shows how the same charting is represented by the two systems.

6 E D 3 1	C 4 7 8
5 3 2 A	1 B 4 E

16 55 54 13 11 63 24 27 28 75 34 72 31 81 42 43 45.

Anatomy of individual teeth

A collection of extracted teeth in good condition is a great help in learning anatomy, and preparing for such items in examination spotter and oral tests (Figure 12.9).

Permanent incisors

Incisors have one root and flattened chisel-shaped crowns. The upper crowns are much wider than their lower counterparts.

The upper lateral incisor crown is smaller than the upper central; but the lower lateral crown is slightly larger than the lower central.

The palatal surface of upper incisors is often raised into a small mound near the cervical margin. It resembles a miniature cusp and is called the **cingulum**.

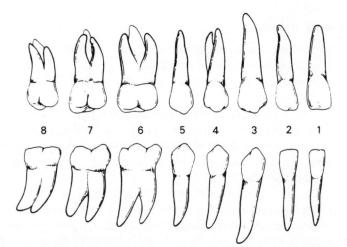

Figure 12.9 *Upper and lower permanent teeth.*

Permanent canines

These have large conical crowns and one long root. The upper canine is larger than the lower and has the longest root of the whole dentition.

Premolars

The upper first premolar has two roots, one buccal and one palatal. The remaining premolars have one root. Each premolar has two cusps, one buccal and one palatal or lingual (Figure 12.10).

The cusps of upper premolars are almost equal in size to each other and are much bigger than those of the lowers. The lingual cusp of lower premolars is much smaller than the buccal cusp.

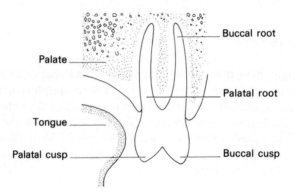

Figure 12.10   *Upper first premolar.*

Permanent molars

Upper molars have three roots, two buccal and one palatal. The buccal roots are mesial and distal.

Lower molars have two roots, one mesial and one distal (Figure 12.11).

Upper molars have four cusps, two buccal and two palatal. Their crowns are characterized by an oblique ridge which runs from the mesio-palatal cusp to the disto-buccal cusp. Upper first molars often have an extra cusp on their mesio-palatal surface. This is called the **cusp of Carabelli**.

Lower first molars have five cusps, three buccal and two lingual. Lower second molars have four cusps, two buccal and two lingual.

First molars are the largest teeth of all. Third molars vary in size and number of roots and cusps. Usually they are the smallest molars and their roots are often fused together.

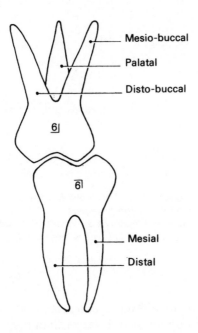

Mesio-buccal

Palatal

Disto-buccal

6|

6|

Mesial

Distal

Figure 12.11 *Upper and lower permanent first molars.*

Deciduous teeth

Deciduous teeth in general resemble their corresponding permanent teeth but there are some important differences:

1 Deciduous teeth are much smaller. Consequently there is adequate space for the front teeth and crowding is uncommon.
2 Deciduous crowns are whiter. The permanent successors are naturally darker in colour and many parents mistakenly believe that their children are not cleaning them properly.
3 Pulp chambers of deciduous teeth are relatively larger, and their enamel is much thinner. This allows decay to reach the pulp much more rapidly.

Deciduous incisors and canines are smaller versions of their permanent successors.

Deciduous molars have the same number of roots as permanent molars but differ in other respects:

1 The crowns of deciduous molars are more bulbous.
2 To provide space for the developing premolars, the roots of deciduous molars are more divergent than those of permanent molars (Figure 12.12).
3 Deciduous second molars resemble miniature first permanent molars; but the shape of deciduous first molars is much less typical, having a pronounced mesio-buccal bulge.

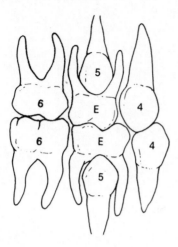

Figure 12.12 *Deciduous 2nd molars and unerupted 2nd premolars.*
Source: *A Textbook of Orthodontics*, (3rd edn).
T.D. Foster, Blackwell Science Ltd, Oxford.

Occlusion of the teeth

When the upper and lower teeth are closed together, they are said to be in **occlusion**. The arch of the upper teeth is larger than the lower; thus upper teeth overlap the lowers on the buccal side. Lower buccal cusps accordingly bite into the fissure between upper buccal and palatal cusps (Figure 12.13).

At the midline the mesial edges of upper and lower central incisors form one straight vertical line. As lower central incisors are much narrower than uppers, all the remaining lower teeth occlude with two upper teeth – their corresponding upper tooth and the one in front, as shown in Figure 12.13.

From this diagram of **normal occlusion** it is clear that:

1 The mesial cusp of the upper first molar bites into the fissure between mesial and distal cusps of the lower first molar.
2 The lower canine bites in front of the upper canine.
3 The mesial edges of the upper and lower central incisors form one straight vertical line.

Functions of the teeth

Incisors and canines are for cutting up food into smaller pieces ready for chewing.

Premolars and molars are for chewing; their cusps grind the food into a soft mass suitable for swallowing.

Teeth are also necessary for clear speech and good appearance. People who lose all their teeth and do not wear dentures may have slurred speech and an aged appearance.

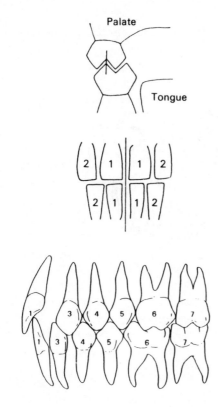

Figure 12.13 *Normal occlusion.*
Source: *A Textbook of Orthodontics*,
(3rd edn). T.D. Foster, Blackwell
Science Ltd, Oxford.

The skull

The skull or **cranium** consists of an upper hollow rounded part
housing the brain; and a lower part which forms the skeleton of the
face and contains the jaws (Figure 12.14).

The skull is a very complex structure and it is unnecessary for
nurses to know its anatomy in minute detail. However, a skull is
usually present on the National Certificate oral examination table and
candidates should know the names and functions of parts considered
relevant to their work.

The **frontal**, **parietal**, **temporal** and **occipital** bones, forming part of
the protective shell for the brain, are thin plates which interlock with
each other like a jigsaw puzzle. The facial skeleton contains bones
forming the eye sockets, cheeks, nose and jaws.

Nerves supplying the face, jaws and teeth leave the brain through
holes in the base of the skull. Each hole is called a **foramen**. Nerves
supplying the rest of the body arise from the spinal cord. This leaves
the brain through the **foramen magnum** and occupies a canal running through the entire length of the spine. The foramen magnum
(Figure 12.15) is a large hole in the base of the skull, and its lower

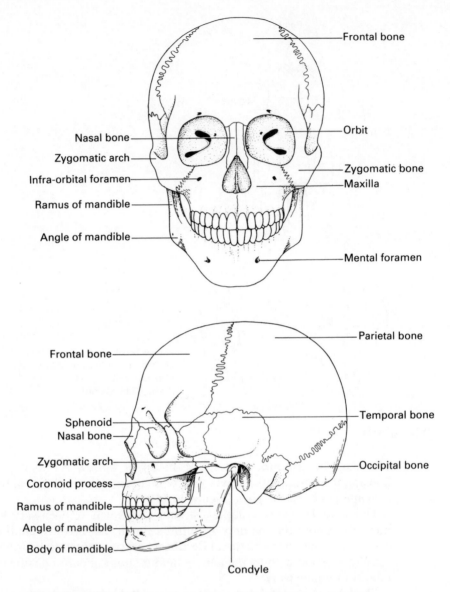

Figure 12.14   *The skull.*
Source: *Clinical Anatomy*, (9th edn). H. Ellis, Blackwell Science Ltd, Oxford.

sides form a joint with the top of the spine to permit movement of the head.

The upper jaw is called the **maxilla** and the lower is the **mandible**. The outer layer of compact bone is much thinner in the maxilla than the mandible; the importance of this will be seen in Chapter 13. Both jaws contain holes for the passage of nerves and blood vessels which supply the teeth and soft tissues of the face and mouth; they, too, are described in Chapter 13.

Maxilla

The maxilla is fixed to the skull and is immovable. It contains all the upper teeth in its alveolar process. The alveolar process ends at the back of the maxilla in a rounded bulge called the **tuberosity** of the maxilla.

The maxilla consists of two halves – the right and left maxillae. These are joined together below the nose by the hard palate and alveolar process; but they are separated above by the nasal cavity. Each half of the maxilla helps form its respective side of the nose, palate, floor of the **orbit** (eye socket) and front of the cheek bone (Figures 12.14, 12.15).

The **hard palate** forms the roof of the mouth and separates the oral cavity (mouth) from the nasal cavity (nose). Thus the lower surface of the hard palate forms the roof of the mouth, while its upper surface forms the floor of the nose (Figures 12.15, 12.16, 6.3).

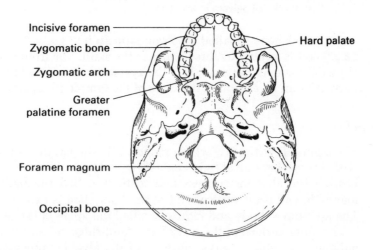

Incisive foramen

Zygomatic bone

Zygomatic arch

Greater palatine foramen

Foramen magnum

Occipital bone

Hard palate

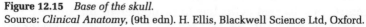

Figure 12.15   *Base of the skull.*
Source: *Clinical Anatomy*, (9th edn). H. Ellis, Blackwell Science Ltd, Oxford.

On either side of the nasal cavity the maxilla is hollow. Each hollow is known as a **maxillary sinus** or **antrum** (Figure 12.16). It is of great practical importance as the floor of the antrum lies just above the roots of the premolar and molar teeth. During extraction of these teeth, the floor may be perforated or a root pushed inside the antrum (Chapter 16). The nasal cavity is continuous with the antrum through a small hole near the top of the antrum. This connection between the air spaces of the antrum and nose gives resonance to the voice. Inflammation of the antrum is called **sinusitis**. It is a common complication of a cold and a cause of toothache in the upper back teeth. Similar sinuses, continuous with the nasal cavity, are present in the frontal, ethmoid and sphenoid bones of the skull.

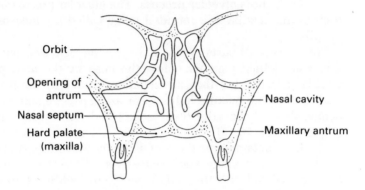

Figurer 12.16   *Facial bones and air spaces in cross section.*
Source: *Basic Anatomy and Physiology for Radiographers*, (3rd edn). M.R.E. Dean & T.E.T. West, Blackwell Science Ltd, Oxford.

The cheek bone is called the **zygomatic arch** (Figures 12.14, 12.15, 12.23) and is formed by three bones of the skull. The front of the arch is part of the maxilla; the side is the **zygomatic bone**; and the back is formed by an extension of the bone of the temple (temporal bone).

Mandible

The mandible is the jaw which moves. It is shaped like a horseshoe with its ends bent up at right angles (Figure 13.3). The horizontal part bearing the alveolar process and teeth is called the **body** of the mandible and each vertical end of the horseshoe is called a **ramus**. The junction of body and ramus is called the **angle** of the mandible.

The outer surface of the body has a faint ridge called the **external oblique line** which marks the base of the alveolar process, and is continuous behind with the front border of the ramus. The inner surface of the body has a similar ridge called the **mylohyoid line** which marks the floor of the mouth (Figure 12.17).

Attached to the ramus are the **muscles of mastication** which close the mouth. Muscles opening the mouth are attached to the body just below the chin and pass down to the **hyoid bone**. This can be felt at the front of the neck just above the larynx (Figure 12.23).

On top of the ramus are two projections: the **coronoid process** in front and the **condyle** behind. They are separated from each other by the **sigmoid notch**. The condyle and base of the skull form the

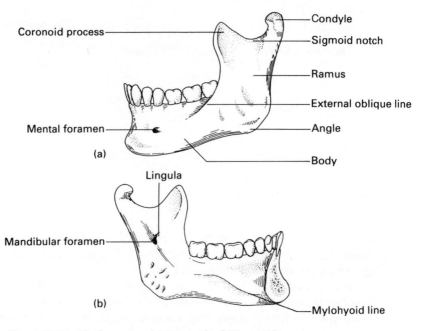

Figure 12.17 *The lower jaw.* (a) Outer side; (b) Inner side.
Source: *Clinical Anatomy*, (9th edn). H. Ellis, Blackwell Science Ltd, Oxford.

temporo-mandibular joint, which allows the lower jaw to move
(Figure 12.18). More details of jaw anatomy are given in Chapter 13.

Movements of the jaws

The only jaw which can move is the mandible. The first movement
involved in eating is a hinge-like opening of the mandible to separate
the incisors. It then moves forward until the incisors can grasp the
food between their cutting edges. The mandible then returns backwards and closes. This produces a shearing action of the incisors
which thereby cut the food into smaller pieces ready for chewing. It is
similar to the cutting action of a pair of scissors.

Chewing is brought about by rotary movement of the mandible
which swings from side to side, crushing food between the cusps of
opposing molars and premolars.

Temporo-mandibular joint

This joint is formed between the condyle of the mandible and the
temporal bone at the base of the skull. When the mouth is shut the

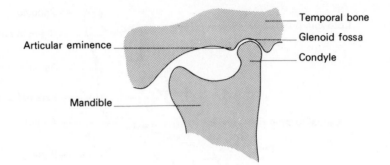

Figure 12.18   *Temporo-mandibular joint.*

condyle rests in a hollow in the temporal bone called the **glenoid fossa**. The front edge of the glenoid fossa is formed into a ridge called the **articular eminence** (Figure 12.18).

Thus the mandibular surface of the joint consists of the condyle; and the temporal surface consists of the glenoid fossa and articular eminence. Between these two surfaces there is a disc of fibrous tissue.

As already described, the first stage of opening the mouth is a hinge-like opening of the mandible to separate the incisors. The condyle remains in the glenoid fossa during this stage.

As the mouth opens further, the condyle slides downwards and forwards from the glenoid fossa along the slope of the articular eminence. When the condyle reaches the crest of the articular eminence, the mouth is open to its fullest extent and the incisors can grasp food between their cutting edges. For the closing movement, which produces the shearing action of the incisors, the condyle returns to its rest position in the glenoid fossa.

Sometimes the condyle slips too far forward and gets stuck in front of the articular eminence. When this happens it cannot move back and the joint is said to be **dislocated**. It is recognized by an inability to close the mouth. It can be treated quite easily by pressing down on the molars to force the condyle downwards and backwards into the glenoid fossa – but a general anaesthetic may be necessary.

The rotary movements of chewing involve alternate forwards and backwards movements of each condyle as the mandible swings from side to side. When the mandible swings to the right, the *left* condyle moves forward and the right stays put. For the return movement to the left, the *right* condyle moves forward while the left returns backwards into the glenoid fossa.

These movements of the condyle can be felt by placing a finger in front of the ear while opening and closing the mandible. They are all produced by the muscles of mastication.

Muscles of mastication

On each side of the skull there are four muscles of mastication (Figure 12.19).

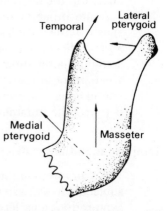

Figure 12.19 *Muscles of mastication.*

1   The **masseter** muscle extends from the zygomatic arch to the outside of the ramus of the mandible (Figures 12.21, 12.23). It closes the mandible.
2   The **medial pterygoid** muscle extends from behind the maxilla to the inside of the ramus (Figure 12.20). It closes the mandible.
3   The **temporal** muscle extends from the side of the head to the coronoid process of the mandible, through the zygomatic arch (Figure 12.23). It closes the mandible and pulls it backwards.
4   The **lateral pterygoid** muscle extends from behind the maxilla to the condyle of the mandible (Figure 12.20). Both muscles acting together pull the jaw forwards. One, acting alone, swings the jaw to the *opposite* side.

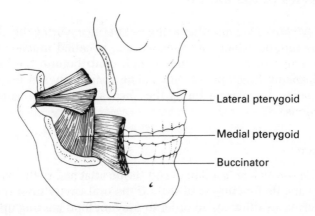

Figure 12.20 *Buccinator and deep muscles of mastication.*

When the teeth are clenched together, the temporal and masseter muscles can be felt by placing a hand on the side of the head and face respectively. They form the superficial layer of the muscles of mastication (Figure 12.23); while the medial and lateral pterygoid muscles form the deep layer (Figure 12.20).

Acute inflammatory conditions sometimes result in a protective spasm of the muscles of mastication. This condition is called **trismus** and its effect is an inability to open the mouth. It occurs most often in acute inflammation of the gum surrounding an erupting lower wisdom tooth (pericoronitis); after surgical removal of these teeth; and in acute inflammation of the parotid gland (mumps). Its purpose is to rest the inflamed part and prevent pain.

Temporo-mandibular disorders

The temporo-mandibular joint and muscles of mastication may be subjected to excessive strain from seemingly trivial causes; and these can produce a variety of effects ranging from spasm of the muscles of mastication to degenerative changes in the joint. They result in a wide range of symptoms but the commonest are pain or tenderness over the joint, clicking noises and restricted movement of the mandible.

The symptoms are most common in young women and people under emotional stress. It often affects people who habitually grind or clench their teeth. Tooth-grinding activity is called **bruxism** and often occurs during sleep. It can be recognized by excessive wear facets on the teeth.

Treatment of these disorders depends on the symptoms and may include tranquillizers, physiotherapy, or an occlusal splint to prop open the occlusion.

Soft tissues of the mouth

The *skin* of the mouth, i.e. the red tissue covering the cheeks, floor of the mouth, palate and tongue, etc., is called **mucous membrane**. It contains many tiny glands which contribute to the lubricating and cleansing functions of saliva. The space between the teeth and the mucous membrane lining the cheeks and lips is called the **buccal sulcus**.

Soft palate

The soft palate is a flap of soft tissue attached to the back of the hard palate. Its function is to seal off the oral cavity from the nasal cavity during swallowing, in order to prevent food passing up into the nose (Figure 7.1). The free edge of the soft palate has a central prolongation called the **uvula**. You can see this for yourself by looking in a mirror with your mouth wide open.

Tongue

The floor of the mouth lies within the arch of the mandible and is occupied by the tongue. The tongue is attached to the floor of the mouth by a thin band of fibrous tissue called the **lingual frenum**. The upper lip is attached to the gum above the central incisors by a similar frenum (Chapter 16).

The functions of the tongue are swallowing, speech, taste and cleansing the mouth. The tongue is a mobile muscular organ covered by a thick layer of mucous membrane on top and a thinner layer below. The thick upper layer is studded with minute projections which give it a rough surface. This helps the cleansing action of the tongue. Situated in these minute projections are **taste buds** which allow us to distinguish sweet, sour, salty and bitter flavours. The lower layer of mucous membrane is so thin that it can very rapidly absorb drugs placed under the tongue. Patients given glyceryl trinitrate tablets for treatment of angina pectoris use them in this way.

The swallowing, speech and cleansing functions are brought about by the muscular activity of the tongue. Swallowing is a complex muscular act described in Chapter 7. It prevents food entering the nasal cavity or larynx instead of the oesophagus (Figure 7.1).

Soreness of the tongue can occur in conditions such as anaemia, vitamin B deficiency and hormonal disturbances. It is associated with a thin, smooth glazed appearance of the normally thick layer of mucous membrane on its upper surface.

Salivary glands

The functions of saliva are covered in Chapter 7. It is produced by the mucous membrane glands, mentioned on page 130, and the salivary glands, which are situated close to the mandible. Saliva passes through tubes, called ducts, from the salivary glands into the mouth (Figures 12.21, 12.22).

The **parotid gland** lies partly over the outside and partly behind the ramus. The duct from the parotid gland passes forward, across the surface of the masseter muscle, and then inwards through the cheek to open into the buccal sulcus opposite the upper second molar. By clenching your teeth, you can not only feel the masseter, but also the parotid duct as it crosses its surface. It feels like a piece of string. Mumps is an acute inflammation of the parotid gland caused by a virus.

The **submandibular gland** lies in the floor of the mouth below the mylohyoid line, against the inner and lower surface of the body near

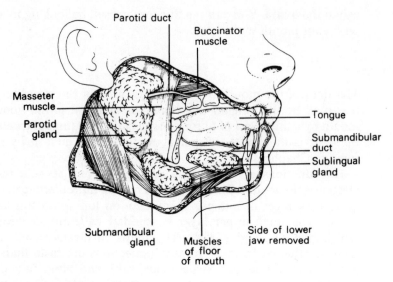

Figure 12.21   *Salivary glands.*

the angle of the mandible (Figures 12.21, 12.22). The submandibular duct passes forward in the floor of the mouth to open at the midline, beside the lingual frenum.

The **sublingual gland** also lies in the floor of the mouth, but above the mylohyoid line and much further forward than the submandibular gland (Figures 12.21, 12.22). There are several sublingual ducts and these open into the floor of the mouth just behind the orifice of the submandibular duct.

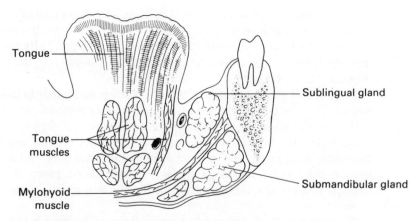

Figure 12.22   *Floor of the mouth in cross section.*
Source: *Clinical Anatomy*, (9th edn). H. Ellis, Blackwell Science Ltd, Oxford.

Muscles of facial expression

The muscles of facial expression can produce an infinite variety of movements and expressions. They form a complex of muscles beneath the skin of the face which may, for the sake of simplicity, be divided into three main groups: muscles of the mouth, eyes and cheeks (Figure 12.23).

The mouth is surrounded by a ring of muscle called the **orbicularis oris**. A similar ring of muscle called the **orbicularis oculi** surrounds each eye. Thin straps of muscle radiate between, and away from, these rings to produce movements of the eyelids, lips, mouth and nose.

The muscle of the cheek is the innermost muscle of facial expression. It is called the **buccinator** (Figures 12.20, 12.21, 12.23) and is attached above and below to the buccal surface of the alveolar process of each jaw. It is continuous behind with the muscular wall of the throat, and in front with the orbicularis oris. Its attachment to the alveolar process determines the extent of the buccal sulcus. Although the buccinator is classified as a muscle of facial expression, it greatly

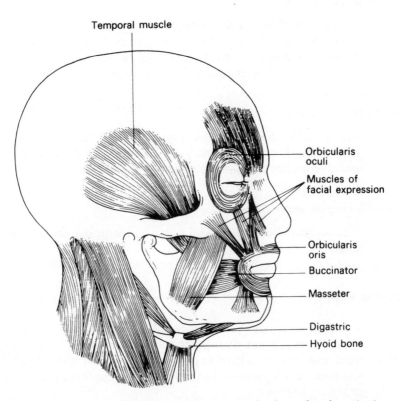

Figure 12.23 *Muscles of facial expression and superficial muscles of mastication.*

assists the muscles of mastication by pressing against the teeth, thereby keeping the food between them during chewing.

Nerve supply of the head

The head is supplied by twelve pairs of **cranial nerves**. They all branch off from the brain, one from each pair supplying the left side, while the other supplies the right.

The nerves which make muscles and glands work are called **motor** nerves, while those which convey pain and other sensation are called **sensory** nerves. For examination purposes, the only ones you need know are the fifth, seventh, ninth and twelfth cranial nerves.

Fifth cranial nerve

This is the most important of all as it supplies the teeth and jaws. It is called the **trigeminal** nerve and is described in detail in Chapter 13.

Seventh cranial nerve

This is called the **facial** nerve and supplies the muscles of facial expression. It also provides taste sensory branches to the anterior (*front*) two-thirds of the tongue and motor branches to the submandibular and sublingual salivary glands.

Ninth cranial nerve

This is called the **glossopharyngeal** nerve. It supplies sensory branches to the throat and posterior (*back*) third of the tongue. A motor branch supplies the parotid gland.

Twelfth cranial nerve

This is called the **hypoglossal** nerve and supplies the muscles of the tongue.

Blood supply

The face, teeth and jaws are supplied by branches of the **external carotid** artery. Veins draining these parts eventually join the superior vena cava. For examination purposes it is unnecessary to learn these blood vessels separately as they generally run alongside their corresponding nerves.

Written examination

Write short notes on:

(a) the maxillary sinus
(b) the inferior alveolar (dental) nerve
(c) temporo-mandibular joint. (November 1994)

Summary

Structure of the teeth and jaws

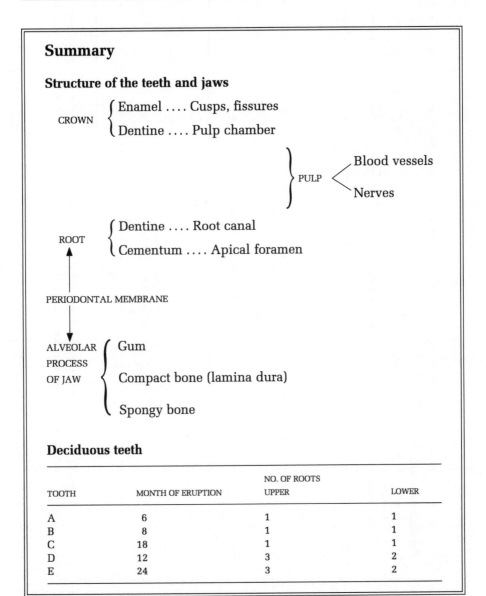

CROWN { Enamel .... Cusps, fissures
          Dentine .... Pulp chamber

PULP < Blood vessels
          Nerves

ROOT { Dentine .... Root canal
         Cementum .... Apical foramen

PERIODONTAL MEMBRANE

ALVEOLAR PROCESS OF JAW { Gum
                            Compact bone (lamina dura)
                            Spongy bone

Deciduous teeth

TOOTH	MONTH OF ERUPTION	NO. OF ROOTS UPPER	LOWER
A	6	1	1
B	8	1	1
C	18	1	1
D	12	3	2
E	24	3	2

Permanent teeth

TOOTH	YEAR OF ERUPTION		NO. OF ROOTS		NO. OF CUSPS			FUNCTION
	UPPER	LOWER	UPPER	LOWER	TOTAL	BUCCAL	LINGUAL OR PALATAL	
1		7	1	1	—	—	—	CUTTING
2	11	8	1	1	—	—	—	
3		9	1	1	—	—	—	
4	9	10	2 Buccal Palatal	1	2	1	1	
5	10	11	1	1	2	1	1	
6		6	3 Mesiobuccal Distobuccal Palatal	2 Mesial Distal	LOWER 5 / Upper 4	3	2	CHEWING
7		12	"	"	4	2	2	
8		18–25	"	"	Variable	2	2	

Surfaces of the teeth

Biting = *occlusal* for back   teeth   Outer = *buccal* for back teeth
     incisal   "   front   "   *labial*   "   front   "
Inner = *palatal*   "   upper   "   Facing front = *mesial* ⎱ *proximal*
      lingual   "   lower   "   Facing back = *distal* ⎰

Charting

Missing	—
Recently extracted	×
For extraction	/
Cavity	○
Filling present	●
Replace filling	◉
Tooth drift	→ ←
Tooth rotation	↺
Retained root	+
Fracture	#

UPPER RIGHT	UPPER LEFT
LOWER RIGHT	LOWER LEFT

FDI two-digit system

Permanent

quadrant 1	quadrant 2
quadrant 4	quadrant 3

18 17 16 15 14 13 12 11	21 22 23 24 25 26 27 28
48 47 46 45 44 43 42 41	31 32 33 34 35 36 37 38

Deciduous

quadrant 5	quadrant 6
quadrant 8	quadrant 7

55 54 53 52 51	61 62 63 64 65
85 84 83 82 81	71 72 73 74 75

Normal occlusion

Lower buccal cusps bite in fissure between upper buccal and palatal cusps.

Mesial edges of upper and lower central incisors form one straight vertical line.

Mesial cusp of upper first molar bites in fissure between mesial and distal cusps of lower first molar.

Every tooth, *except* the lower central incisor and upper third molar, occludes with two opposing teeth.

Maxilla

Contains:

- *Thin* covering of compact bone
- Upper teeth in alveolar process
- Hard palate
- Maxillary sinuses

Mandible

Contains:

- *Thick* covering of compact bone
- Lower teeth in alveolar process of the body
- Condyle on the ramus, forming temporo-mandibular joint with the skull

Temporo-mandibular joint

Mandible ⟷ Temporal bone

Condyle ← Fibrous → Glenoid   Articular
            disc   fossa   eminence

Movements of the mandible

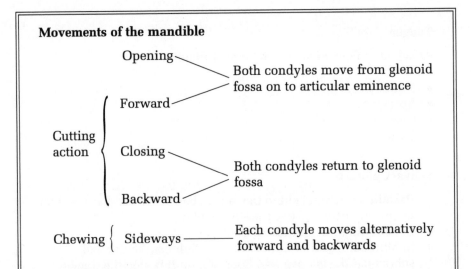

Cutting action
- Opening — Both condyles move from glenoid fossa on to articular eminence
- Forward
- Closing — Both condyles return to glenoid fossa
- Backward

Chewing
- Sideways — Each condyle moves alternatively forward and backwards

Muscles of mastication

MUSCLE	ATTACHMENTS	ACTION
Masseter	1 Zygomatic arch 2 Outside of ramus	Closes jaw
Medial pterygoid	1 Behind maxilla 2 Inside of ramus	Closes jaw
Temporal	1 Side of head 2 Coronoid process	Closes jaw Pulls jaw backwards
Lateral pterygoid	1 Behind maxilla 2 Condyle	Both together: pulls jaw forwards One only: swings jaw to opposite side

Muscles of facial expression

- Orbicularis oris – mouth
- Buccinator – cheek
- Orbicularis oculi – eye

Soft palate

- Flap of soft tissue attached to hard palate
- Seals off nasal cavity from mouth when swallowing

Tongue

Attached to floor of mouth by lingual frenum. Functions:

- Swallowing
- Speech
- Cleansing
- Taste

Salivary glands

1 **Parotid**. Over and behind the ramus, below the ear. Parotid duct opens opposite maxillary second molar.
2 **Submandibular**. At back of floor of mouth.
3 **Sublingual**. Front of floor of mouth. Submandibular and sublingual ducts open into floor of mouth beside the lingual frenum.

Cranial nerves

	SENSORY	MOTOR
5th Trigeminal	*See Chapter 13.*	
7th Facial	Taste (anterior $\frac{2}{3}$ tongue)	Muscles of facial expression Submandibular ⎱ Sublingual ⎰ salivary glands
9th Glossopharyngeal	Throat Posterior $\frac{1}{3}$ tongue	Parotid gland
12th Hypoglossal		Tongue

13   Nerve Supply of the Teeth and Local Anaesthesia

The teeth, jaws and face are supplied by the **fifth cranial nerves**, one for the left side and one for the right. The fifth cranial nerve is also known as the **trigeminal nerve** as it splits up into three divisions: the **ophthalmic**, **maxillary** and **mandibular** nerves (Figure 13.1). The ophthalmic nerve does not supply the teeth and need not be considered further. The maxillary nerve supplies the upper jaw, its teeth and the upper part of the face. It is purely sensory. The mandibular nerve has sensory and motor branches: the sensory branches supply the lower jaw, its teeth and the lower part of the face; the motor branches supply the muscles of mastication. The names of all these branches are easier to understand if you remember that *anterior* means front; *posterior* means back; *superior* means upper; and *inferior* means lower.

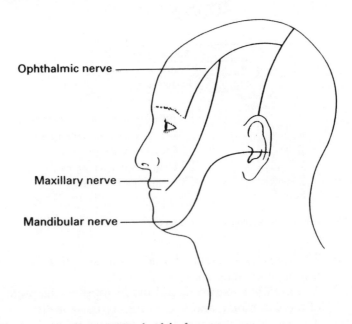

Figure 13.1 *Sensory nerve supply of the face.*
Source: *Clinical Anatomy* (9th edn). H. Ellis, Blackwell Science Ltd, Oxford.

Upper teeth

The nerves supplying upper teeth and gums are the superior dental (alveolar) and palatine branches of the maxillary nerve (Figure 13.2).

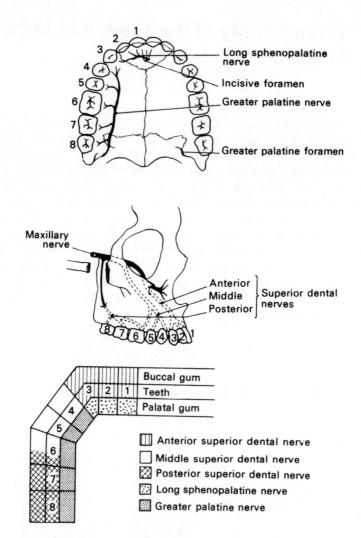

Figure 13.2 *Nerve supply of upper teeth.*

(a) The **anterior superior dental nerve** supplies the incisors and canine, and labial gum of these teeth.

(b) The **middle superior dental nerve** supplies the premolars, part of the first molar, and buccal gum of these teeth.

(c) The **posterior superior dental nerve** supplies the remainder of the first molar, the second and third molars, and buccal gum of these teeth.

(d) The **long sphenopalatine nerve** supplies the palatal gum of the incisors and part of the canine.

(e) The **greater palatine nerve** supplies the palatal gum of the canine, premolars and molars.

Maxillary nerve

The maxillary nerve emerges from the base of the skull and passes forward through the floor of the orbit. Before entering the orbit it gives off its posterior superior dental and palatine branches. Within the orbit it gives off the middle and anterior superior dental nerves. It emerges from the orbit through the **infra-orbital foramen** on the front of the maxilla (Figures 12.14, 13.2), to supply the skin and mucous membrane of the lower eyelid, cheek and upper lip.

The posterior superior dental nerve enters the back of the maxilla to reach its destination.

The greater palatine nerve also passes through the back of the maxilla and reaches the surface of the hard palate through the **greater palatine foramen**, opposite the third molar tooth.

The long sphenopalatine nerve passes through the floor of the nasal cavity to reach the surface of the palate through the **incisive foramen** behind the central incisors (Figures 13.2, 12.15).

The anterior and middle superior dental nerves branch off from the maxillary nerve in the floor of the orbit. They pass down inside the maxilla, in the walls of the maxillary sinus, to reach the teeth.

Lower teeth

The nerves supplying the lower teeth and gum are the inferior dental, lingual and long buccal branches of the mandibular nerve (Figure 13.3). The mandibular nerve passes down from the base of the skull on the inner side of the ramus of the mandible, between the medial and lateral pterygoid muscles, and divides into the above branches.

The **inferior dental (alveolar) nerve** supplies all the lower teeth and enters the mandible through the **mandibular foramen**. This is situated at the centre of the inner surface of the ramus and is guarded on its front edge by a small bony projection called the **lingula** (Figure 12.17). After entering the mandibular foramen, the nerve passes through a canal running inside the mandible, below the apices of the teeth. A branch of the inferior dental nerve emerges on the outer surface of the mandible through the **mental foramen** which is situated below the apices of the premolars (Figures 12.14, 12.17, 13.3). It is called the **mental nerve** and supplies the buccal gum of incisors, canine and premolars, plus the lower lip and chin.

The **long buccal nerve** supplies the buccal gum of the molars. It passes into the gum on the outer surface of the mandible.

The **lingual nerve** supplies the lingual gum of all lower teeth. It passes along the floor of the mouth on the inner surface of the mandible, where it also supplies the anterior two-thirds of the tongue and floor of the mouth.

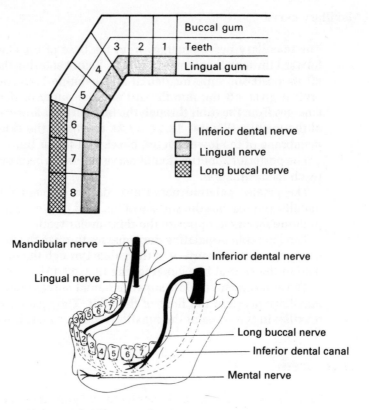

Figure 13.3 *Nerve supply of lower teeth.*

Local anaesthesia

Pain messages passing along a nerve to the brain cause a sensation of pain in the area supplied by that nerve. A local anaesthetic injected into the vicinity of a nerve prevents the passage of such messages, thus producing a temporary local anaesthesia. All perception of pain is lost but other sensations, such as pressure or vibration, are still felt.

Anaesthesia means the complete loss of feeling; whereas **analgesia** means loss of pain only. Thus local anaesthesia should, strictly speaking, be called local analgesia but the former term is in such common use that it will be continued here.

Local anaesthetic drugs

The drugs most commonly used are a 2% solution of **lignocaine** (lidocaine) and a 3% solution of **prilocaine** (*Citanest*). The first local anaesthetic to be introduced was cocaine, but this is a dangerous drug and is no longer used.

A small quantity of adrenaline (1:80,000) is included in anaesthetic solutions in order to prolong the duration of anaesthesia. It achieves this by its vasoconstrictor action which confines the anaesthetic to the injection site for an hour or more. Some practitioners prefer not to use adrenaline on patients with heart disease, high blood pressure and diabetes; or on patients taking drugs for the treatment of mental depression and high blood pressure. In such cases 4% prilocaine without adrenaline can be used for short procedures. If a longer action is required, 3% prilocaine with **felypressin** is used. Felypressin (*Octapressin*) is an alternative vasoconstrictor which does not affect the heart or blood pressure.

Other possible additives are a preservative to prolong shelf life, and a buffering agent to reduce acidity.

Anaesthetic solutions are supplied in cartridges containing sufficient anaesthetic (2 ml) for one injection. A cartridge is a glass or plastic tube sealed at one end with a thin rubber cap and at the other with a rubber bung. A special syringe and needle are required for use with cartridges. When a cartridge is inserted in the syringe, a double-ended needle pierces the thin cap. Solution is injected when the syringe plunger engages the rubber bung and pushes it down the tube.

Surface anaesthetics

Surface anaesthetics anaesthetize the surface of mucous membrane so that a syringe needle can be inserted painlessly. They are used in the form of paste, solution or spray which is applied to the appropriate site a few minutes before an injection is given. 5% lignocaine is commonly used as a surface anaesthetic.

They are also used to minimize the discomfort of superficial scaling, fitting matrix bands, and for preventing sickness when taking impressions.

Types of injection

Methods used to produce local anaesthesia are nerve block, local infiltration, intra-ligamentary and intra-osseous injections (Figure 13.4).

Nerve block

A nerve block is an injection which anaesthetizes the nerve in soft tissue before it enters the jaw to reach the teeth and associated parts. Pain sensations from every part supplied by the nerve are blocked at the site of injection and cannot reach the brain. A nerve block is used when it is necessary to anaesthetize several teeth in one quadrant or where a local infiltration cannot work.

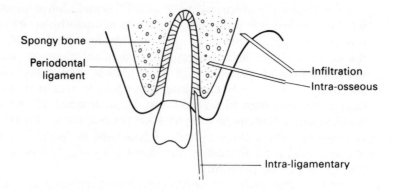

Figure 13.4   *Types of injection.*

The commonest example of this type of injection is the **inferior dental block**. For this injection the anaesthetic solution is injected over the mandibular foramen (Figure 12.17). At this site the inferior dental and lingual nerves are so close to each other (Figure 13.3) that both nerves are anaesthetized together. Thus it has the effect of anaesthetizing all the lower teeth and lingual gum on that side, together with half the tongue as well. Furthermore it anaesthetizes the lower lip and buccal gum of incisors, canine and premolars as these are supplied by the mental branch of the inferior dental nerve. So once the patient confirms the numbness of the lower lip, the dentist knows that all the lower teeth on that side are numb too.

The only part unaffected by this injection is the buccal gum of lower molars; this area of soft tissue is supplied by the long buccal nerve which is too far from the injection site to be affected (Figure 13.3).

Local infiltration

A local infiltration injection is given over the apex of the tooth to be anaesthetized. The needle is inserted beneath the mucous membrane overlying the jaw (Figure 13.4). The anaesthetic soaks through pores in the bone and anaesthetizes the nerves supplying the tooth and gum at the site of injection. Thus the difference between these two types of injection is that a nerve block applies the anaesthetic to the nerve trunk, whereas an infiltration applies it to nerve endings.

A local infiltration injection can only be used where the compact bone is sufficiently thin and porous to allow the anaesthetic to penetrate into spongy bone. Thus it is usually effective for all upper teeth. The compact bone overlying the mandibular premolars and molars, however, is too thick and an inferior dental block is necessary for these. A local infiltration can always be used to anaesthetize gum only as will be seen in the section on injections for extractions.

Intra-ligamentary injection

Some patients, particularly children, find an inferior dental block injection unpleasant, or dislike the numb tongue and lip it produces. An alternative for these patients is an injection directly down the gingival crevice into the periodontal ligament on the mesial and distal sides of the tooth concerned. This is called an intra-ligamentary injection (Figure 13.4). It immediately anaesthetizes the tooth and its buccal and lingual gum, ready for filling or extraction. The cheek, lip and tongue are unaffected, thus preventing the common injury in children of biting or scalding a numb lip or tongue.

A special syringe using a smaller cartridge and needle are required (Figure 13.5). The disadvantages of this injection are that it cannot be used in the presence of gingival infection, and is not always successful on adults. However, it often succeeds as an additional injection where an infiltration or block has failed to work.

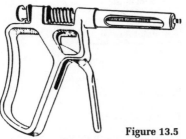

Figure 13.5 *Intra-ligamentary syringe (Ligmaject).*

Intra-osseous injection

An intra-osseous injection is given directly into spongy bone between two teeth. A few drops of anaesthetic are first injected into the gum. This permits painless drilling of a small hole through the compact bone, to allow access for a needle to be inserted directly into spongy bone (Figure 13.4).

This injection provides a relatively short duration of anaesthesia for the tooth, and buccal and lingual gum, on either side of the injection site, but it does not numb the cheek, lip or tongue. This makes it an excellent method for extractions. Other advantages are that it works immediately and rarely fails, thus making it useful where an infiltration or block has been unsuccessful. The disadvantage is that it cannot be used where gingival (gum) infection is present.

The technique is very old but has gained a new lease of life with the introduction of the *Stabident* kit, containing a special drill for perforating the compact bone, and a matching ultra-short needle for injecting directly into spongy bone.

Local anaesthesia for extractions

For extraction it is necessary to anaesthetize not only the tooth, but also its surrounding gum. The injections required will be more readily understood by referring back to the nerve supply of teeth.

Upper teeth

To anaesthetize any upper tooth for extraction a local infiltration injection is given on its buccal and palatal sides (Figure 13.6).

For the second and third molars, some operators prefer to give a posterior superior dental block instead of a local infiltration on the buccal side.

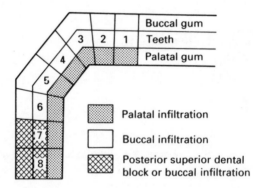

Figure 13.6   *Injections for upper teeth.*

Lower teeth

An inferior dental block injection blocks the lingual as well as the inferior dental nerve. This single injection will therefore suffice for the extraction of premolars, canine and incisors (Figure 13.7).

For molars a local buccal infiltration is required in addition to an inferior dental block.

The compact bone in the incisor region of the mandible is sufficiently thin to allow the use of a buccal and lingual local infiltration, and many operators prefer this to an inferior dental block for anaesthetizing lower incisors.

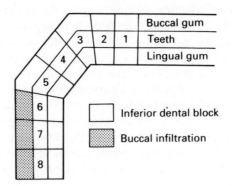

Figure 13.7   *Injections for lower teeth.*

Local anaesthesia for fillings

It is unnecessary to anaesthetize the gum for fillings. Only the injection which anaesthetizes the tooth is given; there is no need for a second injection.

Upper teeth

A local buccal infiltration is enough. A posterior superior dental block is sometimes preferred for the second and third molars.

Lower teeth

An inferior dental block will anaesthetize every lower tooth. For incisors, a local buccal infiltration will do instead.

Preparation for local anaesthesia

A long needle is used for a nerve block. For local infiltration, a short needle is usually preferred. Although needles rarely break during an injection, precautions must still be taken to deal with such accidents. A suitable pair of forceps (e.g. Spencer Wells, Figure 16.6) should always be available to grasp and remove the broken end.

A surface anaesthetic is applied for a few minutes while the syringe is being prepared. The smaller guard at the syringe end of the needle is removed and the needle screwed on to the hub of a sterile syringe. As injection of cold solutions can be painful, the cartridge may first be warmed to body temperature. The thin cap at the needle end of the cartridge is flamed before insertion into the syringe. The injection site is then dried and disinfected. This is done by applying a suitable disinfectant, such as chlorhexidine, on a pledget of cotton wool for 15 seconds. The injection is now given and the needle guard refitted immediately. A glass of mouthwash is provided for the patient, as local anaesthetic solutions have an unpleasant taste.

Nervous patients sometimes faint when a local anaesthetic is given. For this reason they must not be left alone while waiting for the injection to work. Apart from nervousness, patients are liable to faint if the anaesthetic is accidentally injected into a blood vessel. One way of preventing this is to use an **aspirating** syringe (Figure 13.8). With such a syringe, blood will be seen flowing back into the cartridge if the needle has penetrated a blood vessel. If so, it must be withdrawn and reinserted; whereupon the injection can be given if no more blood is seen.

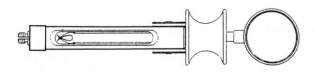

Figure 13.8   *Aspirating syringe.*

Before leaving the surgery, patients must always be warned not to eat or drink on the anaesthetized side, and not to smoke, until the effect has worn off. Otherwise there is a danger that they may burn or bite the numb area without being aware of it.

At the end of the appointment the cartridge and needle are discarded. Empty glass cartridges are put into the sharps bin but normal clinical waste bags are used for plastic cartridges. With the needle guard still in place, the used needle is unscrewed from the syringe and inserted into the sharps bin, ready for incineration.

As mentioned in Chapter 10, a new needle and cartridge must be used for every patient to prevent cross-infection from blood containing HBV, HIV or any other contaminants. Surgery methods of sterilization cannot penetrate the hollow interior of a blood-stained needle. Similarly, a partially used cartridge may also be contaminated with blood as microscopic aspiration takes place even without using aspiration methods.

Needlestick injury

Needlestick injury is the name given to an inoculation injury (Chapter 10) caused by an accidental prick from a syringe needle. It is one of the occupational hazards of dentistry and its effect ranges from nil to potentially dangerous, depending on the circumstances of the accident.

If a nurse pricks herself with a sterile needle, i.e. one which has not yet been used on a patient, there is no danger. The skin puncture should be covered with a waterproof dressing and the needle and cartridge discarded.

But if the needle is not sterile, i.e. has already been used on a patient, then the situation is potentially serious although no harm results in the vast majority of cases. The wound should be squeezed and rinsed under hot running water and then covered with a waterproof dressing. The dentist must be informed and the patient's notes checked for any medical history suggesting the possibility of cross-infection. If there is no relevant history, the wound will probably heal satisfactorily without any complications; but if it becomes red, painful, and swollen, then acute inflammation has occurred and the nurse's doctor may consider antibiotic treatment necessary to treat the infection. The doctor should also be consulted if there is any suspicion that the patient may be an HBV or HIV carrier, e.g. in one of the high risk groups described in Chapter 10.

If needlestick injury occurs from a needle used on a known HBV or HIV carrier the accident must be reported immediately to the dentist, nurse's doctor and the public health authority. Appropriate action can then be taken for careful monitoring and blood sampling to ensure that the disease has not been transmitted to the nurse. Although the risks are alarming, there is little danger in practice. As far as HBV infection is concerned, all nurses should already have been vaccinated and are consequently immune. There is no vaccine available against AIDS, but needlestick injury from such a patient is unlikely to transmit the disease as HIV has a very low infectivity and repeated exposure is usually necessary to contract AIDS.

As with all the other occupational hazards of dentistry, no harm need result if appropriate care is taken. All surgery staff must be vaccinated against HBV and needles handled with very great care to avoid accidental pricks. Needle guards should always be in place. When resheathing needles the risk of injury is greatly reduced if a special resheathing device is used or the needle guard held with a suitable instrument.

If needlestick injury does occur, the reason for it should be analysed and procedures reviewed if necessary to prevent a recurrence.

The same applies to any other instrument which accidentally penetrates the skin of surgery staff. All such injuries should be recorded in the accident book.

All used needles, glass cartridges and other sharp items for disposal must be kept in a special sharps container complying with the British Standard. This is a rigid puncture-resistant container with a secure cover, coloured yellow to indicate that it contains hazardous clinical waste. It should not be filled more than two-thirds full and special arrangements must be made for its incineration, separate from other clinical waste.

Written examination

(a)   List the contents of a typical local anaesthetic cartridge.
(b)   List the ways in which a dental surgeon could anaesthetize a tooth.
(c)   Describe to a patient the effects of a local anaesthetic and
the care required after a restoration has been placed under
local analgesia (anaesthetic). (November 1990)

(a)   The dentist is about to extract an upper first molar tooth.
List the nerves which would need to be anaesthetized.
(b)   Describe the role of the dental nurse in preparing for and
assisting with local analgesia.
(c)   List the possible causes of a 'needlestick' injury and the
action you would take in the event of such an injury. (May
1994)

Summary

Nerve supply of the teeth

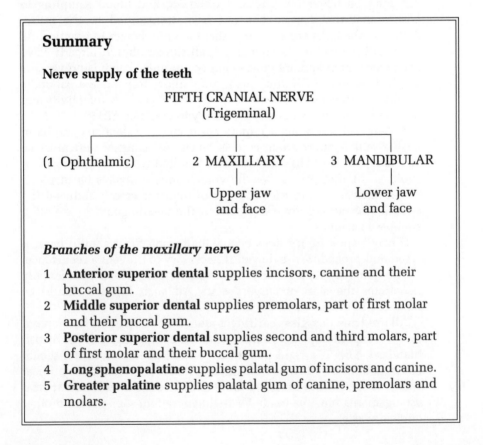

FIFTH CRANIAL NERVE
(Trigeminal)

(1 Ophthalmic)   2 MAXILLARY   3 MANDIBULAR

Upper jaw   Lower jaw
and face   and face

Branches of the maxillary nerve

1   **Anterior superior dental** supplies incisors, canine and their
buccal gum.
2   **Middle superior dental** supplies premolars, part of first molar
and their buccal gum.
3   **Posterior superior dental** supplies second and third molars, part
of first molar and their buccal gum.
4   **Long sphenopalatine** supplies palatal gum of incisors and canine.
5   **Greater palatine** supplies palatal gum of canine, premolars and
molars.

6 **Infra-orbital** supplies skin and mucous membrane of lower eyelid, cheek and upper lip.

Branches of the mandibular nerve

1 **Inferior dental** supplies every lower tooth.
   Mental branch of inferior dental nerve supplies lower lip, chin and buccal gum of incisors, canine and premolars.
2 **Long buccal** supplies buccal gum of molars.
3 **Lingual** supplies all the lingual gum; anterior two-thirds of tongue and floor of mouth.
4 **Motor** nerves to muscles of mastication.

Local anaesthetic drugs

Lignocaine 2% } Adrenaline
Prilocaine 3%   } prolongs anaesthesia

Prilocaine 4% without adrenaline } Heart disease
Prilocaine 3% with felypressin   } High blood pressure
                                 } Diabetes

Surface anaesthetics

Lignocaine 5%
   Used to minimize pain of:

● Injection
● Scaling
● Application of matrices, clamps, etc.

Types of injection

1 **Local infiltration**
   Anaesthetic soaks into bone to reach nerve endings.
   Used mainly for upper teeth.
2 **Nerve block**
   Nerve trunk anaesthetized as it passes through soft tissue before entering jaw.
   Anaesthetizes entire area supplied by nerve.
   Used mainly for lower teeth.

3   **Intra-ligamentary**
    Anaesthetic injected through gingival crevice directly into
    periodontal ligament.
    Anaesthetizes single tooth and its buccal and lingual gum.
    Suitable for filling or extraction.
    Works immediately. Skin and tongue unaffected.
    Requires special syringe and needle.
    Cannot be used in presence of gingival infection.
4   **Intra-osseous**
    Injected directly into spongy bone between two teeth.
    Anaesthetizes both teeth, and their buccal and lingual gum.
    Works immediately; other soft tissues unaffected.
    Suitable for short duration drilling or extraction; and when other
    methods have failed.

Injections for upper teeth

TOOTH	INJECTION FOR FILLING	ADDITIONAL INJECTION FOR EXTRACTION
1	Buccal infiltration	Palatal infiltration
2	" "	" "
3	" "	" "
4	" "	" "
5	" "	" "
6	" "	" "
7	Posterior superior dental	" "
8	block or buccal infiltration	" "

Injections for lower teeth

TOOTH	INJECTION FOR FILLING	ADDITIONAL INJECTION FOR EXTRACTION
1	Inferior dental block or	None
2	buccal infiltration	Lingual infiltration
3	Inferior dental block	None
4	" " "	"
5	" " "	"
6	" " "	Buccal infiltration
7	" " "	" "
8	" " "	" "

Procedure for local anaesthesia

1 Apply surface anaesthetic.
2 Prepare sterile aspirating syringe.
3 Disinfect injection site.
4 Injection – aspirate first.
5 Provide mouthwash.
6 Keep patient under observation.
7 Discard needle and glass cartridge into sharps bin.
8 Warn patient to avoid eating, drinking or smoking on affected side until numbness wears off.

Needlestick injury

Sterile needle

- Cover with waterproof dressing
- Discard needle and cartridge

Unsterile (used) needle

- Squeeze wound to encourage bleeding
- Rinse under hot running water and apply waterproof dressing
- Inform dentist
- Check patient's medical history
- Consult doctor if uncertain or symptoms develop
- Inform public health authority if patient is known HBV or HIV carrier

Record all needlestick and other injuries from sharp instruments in accident book.

14   General Anaesthesia and Sedation

General anaesthesia (GA) is a state of unconsciousness with complete loss of feeling and protective reflexes (Chapter 6). In the dental chair it is used mainly for short procedures such as extractions and the incision and drainage of abscesses.

Sedation is a state of conscious relaxation which enables prolonged treatment to be carried out under local anaesthesia (LA). It is used for patients who are otherwise too nervous to tolerate dental treatment. The patient remains conscious and completely relaxed throughout and retains all protective reflexes against blockage of the airway. It is used mainly for long procedures such as fillings.

Mentally or physically handicapped patients, and others who are too unco-operative to accept short GA or prolonged sedation techniques, can be treated in suitably equipped dental premises under **endotracheal anaesthesia**. This is the general anaesthetic method normally used in hospitals.

Legal aspects

Dentists are legally entitled to use GA and sedation for patients but are required to maintain proper standards of practice for the safety of patients. Deaths have occurred in the dental surgery under GA, causing great concern to the public, as well as to the medical and dental professions.

The General Dental Council has a duty, under the Dentists Act, to protect the public by ensuring that dentists are adequately trained for GA, sedation and resuscitation. The GDC accordingly issues clear guidelines for these procedures. They specify the following conditions which should be fulfilled in dental practice.

1   GA should be avoided in dental practice if at all possible.
2   Before GA or sedation procedures, a full medical history must be taken and precise written pre- and post-operative instructions given. Adequate records of the procedure, made at the time, must be kept.
3   General anaesthetics must not be given by a dentist acting as both operator and anaesthetist.
4   The anaesthetic must be given by a second medical or dental practitioner who is appropriately trained and experienced, and who remains responsible for the patients until they are fit to return

home. The dentist and the anaesthetist must each have an adequately trained dental nurse to assist them; and the facilities for advanced life support (pp. 180, 194) must be present.

5 Suitably experienced dentists may use sedation techniques and act as operator, provided that a suitably trained nurse is present throughout. The training and experience of such nurses must enable them to be efficient members of the dental team, capable of monitoring the clinical condition of the patient and assisting in case of emergency.

6 Sedation is defined as a state which enables treatment to be carried out, but with the patient conscious enough to respond to command throughout the procedure. Only one drug should be used for intravenous sedation. Children should not be given intravenous sedation.

7 Neither GA nor sedation should be used unless proper equipment and facilities for their administration; monitoring of patients' condition; resuscitation; and recovery are readily available with both the dentist and staff trained and practised in their use.

8 Patients must not be left unattended in the recovery room, or allowed to return home without an escort. The anaesthetist or dentist must specify the patient as fit for discharge.

Any failure to comply with these conditions would be regarded as serious professional misconduct and render the dentist liable to be removed or suspended from the Dentists Register. Nurses should specially note the requirements relating to themselves in paragraphs 4 and 5.

In this respect, special post-certification courses in general anaesthetic nursing and conscious sedation are available for qualified nurses. They include inhalational and intravenous anaesthesia and sedation, monitoring the patient's condition and resuscitation procedures.

In view of their strict legal obligations, many dentists enlist the services of a specialist anaesthetist for GA in their practice; or refer their patients to clinics specially equipped and staffed for this purpose.

General anaesthesia

The drugs most commonly used for GA in the dental chair are nitrous oxide, halothane and methohexitone.

Nitrous oxide

Nitrous oxide (N_2O) is a gas supplied in blue cylinders and is the most widely used general anaesthetic in dentistry. It is administered together with oxygen through a nasal inhaler so that the mouth can be left uncovered throughout the operative procedure.

Air contains 20% oxygen and every anaesthetic mixture must contain at least this amount. Any reduction of the oxygen content below 20% is dangerous. Although nitrous oxide is a strong analgesic, it is a weak anaesthetic; and this means that it cannot produce adequate anaesthesia when given with 20% oxygen. An additional anaesthetic agent is accordingly used with nitrous oxide to allow provision of a normal amount of oxygen and permit maintenance of safe smooth anaesthesia with adequate time for careful complete surgery. Additional agents used for this purpose include halothane and methohexitone.

Nitrous oxide and halothane

Halothane (*Fluothane*) is a colourless liquid supplied in a dark bottle. Before use it is poured into a vaporizer bottle attached to the anaesthetic machine. The flow of nitrous oxide vaporizes some halothane and the patient receives a mixture of nitrous oxide, halothane and at least 30% oxygen.

The advantages of halothane are that it allows the use of at least 30% oxygen; provides safe, smooth anaesthesia; and gives the operator ample time to complete all the procedures normally performed under GA in the dental chair.

A disadvantage of halothane is that repeated use may severely, or even fatally, damage the patient's liver. Patients must always be questioned to ascertain whether halothane has been given previously or if reactions to halothane have occurred. Patients with a history of jaundice or fever following the administration of halothane must not be given it again. Patients with no history of adverse reactions to halothane should not be given it again within a period of three months. If a second anaesthetic is necessary, the patient is given enflurane or isoflurane instead.

Enflurane

Enflurane (*Ethrane*) is a colourless liquid which is used in a vaporizer bottle in the same way as halothane. It is only half as powerful as halothane so is only used when halothane cannot be given. Enflurane is unsuitable for epileptic patients.

Isoflurane (*Forane*)

This is similar to enflurane but has the advantage of giving a much more rapid recovery. It is used as an alternative to enflurane for epileptic patients.

Methohexitone

Methohexitone (*Brietal*) is injected into a *vein* (intravenous injection) to produce instantaneous anaesthesia. This alone will suffice for a very short operation such as a simple extraction. For longer procedures, anaesthesia is maintained with nitrous oxide and at least 30% oxygen, together with halothane if necessary. It is used for patients who are difficult to anaesthetize by inhalational methods. Struggling is thereby prevented and damage avoided. Apart from resistant patients it is also used extensively for very nervous adults and older children. Patients lose consciousness immediately after injection, and are thereby spared the unpleasant experience of placement of the nasal inhaler and a relatively slow loss of consciousness.

Propofol

Propofol (*Diprivan*) is injected intravenously as an alternative to methohexitone. It produces a more rapid recovery than methohexitone.

Endotracheal anaesthesia

As mentioned in the introduction to this chapter, some patients are too physically or mentally handicapped to be controllable throughout prolonged dental treatment. However, they can be treated successfully in suitably equipped dental premises under endotracheal anaesthesia. This is the method normally used in hospitals and involves delivery of the anaesthetic mixture directly into the lungs through a **nasotracheal tube**. The anaesthetist passes the tube through a nostril, along the floor of the nose, into the nasopharynx. From here, using a special instrument called a **laryngoscope**, the tube is guided by direct vision through the larynx and into the trachea. The oropharynx can then be packed with gauze to prevent any foreign bodies, blood, saliva or debris entering the airway.

The first step in such a procedure is the injection of an intravenous anaesthetic, such as methohexitone, to produce immediate unconsciousness. A short-acting muscle relaxant, such as *Scoline* or *Tracrium*, is then injected. This paralyses all the muscles and allows the nasotracheal tube to be passed into the trachea without evoking the natural reflexes which prevent such invasion of the airway. A normal general anaesthetic mixture of nitrous oxide, halothane and oxygen can then be administered.

The effect of the muscle relaxant lasts for a few minutes, and during this time natural breathing is impossible as all the respiratory muscles have been paralysed. The anaesthetist accordingly applies artificial respiration by squeezing the reservoir bag on the anaesthetic machine. This pumps the anaesthetic into the patient's lungs in the same way as natural breathing. As soon as the effect of the muscle relaxant has worn off, natural breathing resumes. The anaesthetist often gives an injection of **atropine** beforehand to inhibit the secretion of saliva and mucus. This gives the operator a dry field of work and helps prevent fluids entering the airway.

The advantages of endotracheal anaesthesia are that it gives the anaesthetist complete control over the airway, with no danger of obstruction, and allows use of any resuscitative measures which may be needed; while for the operator, it provides perfect anaesthesia with a clean, dry field of work for as long as required.

The disadvantages are that it requires the services of a specialist anaesthetist, and the patient may suffer from a sore throat and muscle pains afterwards. Adequate recovery facilities are also necessary as it may be an hour or so before the patient is fit enough to be taken home.

Stages of anaesthesia

Short procedures such as extractions are usually done with nitrous oxide and halothane. Only a few minutes elapse between administration of this anaesthetic to a conscious patient and the state in which anaesthesia is deep enough for extractions to be performed. In this brief period the patient passes through three stages:

1 Analgesia
2 Delirium
3 Surgical anaesthesia

Analgesia

The first few breaths of gas render the still-conscious patient incapable of feeling slight pain – a state known as analgesia. A sense of touch and hearing remain, though, and extractions cannot be performed at this stage.

Delirium

The patient is unconscious but not relaxed. Breathing is irregular and struggling may occur.

Surgical anaesthesia

This is the stage at which the operation is performed, and the anaesthetic is maintained at this depth throughout. It is recognized by relaxation of the limbs and the onset of automatic regular nasal breathing.

If anaesthesia becomes too deep the patient's breathing will weaken and then stop. This is the final stage of anaesthesia, known as **failure of respiration**. It must be remedied immediately by providing the patient with oxygen. The ways in which this can be done are discussed later in the chapter.

Care of the patient

Anaesthetic history

Certain questions are asked in order to ascertain the patient's suitability for a general anaesthetic:

(a) Details of previous anaesthetic reactions; recent halothane
(b) General health – condition of heart and chest, nasal blockage, other illnesses, drugs prescribed
(c) Pregnancy – special care is required if GA is necessary
(d) Allergies
(e) Family history of problems with anaesthetics

Anaesthetic appointment

Having signed a consent form for the treatment and GA, an appointment is given for the patient to arrive 15 minutes before required in the surgery. This allows time for the patient to be made ready for the anaesthetic and relax a little before entering the surgery.

Instructions are given, verbally and in writing, for the patient to:

(a) Abstain from food and drink for *at least* four hours before the appointment.
    This is to prevent vomiting during the anaesthetic which can result in a dangerous blockage of the airway.
(b) Be accompanied by a responsible adult to look after the patient until recovery is complete.
(c) Not to drive any form of vehicle, operate machinery or take alcohol for 24 hours after the anaesthetic.
    This amount of time is necessary for complete recovery from the effects of anaesthesia. Alcohol prolongs this time.
(d) Not to wear any jewellery, contact lenses, a wrist watch, nail varnish or facial cosmetics.
    These may mask vital signs (page 167) or hinder the use of monitoring or resuscitation equipment.
(e) Notify the surgery beforehand if suffering from a cold or other infection. Anaesthetics are not given if the nose is blocked. The appointment can be changed for a later date when the patient has recovered.

Patients are warned that the appointment will be cancelled if any instructions are disobeyed.

Before anaesthesia

The nurse checks that instructions given with the appointment have been obeyed. If the patient has a cold, or has not obeyed instructions, the nurse must inform the anaesthetist. Before admission to the surgery, patients are requested to:

(a)   Remove excess outer clothing
(b)   Use the toilet
(c)   Loosen tight clothing which could interfere with freedom of respiration, e.g. collar, belt, etc.

Pulse and blood pressure are recorded; and for intravenous anaesthesia the patient may be weighed, as the dose depends on body weight.

During anaesthesia

In addition to passing the dentist or anaesthetist anything they require, and assisting as directed, the nurse must carefully watch the patient. Immediate assistance can thereby be rendered if the patient should start struggling or tend to slip out of the chair. GA demands the undivided attention of anaesthetist and dentist, while the nurse plays an invaluable part in being ready to help in any situation that may arise.

After anaesthesia

In order to maintain a clear airway and prevent injury, the patient's head is held and the mandible supported until consciousness occurs. The nurse then provides a mouthwash; cleans any blood off the face; and helps the patient to a couch or seat by a spittoon in the recovery room, attended throughout by a nurse. When the patient has fully recovered and bleeding has ceased, the dentist or anaesthetist authorizes the escort to accompany the patient home. Then, if an indwelling intravenous needle was used, the nurse removes it and applies a dressing.

Before leaving the premises, however, verbal and written advice is given on the prevention of bleeding and after-pain (Chapter 16). Patients are warned not to drive a vehicle or operate machinery for 24 hours after the anaesthetic; or to drink any alcohol. It can take several hours for the effects of an anaesthetic to wear off, and throughout that time the patient is under the influence of drugs. Driving under the influence of drugs is not only an offence, but may invalidate a driver's insurance. Alcohol makes matters worse by prolonging the effect of the anaesthetic, and may also help cause post-operative bleeding.

Preparation and procedure

1 All the forceps, gags, props and other instruments required are sterilized. To avoid burning the patient, the nurse must check to ensure that they are cool enough. Then they are set out, together with mouth packs, swabs, monitoring and resuscitation equipment, out of sight of the patient.

 The anaesthetic machine is checked to ensure that it is in correct working order, with full nitrous oxide and oxygen cylinders. Spare cylinders should be at hand in case one becomes empty during administration. Nitrous oxide cylinders are light blue; oxygen cylinders are black with a white top. All cylinders, on or off the machine, must be fitted with the correct labels denoting whether they are full, in use, or empty.

 The halothane vaporizer is filled and, if intravenous agents are used, sterile disposable syringes and needles are provided and anaesthetic solutions prepared.

 The monitoring equipment and suction apparatus are also checked to ensure they work satisfactorily.

 The patient's notes and X-rays are checked to see that they are correct.

2 The patient is then brought into the surgery and seated with hands clasped together in the lap. Any tight clothing round the neck is loosened, spectacles, dentures or orthodontic appliances removed, and a large bib is provided.

3 The anaesthetist then places the mask in position and induction is commenced. Silence is essential at this stage as hearing is the last sense to be lost.

 If the anaesthetist decides on an intravenous induction the nurse prepares the patient's arm, or back of the hand, for injection. This involves rolling up the sleeve and swabbing the injection site with a skin disinfectant; then applying pressure above the elbow, manually or with a tourniquet, to make the vein stand out and facilitate injection. An indwelling **cannula** or butterfly needle (Figure 14.2) is used. This is a special needle which is taped into place and remains in the vein for the duration of anaesthesia. It allows further injections of anaesthetic or resuscitation drugs to be given without delay.

 The anaesthetist informs the dentist when the patient is in the stage of surgical anaesthesia, ready for extractions to be performed.

4 The nurse switches on the operating light and the dentist inserts a

prop (Figure 14.1) between the teeth in order to keep the mouth open during anaesthesia.

5   The nurse hands the dentist a **mouth pack** which is used to prevent blood or debris entering the airway. The end of the pack is used to block off the floor of the mouth alongside the tongue where the extractions are to be done; the middle part is used to pack the space between the top of the tongue and hard palate to prevent the tongue falling back and blocking the airway; and the remainder is left hanging out of the mouth so that it can be withdrawn immediately if necessary.

   If the chair has been tilted to a horizontal position, protection must be provided for the patient's eyes.

6   The nurse hands the dentist the appropriate forceps and holds a **kidney dish** into which the extracted teeth and discarded forceps are placed. If it is necessary to extract any teeth covered by the prop, a new one is inserted on the opposite side and the old one withdrawn. Alternatively a **Fergusson gag** (Figure 14.1) may be used. This is essentially an adjustable prop used to force open the mouth and keep the jaws apart. Throughout this procedure the nurse must be ready to provide suction, swabs or new mouth pack to clear away the copious flow of blood which occurs during extractions under GA; and must also check that the correct number of teeth are removed and account for every one of them as they are placed in the kidney dish.

7   When the operative procedure is completed the dentist informs the anaesthetist, who stops the anaesthetic and, if treatment was in an upright position, supports the patient's head until conscious. Supine patients are tipped on to one side with their head slightly down to maintain a clear airway. The nurse then takes

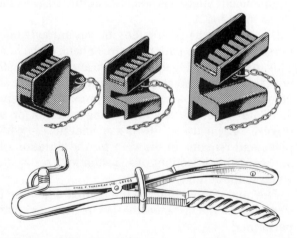

Figure 14.1 *Props and Fergusson gag.*

over as described before on the care of the patient after anaesthesia.

8   After each case all used instruments and dishes are cleaned of
blood, sterilized, and everything made ready again for the next
patient. All used sharps and other disposables are put in the
correct containers. The disposal of clinical waste is described in
Chapter 10.

9   The surgery must be well ventilated during GA as the patient's
exhaled air contains waste anaesthetic gases. These pollute the air
in the surgery and are reinhaled by the staff. If GA sessions are
held frequently a scavenging system to remove waste gases and
other pollutants is necessary to safeguard staff health. A simple
method is the use of a special scavenging nasal mask; but for
surgeries devoted mainly to GA sessions, installation of an
appropriate air-conditioning system is preferable.

It is obvious from this account that nurses have an extremely busy
time during GA sessions. Four qualified dental nurses are required:
one in the recovery room; one assisting the dentist; one assisting the
anaesthetist; and another preparing the instruments. Arrangements
must also be made to ensure that messages, enquiries and telephone
calls are dealt with by reception staff to prevent any interruption or
delays to proceedings in the surgery. Nurses have an indispensable
role in ensuring that the entire procedure runs smoothly, efficiently
and with the maximum consideration for the patient's comfort.

Choice of anaesthesia

When extractions are necessary the dentist decides whether they
should be performed under LA or GA. Many factors are considered in
reaching a decision.

The patient's general health

General anaesthesia in the dental chair may be dangerous for patients
suffering from certain diseases or taking certain drugs. In such cases it
is preferable to use LA. Alternatively the patient can be referred to
hospital if GA is necessary.

Conditions which can make GA hazardous are disorders of the
heart, circulation and respiration; anaemia, diabetes, liver and kidney
disease. Some patients of African or Caribbean origin have a hereditary type of anaemia called **sickle cell disease** and tests must be done
to exclude this before GA is given. The test result is shown on a card
which is carried by these patients and shown to any dentist treating
them. Drugs which may affect GA are corticosteroids and some used
for the treatment of mental depression and high blood pressure.

Administration of drugs should be avoided whenever possible during pregnancy. If treatment is necessary, LA is preferable to GA or sedation. In all cases of doubt, the patient's doctor is consulted before GA is used.

Acute infection

Local anaesthesia can be dangerous in the presence of acute infection as it may spread the infection to healthy parts. It is also less likely to work properly.

Difficult extractions

Extractions liable to take some time are performed in the dental chair under LA, or in a hospital operating theatre under GA.

Multiple extractions

General anaesthesia is often preferred for multiple extractions as they can be completed in fewer visits than for LA.

Children

Young children and very nervous patients are best treated under GA or sedation.

Emergency extractions

Patients presenting as emergencies with severe toothache are best treated under LA. This can be given to people who have recently eaten or are medically unfit for GA.

If LA is unsuitable, e.g. acute alveolar abscess, GA can only be given if conditions are suitable: an anaesthetist is available; the patient has fasted beforehand, and is not suffering from a cold or other condition which could cause difficulties under GA.

Patient's preference

Whenever possible the dentist accedes to patients' wishes in the choice of anaesthesia, provided it is safe and practicable.

No anaesthetist available

In these cases LA is used. A dentist who is working single-handed cannot accept the dual responsibility of anaesthetist and operator. It is potentially dangerous and is regarded as serious professional misconduct by the General Dental Council. If LA is unsuitable there are alternative ways of relieving pain and controlling infection until an anaesthetist is available.

Monitoring patients

Throughout any procedures under GA or sedation, it is essential to ensure and check that the circulation is adequately oxygenated. This is done by observing and recording the patient's vital signs: colour, breathing, pulse and blood pressure. This is called monitoring. Records must also be kept, at the time, of drugs given and monitoring procedure.

Colour

A patient's colour can be observed by watching the face, fingers, lips or ears. It indicates the state of oxygenation of the blood.

A pink colour is normal. A purple tinge (**cyanosis**) denotes deficient oxygenation, while pallor and sweating denote a more severe deficiency. Any such changes require immediate identification and treatment of the cause.

Breathing

Regular chest movements show that a patient is breathing but they are easier to feel than see. Placing a hand on the chest or upper abdomen, or watching for chest movements, can confirm normal respiration. Watching the reservoir bag on an anaesthetic machine also indicates the breathing pattern.

Pulse

Feeling the wrist, neck or temporal pulse will indicate the rate, regularity and strength of the heart beats. The neck (carotid) pulse is found beside the top outer edge of the larynx. The temporal pulse is felt on the zygomatic arch (page 126) immediately in front of the ear.

Blood pressure

The pulse gives some indication of blood pressure but is accurately measured with a **sphygmomanometer** and stethoscope. The sphygmomanometer comes with an inflatable cuff which is fitted on the upper arm. When inflated it stops the flow of blood through the artery on the inner side of the arm opposite the elbow. This area (the *antecubital fossa*) is the central depression seen between the upper arm and forearm; and it is on here that the stethoscope is placed. When the cuff is slowly deflated, blood starts flowing again and this can be heard through the stethoscope. The reading on the instrument scale at which the first sound is heard is noted. This is called the *systolic* pressure and denotes ventricular contraction. As deflation of the cuff is slowly continued, the sound increases to a maximum and then disappears. Another reading taken and noted at this point is called the *diastolic* pressure, denoting ventricular relaxation between heart beats. The cuff is then deflated and removed until a further blood pressure check is required. Sphygmomanometer readings are still measured in units of millimetres of mercury (mm Hg) even though mercury is not often used in modern equipment. Average readings for a healthy young adult are 120/80 for systolic/diastolic pressures.

Continuous monitoring equipment

Traditional methods of monitoring patients' vital signs by observation, feeling the pulse, and checking blood pressure can be supplemented, but not replaced, by modern electronic devices giving a continuous readout which are standard equipment in hospitals.

Dentists cannot be expected to have access to all such devices but a sphygmomanometer, a **pulse oximeter**, an **electrocardiogram** and a **capnograph** must be available during the administration of GA. For intravenous sedation, only a sphygmomanometer and pulse oximeter are required.

A pulse oximeter is a small portable device with a special illuminated probe on the end of a long lead. The probe clips on to the patient's finger or ear lobe. It detects the colour of the blood and enables the instrument to display readings of the rate and regularity of the pulse, and oxygenation of the blood. It can also sound an alarm if any readings differ from a predetermined range. A pulse oximeter is regarded as essential equipment in the surgery and recovery room for GA and intravenous sedation.

An electrocardiogram (ECG) is a device which provides a range of information on heart function from leads attached to the chest. It is essentially a heart monitor with a screen displaying the rate, strength, regularity and rhythm of the heart beats. It also has an audible alarm facility. A capnograph is a carbon dioxide monitor.

Whichever method or instrument is used for measuring pulse and blood pressure, the recordings are noted before and during the procedure. This allows any significant changes to be drawn to the attention of the dentist or anaesthetist.

The GDC requires dental nurses to be adequately trained and experienced for assisting with treatment under GA and sedation. This means that they must know how to monitor a patient's condition with the available equipment; and understand the significance of their findings.

Conscious sedation

Normally in the dental surgery, GA is confined to short procedures such as extractions. Long procedures such as fillings are done under LA. However, some patients are too nervous or otherwise unco-operative to tolerate LA. In such cases sedation techniques may be used to permit prolonged painless operating time on a relaxed patient.

The patient's fear is overcome, and a state of conscious relaxation achieved, by administering a sedation drug intravenously or by inhalation. The relaxed patient is then able to accept LA without anxiety or resistance, while the dentist can painlessly complete whatever treatment is necessary on a relaxed and co-operative patient without any stress for all concerned.

The advantages of sedation techniques are:

1 Patients remain conscious and co-operative throughout.
2 Patients retain their protective reflexes against blockage of the airway.
3 There is no need for a long period of starvation beforehand.
4 A separate anaesthetist is not required. However, as already described, there are strict legal requirements concerning the experience and training of all surgery staff involved.

Although protective reflexes remain active during sedation, small mouth packs may be used to prevent irritation from debris and spray during the dental treatment. Rubber dam should be used if possible. Props may be used to prevent discomfort from keeping the mouth open for a long time.

Dentists are expected to use conscious sedation in preference to GA whenever possible. As already described for GA (page 161), a full medical and anaesthetic history must be taken to assess patients' fitness for the procedure. Written consent to sedation, LA and the dental treatment must be obtained; and verbal and written pre- and post-operative instructions given when the appointment is made. Patients must not be suffering from a cold at the time of the appointment and must be accompanied by a responsible adult.

Oral sedation

Some people are so frightened of dental treatment that they are unable to sleep beforehand or co-operate adequately in the dental chair. Such patients can be relieved of their anxiety by use of the tranquillizer drugs mentioned in Chapter 11. This is called **premedication** and may be used before any form of dental treatment, with or without LA, GA or conscious sedation.

Drugs used to reduce anxiety prior to treatment in the dental chair are taken by mouth (oral sedation). Diazepam (*Valium*), taken the night before, allows a sound sleep; and temazepam, taken an hour before treatment, facilitates the initial conscious sedation procedures of intravenous injection or the placement of an inhalation mask.

Inhalation sedation

Although nitrous oxide alone is a weak anaesthetic which requires oxygen deprivation to produce unconsciousness, it is a powerful analgesic and this property is utilized in a technique known as **relative analgesia** (RA).

Sedation and analgesia are obtained by continuous inhalation of nitrous oxide and *at least* 30% oxygen. If the degree of analgesia is insufficient to prevent pain, the patient remains sufficiently sedated to accept LA.

Patients are usually seated in the supine position and given 100% oxygen for about two minutes at the start and finish of the procedure.

The advantages of RA are that patients may have a light snack up to two hours beforehand; recovery is rapid (about 15 minutes); electronic monitoring equipment is not required but pulse and respiration must still be checked. It is the safest and simplest form of sedation, and is the most suitable method for children.

The disadvantages are that it requires a special RA machine, which prevents less than 30% oxygen and more than 50% nitrous oxide from being given. It also necessitates a scavenging system for exhaled nitrous oxide. In common with most other types of drug treatment, RA should not be given in the first three months (trimester) of pregnancy.

Intravenous sedation

A single tranquillizer such as midazolam (*Hypnovel*) or diazepam (*Diazemuls*) is injected intravenously. Although it does not produce anaesthesia or analgesia, it relaxes the patient sufficiently to accept LA. Midazolam is the generally preferred drug as it is more potent than diazepam and gives a quicker recovery. Intravenous (IV) sedation also produces **amnesia** (loss of memory of the procedure). A light meal is allowed, not less than two hours beforehand.

The injection is usually given into an arm or hand vein and the needle remains in the vein throughout the procedure (indwelling needle). To give the injection, the arm is immobilized by strapping it to an arm board attached to the dental chair. A special needle called a butterfly cannula (Figure 14.2) is used. It has flanges to facilitate insertion of the needle (**venepuncture**) and allow it to be taped to the skin; and a flexible tube into which the syringe nozzle fits. This enables additional injections to be given immediately at any time if more sedation or resuscitation drugs are required.

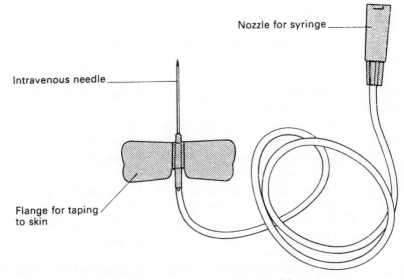

Nozzle for syringe

Intravenous needle

Flange for taping to skin

Figure 14.2   *Butterfly intravenous needle (butterfly cannula).*

The onset of sedation is recognized by slurring of the speech and difficulty in touching the end of the nose.

Monitoring the vital signs is essential throughout and appropriate equipment should be available, together with a resuscitation kit. A specific requirement in such a kit for IV sedation is the drug fluma- zenil (*Anexate*) which is an emergency antidote to an overdose of these IV sedation agents. IV sedation is not given during pregnancy or breast-feeding.

Recovery takes up to an hour and, as for GA and RA, the patient must not be left unattended in the recovery room. When the dentist has confirmed that the patient is fit to leave, verbal and written instructions are again given for the patient not to drive, operate machinery or take alcohol for 24 hours.

The nurse's duty

Dentists are only allowed to use sedation techniques and act as operator if a suitably trained and experienced nurse is present throughout. Such nurses must be able to assist the dentist in the preparation and use of sedation agents and equipment. They are required to monitor a patient's condition throughout the procedure and warn the dentist of any impending problems. They are also required to assist efficiently and speedily in any emergencies such as respiratory failure, cardiac arrest or other types of collapse. They must know the uses of all the contents of an emergency kit so that no time is lost in successfully instituting whatever resuscitation measures are needed.

These duties may be listed as follows:

1   Check that instructions given previously have been obeyed and that the patient is still fit for sedation.
2   For RA, check the machine for correct functioning and cylinder labelling; and have spare nitrous oxide and oxygen cylinders available.
3   For IV sedation, lay out an arm board, syringes, drug ampoules, venepuncture needles, wipes and dressings.
4   Have monitoring and resuscitation equipment ready and check for correct functioning.
5   Lay out props, mouthpacks, LA equipment and all the dental instruments and materials required.
6   For RA, a soothing patter reassures and calms the patient.
7   For IV agents, immobilize and prepare the patient's arm for venepuncture.
8   Throughout procedure: check the patient's pulse and observe the respiration rate, colour and eye signs.
9   Inform the dentist immediately of any changes in the patient's condition.
10   Be prepared, under the dentist's direction, to render immediate assistance in resuscitation procedures.
11   On completion of treatment, assist the patient to a couch in the recovery room, and stay there to monitor and safeguard recovery until the dentist allows the patient to return home with an escort. Before leaving, remove the indwelling needle and apply a dressing; and give written and verbal post-operative instructions: not to drive, operate machinery or take alcohol for 24 hours (remainder of the day for RA patients).

Although no special qualifications are necessary for nurses to comply with all these requirements, they can prove their competence by attending a course and passing the examination for the NEBDN conscious sedation certificate.

Excessive fear of dental treatment is the most common reason for using sedation. Nurses should be constantly aware of such patients' anxiety and do everything possible to show them that they understand how they feel. A sympathetic and soothing manner will in itself make the whole procedure less stressful for the patient. Technical expertise alone is not sufficient for treating nervous patients. They require the extra support of nurses who realize that what is a routine day's work for them, is a terrifying ordeal for a frightened patient. The nurse must be caring, compassionate, calm and approachable; and at all times regard the patient as the most important person in the practice.

Anaesthetic emergencies

If breathing stops (respiratory failure), air cannot enter the lungs and death will occur in a few minutes. The heart continues beating during these critical few minutes as there is still some residual air in the lungs. It only lasts a few minutes though; after which the heart itself stops beating (cardiac arrest) and death is imminent.

Respiratory failure can occur during GA or sedation and may be caused by blockage of the airway or an overdose of anaesthetic or sedation agent.

Blockage of the airway

Blockage of the airway is caused by obstruction of the entrance to the larynx by the tongue or foreign body. It is recognized by the patient's face becoming very blue, congested and clammy; and a rise in pulse rate and blood pressure. There may also be snoring or wheezing.

If the tongue is displaced backwards during anaesthesia or sedation it blocks the laryngeal entrance. Fortunately this can be easily remedied by pulling the jaw forward, as the base of the tongue is attached to the mandible and moves with it. However, this type of obstruction is normally prevented by the anaesthetist's finger held behind the angle of the mandible, thus making it difficult for the jaw to be accidentally pushed backwards by the operator.

Blockage by a foreign body is an extremely serious matter as it must be located and removed before respiration is possible again. Before searching for a foreign body, the patient is laid flat with the head lower than the feet; this is called the head-down position. 100% oxygen is then given.

The foreign body may be a mouth pack, mouth prop, extracted tooth, small instrument, clotted blood or vomited food. The purpose of a mouth pack is to prevent foreign bodies getting past it but these accidents do sometimes occur. Packs and props have a long piece of tape or chain attached which is left dangling out of the mouth, and allows them to be removed easily if they slip backwards and obstruct the airway. Any other foreign bodies are found by feeling behind the tongue with a finger or using the anaesthetists's laryngoscope; and removed immediately, using forceps or suction as necessary.

If these measures fail to relieve an obstruction, the last resort is to surgically open the airway below the obstruction. This is most simply and rapidly done in an emergency by performing a **cricothyrotomy**. A special instrument from the emergency kit called a **cricothyroid cannula** is used. It consists of a hollow needle which is inserted through the neck into the lower part of the larynx (Figure 14.3). An oxygen supply can then be connected to the needle.

Whatever method is used to clear the airway, the essential factor is speed. Respiration cannot occur while the airway is blocked, so delay in removing an obstruction may be fatal.

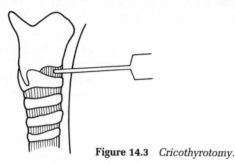

Figure 14.3   *Cricothyrotomy.*

Overdose of anaesthetic

An overdose of a powerful anaesthetic or sedation agent can cause respiratory failure by paralysing the respiratory muscles. The patient is then unable to get enough oxygen despite an adequate amount in the anaesthetic mixture. This lack of oxygen is called **anoxia** and its early stages are indicated by cyanosis. If remedial measures are not taken, breathing will continue to weaken until it stops altogether. The face becomes ashen-grey and the pupils dilate. This will be followed by cardiac arrest unless oxygen can be introduced into the blood.

Resuscitation

If collapse occurs, the dental chair is tilted fully backwards into a head-down supine position; administration of the anaesthetic or sedation drug is stopped and replaced by 100% oxygen. Whether due to an overdose of anaesthetic, or failure of breathing to recommence immediately a blocked airway is cleared, the pulse must first be checked to see if the heart is still beating. The benefit of a pulse oximeter and/or ECG will be realized at this stage.

If the heart is still beating, the lungs must be filled with oxygen artificially. This takes precedence over anything else. All dental nurses must know how to perform **artificial respiration** as they may have to assist in an emergency in the dental surgery or elsewhere.

Methods used in the dental surgery are oxygen inflation and air inflation. Nurses should also know how to perform expired air (mouth to mouth) respiration.

Oxygen inflation

The airway is cleared and the anaesthetist inserts an **oro-pharyngeal (Guedel) airway**. This is a tube which curves over and behind the tongue, and prevents the tongue falling back and blocking the airway again (Figure 14.4). The advantage of inserting such an airway is that it keeps the patient's airway open in whatever position the patient is placed, and frees one pair of hands from manually supporting the mandible to maintain a clear airway.

The dental chair is adjusted so that the patient is horizontal. The nasal mask is replaced by a full face mask and the anaesthetic machine adjusted to give 100% oxygen. The anaesthetist squeezes the reservoir bag to inflate the lungs and then allows expiration to occur passively, after which the lungs are again inflated with oxygen. This process is continued until natural breathing commences.

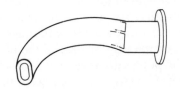

(a)

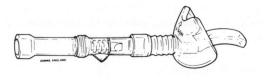

(b)

Figure 14.4 *Airway tubes.*
(a) Oro-pharyngeal (Guedel) airway;
(b) Brook airway.

Air inflation

This is used if oxygen is not immediately available from an anaesthetic machine. A special item of equipment called a **manual pulmonary resuscitator** (e.g. *Ambu Bag*) is required. It consists of a rubber air bag attached to a full face mask.

The technique is virtually the same as oxygen inflation, and a

Guedel airway is inserted if available. The mask is applied and the bag squeezed, thus inflating the lungs with air. Passive expiration then occurs and the sequence is repeated until natural breathing resumes. The resuscitator can be connected to an anaesthetic machine or oxygen cylinder but this is not essential in an emergency. Air alone can save the patient.

A manual pulmonary resuscitator and cylinder of oxygen should be present in the surgery at all times, and in the recovery room whenever GA or sedation is used.

Expired air respiration

If oxygen or air inflation equipment is not available, expired air respiration (EAR) is used. This is commonly known as mouth to mouth respiration. It can be performed anywhere, without any physical effort or special equipment.

The technique is similar to the previous methods except that air is breathed directly into the patient's mouth. The head is tilted backwards and the chin lifted to hold the mandible forward and maintain the airway; while the nostrils are pinched together to prevent the escape of air intended for the lungs (Figures 14.5, 6.4).

The first breath will inflate the lungs with air and make the chest rise. Take your mouth away and allow the chest to fall as passive expiration occurs, but maintain the sealing of the nose and the position of head and chin. The procedure is repeated for a total of ten breaths, and the pulse is checked again. This sequence of ten inflations and a pulse check is continued until natural breathing recommences.

A useful aid for any person giving EAR is a **Brook airway** (Figure 14.4). This is a tube which fits in the patient's mouth and air is blown through it. There is a valve to prevent the patient's expired air reaching the operator, which is particularly valuable when the patient's mouth is soiled with blood or vomit. Alternatively a full face mask can be placed over the patient's face and air blown through the inlet tube (Figure 14.6).

External cardiac compression

If there is no pulse, the heart has stopped beating (cardiac arrest) and death will occur within three minutes. But if *immediate* action is taken to make the heart beat artificially, by external cardiac compression (ECC), recovery is still possible. Cardiac arrest is recognized by absence of pulse, ashen-grey waxy pallor, and widely dilated pupils which do not react to light.

With the dental chair horizontal, or the patient supine (flat on the back) on the floor, pressure is exerted on the base of the breast bone by pressing down with two hands, one on top of the other (Figure 14.7).

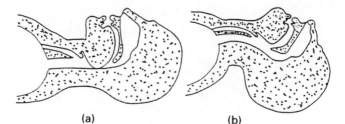

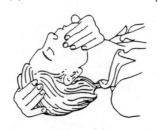

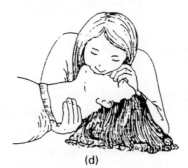

Figure 14.5 *Expired air respiration.*
(a) Airway blocked by tongue;
(b) Head tilt prevents blockage by tongue;
(c) Head positioned to keep airway open;
(d) Mouth to mouth method.
Source: *Emergency Procedures and First Aid for Nurses* (2nd edn). M. Skeet, Blackwell Science Ltd, Oxford.

This squeezes the heart and makes the blood circulate (Figure 5.6). It is done 80 times a minute and EAR is continued at the same time.

The anatomy and physiology on which these resuscitation measures are based is covered in Chapters 5 and 6. The combination of artificial respiration and ECC is called **cardiopulmonary resuscitation** (CPR).

Emergency procedure

A state of preparedness is necessary for meeting dental emergencies associated with respiratory failure and cardiac arrest. A sterile, ready-

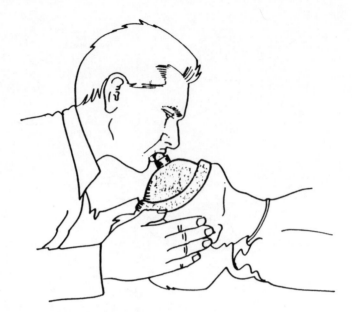

Figure 14.6 *EAR using face mask.*
Source: *Lecture Notes on Anaesthetics.* Lunn, Blackwell Science Ltd, Oxford.

for-use, emergency kit must be immediately available every time GA or sedation is undertaken. Essential items are:

1 An efficient suction apparatus for clearing a blocked airway
2 Oro-pharyngeal (Guedel) airways
3 Cricothyrotomy outfit
4 Full face mask for anaesthetic machine
5 Manual pulmonary resuscitator
6 Resuscitation drugs
7 Syringes and needles for injection of drugs
8 An extra non-electric suction apparatus, manual pulmonary resuscitator and cylinder of oxygen should also be part of the recovery room equipment.

The object of treatment is to restore the supply of oxygenated blood to the brain *without delay.* The first step is to lay the patient flat, stop the administration of anaesthetic or sedation agent, change over to 100% oxygen and clear the airway. This is done by removing all packs and props from the mouth, supporting the jaw with the neck extended, pulling the tongue forward and using suction to remove any obstruction. If natural breathing then recommences automatically, GA may be continued and the operation completed; while the patient remains unaware that anything has happened. If blockage of the airway is caused by vomiting, the above procedure is repeated but the anaesthetic is not resumed.

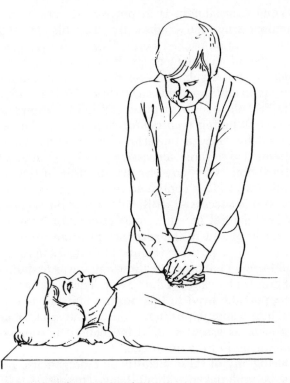

Figure 14.7 *External cardiac compression.*
Source: *Lecture Notes on Anaesthetics.* Lunn, Blackwell Science Ltd, Oxford.

Having cleared the airway, artificial respiration is begun immediately if natural breathing has not resumed. With the patient in the supine position, in the chair or on the floor, oxygen inflation is commenced. If oxygen is not immediately available, air inflation is used. Time must not be wasted fetching a new oxygen cylinder. Once artificial respiration is already under way, however, somebody else can get an oxygen cylinder and connect it to the anaesthetic machine or direct to the manual pulmonary resuscitator. Emergency medical assistance (999) is summoned at the same time.

If respiratory failure progresses to cardiac arrest, ECC is carried out together with artificial respiration. One person does ECC while another inflates the lungs with oxygen or air. Five chest compressions are followed by one inflation of the lungs, and this procedure is continued until help arrives.

If no second person is available, dial 999 and commence a CPR sequence of 15 chest compressions followed by two lung inflations. To summon assistance quickly the nurse must have the telephone numbers of the nearest ambulance, hospital casualty department and doctor, clearly printed, by the telephone.

While resuscitation is in progress it may be decided to inject a stimulant drug such as adrenaline. For this reason the emergency kit must contain prepacked sterile disposable syringes and needles, and ampoules of stimulant drugs. It must be emphasized, though, that drugs are not a substitute for manual resuscitation. They are only given as an additional measure while CPR is already being performed.

If CPR fails to restore a pulse and an ECG shows that the heart beats are just fluttering (*ventricular fibrillation*), the heart beat may be restored by using a powerful electric shock device called a **defibrillator**. Up to three successive shocks are attempted while ECC is stopped and everybody else stands clear. If this fails to restore the circulation, CPR is continued until expert medical assistance takes over. If it is successful, artificial respiration is continued.

When natural breathing and circulation return, an unconscious patient is placed in the **recovery position** until medical assistance arrives. In this position (Figure 14.8) the patient lies prone with the head turned to one side to allow any fluids to drain out of the mouth and prevent blockage of the airway. The arms and legs are positioned to support the head in this posture and prevent the patient rolling back into a supine position. Constant attendance and monitoring of vital signs is essential until the patient is removed to hospital or pronounced fit to return home.

During any of these anaesthetic emergencies, remedial measures must be undertaken without delay. The patient's life depends on it. The GDC accordingly requires all staff involved in GA and sedation to be fully trained and experienced. Dentists must be specially trained in resuscitation, venepuncture and the use of monitoring and resuscitation equipment. For GA this includes a sphygmomanometer, pulse oximeter, ECG, capnograph and defibrillator. For IV sedation a manual pulmonary resuscitator, oxygen cylinder, sphygmomanometer and a pulse oximeter are required. A manual pulmonary resuscitator, oxygen cylinder and suction apparatus are also required in the recovery room. Dentists and nurses must know how to use their monitoring equipment and understand the significance of its readings; how to use resuscitation equipment; the functions and use of all contents of the emergency kit; and how to be proficient at CPR. Special courses covering these requirements should be attended

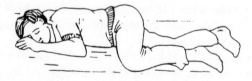

Figure 14.8 *Recovery position.*
Source: *Emergency Procedures and First Aid for Nurses* (2nd edn). M. Skeet, Blackwell Science Ltd, Oxford.

regularly, together with frequent resuscitation drill, against the clock, in the surgery.

Other causes of collapse

Apart from the anaesthetic emergencies covered in this chapter, other medical emergencies can occur in dental practice, irrespective of the type of treatment undertaken, and not necessarily related to it. However, the general principles of resuscitation apply to any cause of collapse and these are covered in Chapter 15.

Written examination

A patient has been given an appointment to have a tooth extracted under a general anaesthetic.

What instructions should be given? Explain why each is important.

Briefly describe how you would care for the patient once the tooth is extracted, until the patient is ready to go home. (May 1983)

A patient attends the surgery for intravenous sedation. What are the duties of the DSA? (May 1987)

Summary

General anaesthetic drugs

1   Nitrous oxide and oxygen
2   Halothane ← vaporized by flow of nitrous oxide
3   Enflurane ← recent use of halothane; unsuitable for epileptics
4   Isoflurane → alternative to enflurane; more rapid recovery; suitable for epileptics
5   Methohexitone ← IV injection
    (a)   Induction of resistant adults and nervous patients
    (b)   Single anaesthetic for short simple procedures
6   Propofol → alternative to methohexitone; quicker recovery

Endotracheal anaesthesia

- Prolonged procedures on difficult or handicapped patients
- Normally used in hospitals
- Anaesthetic gases delivered direct to lungs through nasotracheal tube
- Anaesthetist has complete control of airway

1 Injection of atropine → reduces saliva and mucus production → gives operator clean dry field.
2 Injection of methohexitone → immediate unconsciousness.
3 Injection of muscle relaxant → *Scoline, Tracrium*.
4 Anaesthetist inserts nasotracheal tube – using laryngoscope.
5 Artificial respiration necessary until effect of muscle relaxant wears off.
6 Oro-pharynx packed → complete protection of airway.
7 Operation begins.
8 Recovery time may be prolonged – depending on duration of anaesthetic.
9 Patient may have post-operative sore throat and muscle pains.

Stages of anaesthesia

1 Analgesia
2 Delirium
3 Surgical anaesthesia → regular nasal breathing, operation performed
4 Respiratory failure ← overdose of anaesthetic; blockage of airway

Care of patient

1 Anaesthetic history
   (a) Previous anaesthetics
   (b) General health
   (c) Pregnancy
2 Anaesthetic appointment
   (a) Patient's consent
   (b) No food or drink for at least four hours beforehand
   (c) Accompanied by adult
   (d) Forbidden to drive, operate machinery, or drink alcohol
   (e) No jewellery, nail varnish, cosmetics, wrist watch, contact lenses

3 Before anaesthetic
   (a) Check instructions obeyed; if not, inform anaesthetist
   (b) Remove excess outer clothing
   (c) Use toilet
   (d) Loosen tight clothing
   (e) Remove spectacles, dentures or orthodontic appliances
4 During anaesthesia → watch patient carefully
5 After anaesthetic
   (a) Support patient's head
   (b) Mouthwash
   (c) Clean face
   (d) Assist out to recovery room. Must not be left unattended.
   (e) Advice on after-care

Preparation and procedure

1 Sterilize, lay out and allow to cool:
   (a) Mirrors, probes, tweezers
   (b) Forceps, elevators, props and gags
   (c) Mouthpacks, swabs, kidney dishes
   (d) IV drugs and injection equipment
   (e) Emergency kit
2 Check anaesthetic machine; have labelled spare cylinders ready: nitrous oxide (light blue); oxygen (black with white top)
   • Check monitoring equipment
   • Check patient's notes and X-rays
3 Patient admitted; may be weighed (for IV drug); tight clothing loosened, spectacles and dentures removed; bib fitted
   Pulse and blood pressure recorded
4 Anaesthetic commenced
5 Prop and pack inserted; extractions performed
6 Head and jaw supported while unconscious
7 Patient assisted to recovery room; nurse in attendance; resuscitation facilities. Indwelling needle removed when patient discharged with post-operative instructions
8 Equipment and instruments made ready for next patient

Indications for local anaesthesia

- Disease of heart, blood, circulation, respiration, liver, kidney; diabetes
- Patients with sickle cell disease
- Drug therapy: corticosteroids, mental depression, high blood pressure

- Pregnancy
- Nasal blockage (common cold)
- Difficult extractions
- Emergency extractions
- Patient's preference
- No anaesthetist available

Indications for general anaesthesia

- Acute infection
- Multiple extractions
- Young children
- Nervous patients
- Patient's preference

Sedation

- Oral: diazepam (*Valium*); temazepam ← pre-operative anxiety
- RA: nitrous oxide and oxygen (at least 30%)
- IV: diazepam (*Diazemuls*); midazolam *Hypnovel*)

Advantages

- Prolonged operating time under LA on relaxed patient
- Patient conscious and co-operative
- Protective reflexes retained → fasting unnecessary
- Amnesia

Preparation and procedure

1 Lay out LA equipment; aspirator tubes; materials and instruments for the dental procedure
2 RA: check machine; spare labelled cylinders
3 IV: lay out arm board, venepuncture wipes, syringes and drug ampoules
4 Have monitoring equipment and emergency kit ready
5 Throughout procedure, check vital signs: colour, breathing, pulse
6 Inform dentist immediately of changes in patient's condition
7 Be prepared, under dentist's direction, to render immediate assistance in resuscitation procedures
8 When treatment is finished, keep patient under continuous observation in recovery room until fit to return home with escort
9 Forbid patient to drive, operate machinery or drink alcohol for next 24 hours

Monitoring

Colour: pink → normal
              blue (cyanosis) ← oxygen deficiency
              ashen-grey ← respiratory failure → cardiac arrest

- Pulse: wrist, temporal, carotid; pulse oximeter
- Breathing: chest movements, reservoir bag
- Blood pressure: sphygmomanometer and stethoscope
- Heart: ECG

Anaesthetic emergencies

Caused by:
1 Blockage of the airway.
   (a) Backward displacement of tongue → pull jaw forward.
   (b) Foreign body ← mouthpack, prop, tooth, small instrument, blood clot or vomited food. Must be located and removed before breathing can be restored. Cricothyrotomy as last resort
2 Overdose of anaesthetic or sedation agent

Resuscitation

1 Stop anaesthetic and lay patient flat. Switch to 100% oxygen.
2 Clear the airway → loosen tight clothing, suction
3 Check breathing and pulse
4 Pulse but no breathing: artificial respiration → inflate lungs with oxygen or air (manual pulmonary resuscitator), or EAR (Brook airway); summon help (999)
5 Check pulse every ten inflations
6 No pulse: 2 operators CPR → 1 inflation/5 compressions
                  1   "   "   2   "   15   "
7 Continue until medical assistance arrives
8 Recovery position when pulse and breathing restored
9 Constant nursing attendance until fully recovered
10 Regular drill, against clock, for all staff

Emergency kit

1 Suction
2 Oro-pharyngeal (Guedel) airways
3 Cricothyrotomy outfit
4 Full face mask
5 Manual pulmonary resuscitator
6 Syringes, needles, IV cannulas
7 Resuscitation drugs and oxygen

15 Collapse

Collapse is a term which covers various forms of prostration. They often involve loss of consciousness and range from a simple faint to breathing difficulties, convulsions, chest pain and other medical emergencies. Some causes of collapse in the dental surgery are:

1 Fainting
2 General anaesthesia and sedation
3 Adverse drug reactions
4 Respiratory obstruction
5 Diabetes
6 Epilepsy
7 Heart attack
8 Stroke

The first four causes on this list are directly associated with dental treatment. The remainder can happen anywhere, at any time, and their occurrence in a dental surgery is usually fortuitous. Treatment of these conditions, whatever the cause, follows the resuscitation methods described and illustrated in Chapter 14. Nurses should refer back to it for details.

Fainting

Causes

Fainting is loss of consciousness caused by a reduced blood supply to the brain. The medical term for fainting is **syncope**. It is the commonest cause of unconsciousness in dental patients and is almost invariably a psychological effect brought about by fear, and often aggravated by pain, injection of local anaesthetic, sight of blood or hunger. Fear brings about a change in the distribution of blood, resulting in a diversion of blood from the brain to the abdomen. A similar effect is produced by excessive heat or standing still for a long period; commonly shown by fainting among crowds or on parade grounds.

Symptoms and signs

Symptoms are effects noticed by the **patient**.
Signs are effects noticed by the **practitioner**.

The patient may complain of feeling faint, hot and thirsty. These are the symptoms. Simultaneously, the signs of fainting are apparent: the skin becomes very pale and clammy; pulse feeble; shivering, sighing and dilation of the pupils may occur; and unconsciousness supervenes.

Treatment

As the condition is caused by insufficient blood reaching the brain it is simply treated by lowering the patient's head below the level of the feet, thus increasing the blood supply to the brain. In the dental chair this may be achieved by tilting the chair backwards beyond the horizontal position. A patient falling to the ground is automatically treating the faint correctly by assuming a horizontal position. Should this occur, however, the patient should be lifted on to something more comfortable, such as a couch in the recovery room. Recovery always occurs within a few minutes and a glass of water is generally appreciated.

Patients who have fainted must be kept under continual observation all the time they are on the premises. This is to prevent them slipping out of the chair and injuring themselves while unconscious, or in case they faint again. Furthermore, patients must not be allowed to leave the premises until the dentist is satisfied that they are fit to do so.

Prevention

A dental nurse can do much to prevent fainting by inspiring confidence in the patient, ensuring that excessive clothing is removed, and keeping the surgery properly ventilated.

General anaesthesia and sedation

Collapse during GA or sedation is usually caused by blockage of the airway or an overdose of the drugs used; and is covered in Chapter 14. Two other causes are fainting and drug reactions.

Fainting under general anaesthesia

Patients seated upright in the dental chair during GA sometimes show signs of fainting – pallor, clammy skin and feeble pulse. There may be no apparent cause for this but it can lead to a very dangerous situation if it is not recognized at once. Unlike a simple faint, patients cannot treat this condition by falling to the ground. As long as they remain seated in an upright position the blood supply to the brain is impaired. Respiratory and cardiac arrest will then follow unless immediate action is taken.

Fortunately it can be treated quite easily. The chair is tipped backwards beyond the horizontal position, the anaesthetic is stopped and 100% oxygen administered; whereupon recovery rapidly occurs and the anaesthetic may then be resumed.

This is the reason why most anaesthetists prefer their patients to be seated in the supine position for GA in the dental chair.

Adverse drug reactions

Adverse reactions to drugs may be the result of allergy, corticosteroid therapy or drug interactions. They can produce a severe state of shock and prompt treatment is essential, starting with the *standard resuscitation procedure*, as follows.

The patient must be laid flat, with a clear airway, and oxygen given. Medical assistance is summoned and preparations made for CPR in case the patient's condition deteriorates before help arrives. None of these reactions need happen, however, if a careful medical history is taken beforehand.

Allergic reactions

Allergy and anaphylactic shock are covered in Chapter 9. A possible cause in dental practice is administration of penicillin, or one of its derivatives such as amoxycillin. It may also be caused by some constituents of anaesthetic agents, the use of latex gloves, and some dental materials. The symptoms and signs depend on the severity of the reaction but may include:

- Flushing and swelling of the face
- Generalized itching, especially hands and feet
- Difficulty in breathing
- Pallor
- Rapid feeble pulse
- Low blood pressure
- Loss of consciousness (*anaphylactic shock*)

Respiratory failure and cardiac arrest can occur within minutes of the onset of anaphylactic shock. Emergency treatment is an injection of adrenaline and the standard resuscitation procedure just described. Less severe allergic reactions may be treated by injection of hydrocortisone. These drugs are standard components of an emergency kit.

Corticosteroid therapy

Past or present medical treatment with corticosteroid drugs reduces the ability to react to stress and may result in collapse under GA or during prolonged minor oral surgery under LA. Such patients should carry a steroid therapy card provided by their doctor and show it to the dentist before any treatment is given.

The signs and symptoms are similar to those of fainting. Treatment is standard resuscitation procedure and IV injection of hydrocortisone. This cause of collapse can be prevented by an injection of hydrocortisone half-an-hour before treatment.

Drug interactions

Some of the drugs used for treatment of mental depression or high blood pressure can react with drugs used for GA and cause the patient to collapse. Although there is little risk under LA, a preparation which does not contain adrenaline (such as prilocaine with felypressin) is sometimes preferred.

Respiratory obstruction

Respiratory obstruction is caused by blockage of the airway and was covered in Chapter 14 for such occurrences during GA and sedation. However, it may occur as a result of any form of dental treatment, or be unrelated to it. The obstruction may be total or partial, involving the upper or lower airway. The dividing line between the upper and lower airway may be regarded as the bottom of the trachea.

The most common form of respiratory obstruction is *asthma* which causes partial obstruction of the lower airway. Partial obstruction of both the upper and lower airway may occur in anaphylactic shock, which is described under allergic reactions. The administration of oxygen and appropriate drug treatment leads to recovery in these conditions.

Total obstruction of the upper airway is a life-threatening emergency, giving only a few minutes to restore oxygenation of the blood before cardiac arrest, brain damage and death ensue. The most common example is inhalation of a foreign body.

Asthma

This is a very common condition, often of allergic origin, in which recurrent spasm of the bronchi results in an inability to breathe properly. Attacks cause wheezing as the sufferer gasps for air. Asthmatic patients normally carry an inhaler containing a drug called salbutamol (*Ventolin*) which relaxes bronchial spasm and aborts the attack. The stress of dental treatment can precipitate an attack and is overcome, in most cases, by the patient's inhaler.

Sometimes a more severe attack occurs and the patient becomes very distressed. Normal resuscitation procedure involves laying patients flat, but in cases of breathing difficulty they are more comfortable if kept upright in the dental chair. Oxygen is given and the patient's inhaler used. If there is no improvement, medical assistance is summoned. If unconsciousness supervenes, the dental chair is tilted backwards but the backrest is kept upright and the leg and foot rest kept straight. This helps respiration and circulation. An injection of salbutamol, adrenaline or hydrocortisone may also be given.

Inhaled foreign bodies

Blockage of the airway by a foreign body was described under anaesthetic emergencies in Chapter 14. However, it can occur in a conscious unsedated patient during any dental procedure, and is nonetheless dangerous. If the airway of a conscious patient cannot be cleared as described in Chapter 14, the dental chair is moved to an upright position. This allows the patient to bend forward and cough it clear.

If this is unsuccessful, the **Heimlich manoeuvre** (Figure 15.1) is tried. With the patient standing, grasp the patient's abdomen from behind with both your arms. Clench the fist of the innermost hand and, with the other on top, apply a sudden forcible squeeze to the upper abdomen in an upward and backward direction. This forces the diaphragm upwards and may blast the obstruction clear. This man-

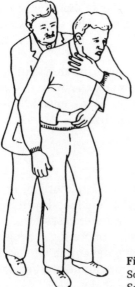

Figure 15.1 *Heimlich manoeuvre.*
Source: *Lecture Notes on Anaesthetics*. Lunn, Blackwell Science Ltd, Oxford.

oeuvre should not be used on small children, pregnant or very obese patients. Small children may be supported head down and slapped on the back to free an obstruction.

If after a few attempts the upper airway remains blocked, and the assistance of an anaesthetist is not immediately available, the last resort is to perform a cricothyrotomy (Figure 14.3).

Sometimes a foreign body does not obstruct the upper airway but, as mentioned in Chapter 6, it may get through the larynx into the lower airway without causing any immediate alarming symptoms. If a small object such as a crown, root reamer, or extracted tooth is missing and cannot be found after searching inside and outside the mouth, it must be assumed that it may have been inhaled or swallowed. Coughing suggests that the body was inhaled rather than swallowed.

The latter possibility is usually harmless as the foreign body should pass through the entire alimentary canal and out through the anus. Inhalation is an extremely serious event which can cause inflammation of the lung (pneumonia) or a lung abscess. Patients are accordingly referred to hospital for X-rays of the chest to check the presence and location of any such foreign body.

Diabetes

Diabetic patients collapse if the amount of sugar in their blood falls below normal. This condition is called **hypoglycaemia** and is caused by inadequate food intake. It is the commonest cause of collapse in diabetics and can happen if food is not taken because GA is necessary; the patient is kept too long at the surgery, beyond the next mealtime; or the patient is unable to eat following dental treatment.

Hypoglycaemia is characterized by:

- Sudden onset
- Profuse sweating
- Disorientation
- Drowsiness or restlessness
- Slurred speech and drunken attitude
- Palpitations with a rapid feeble pulse
- Unconsciousness

If the condition is recognized before unconsciousness occurs, it can be treated quite easily by giving the patient some sugar. Four lumps of sugar, or some chocolate, biscuits or jam will suffice. If unconscious, standard resuscitation procedure is followed, together with the injection of a glucose preparation. This is a normal constituent of the emergency drugs kit.

This form of collapse can be prevented by taking a careful medical history. It would then be known beforehand that the patient was a diabetic; and the patient's doctor would be consulted before undertaking dental treatment. Appropriate dietary arrangements and appointment times could then be made to prevent hypoglycaemia.

Epilepsy

Patients can often tell when an epileptic fit (*grand mal*) is imminent. It is characterized by sudden loss of consciousness and convulsions. The patient may froth at the mouth, bite the tongue and go blue in the face. There may also be urinary incontinence.

Recovery occurs spontaneously and no treatment is required, unless the airway is blocked by a denture or vomit. Mobile equipment should be moved out of range to avoid further injury to the patient during convulsions.

When the fit is over, the patient is placed in the recovery position until conscious, kept under observation and not allowed home until fully recovered.

Rarely, a very serious bout of continuous convulsions occurs (*status epilepticus*), requiring medical assistance and the injection of diazepam or midazolam to bring the patient under control.

Heart attack

This is recognized by the sudden onset of a severe crushing pain across the chest, perhaps radiating to the shoulder and left arm, or into the neck and jaw. It is caused by coronary artery disease and, as explained in Chapter 5, it may be an attack of angina pectoris; or the far more serious condition of coronary thrombosis which causes a sudden complete blockage of a coronary artery. Complete blockage means that the portion of heart muscle supplied by the blocked artery cannot survive or function any longer – a condition called myocardial infarction (Chapter 9). Whatever the cause, the heart may stop beating altogether.

Angina pectoris

Chest pain is usually brought on by physical exertion or emotional stress. In most cases it only lasts for a few minutes. Patients with a history of angina usually carry tablets of glyceryl trinitrate for their condition; but they should also be available in the emergency drug kit. If rest and the placement of a glyceryl trinitrate tablet under the tongue do not provide rapid relief of pain, the patient should be treated as for myocardial infarction.

Myocardial infarction

The pain of myocardial infarction is far more severe and prolonged than angina pectoris. The patient may collapse and cardiac arrest can occur. Nausea and vomiting are common and there is a consequential risk of blockage of the airway. The skin is pale and clammy, pulse weak, blood pressure low and breathing shallow. The following treatment is applied:

1 Summon medical assistance (999) immediately.
2 Allow the patient to rest comfortably with the dental chair upright and legs horizontal. This facilitates breathing.
3 Ensure a clear airway.
4 Keep patient still and warm.
5 Have suction ready in case of vomiting.
6 Be prepared to undertake CPR.
7 If a relative analgesia machine is available, this can be of great benefit while awaiting the arrival of medical assistance. It provides the patient with plenty of oxygen and the nitrous oxide relieves the pain. Aspirin may also be given.

Cardiac arrest

This is the most serious complication of collapse. It may follow angina pectoris, myocardial infarction, or any of the other types of collapse covered in this chapter and in Chapter 14.

The signs of cardiac arrest are:

1 Sudden unconsciousness
2 Absence of breathing and pulse
3 Dilated pupils
4 Deathly appearance; depending on the cause, it may be:
    (a) very blue
    (b) very grey
    (c) very pale

Treatment is by *immediate* institution of CPR and the summoning of emergency medical services.

Stroke

A stroke is a very serious form of collapse which may be fatal. It is caused by a sudden interruption of blood supply to the brain, caused by the rupture of a blood vessel, or thrombosis. The patient loses consciousness and is partially paralysed.

If it occurs in the dental surgery the patient is kept in a horizontal position with a clear airway. Oxygen is given and medical assistance obtained.

Management of collapse

Treatment of fainting has already been described and recovery occurs rapidly. Many other types of collapse simulate fainting but do not respond to simple treatment. In such cases, even though the cause of collapse may be unknown, immediate action is necessary to maintain a clear airway and treat any subsequent respiratory or cardiac arrest. Practical details of these resuscitation methods are described and illustrated in Chapter 14 on GA and sedation.

The fundamental principles of resuscitation are to summon medical assistance and maintain the oxygenation and circulation of the blood. This has priority over anything else and may be memorized as **ABC**:

A for airway, **B** for breathing, **C** for circulation

A   First check for, and maintain, a clear **A**irway
B   Second monitor **B**reathing and give artificial respiration if required
C   Third check the **C**irculation by feeling the pulse and give CPR if absent

This procedure is called **basic life support** and can keep a patient alive, in the absence of an anaesthetist or other medical assistance, by oxygenating and circulating the blood. However, it is unlikely to restore spontaneous heart function. It must accordingly be continued without interruption until help does arrive. Meanwhile, it will help if an IV cannula is inserted and kept in place, ready for the subsequent injection of drugs required.

Once medical help is available, *advanced life support* is initiated. This may involve the administration of stimulant drugs and use of a defibrillator, followed by transfer to hospital.

Treatment

The patient is placed in a supine position with feet raised above the level of the head. The mandible is supported to keep the airway clear and loose dentures are removed. Exceptions to use of the supine position are advanced pregnancy and patients with breathing difficulties. They should be treated with the chair in a semi-upright position.

Oxygen or air-inflation equipment must be at hand in case CPR is needed; and timed records are kept of pulse, respiration and any drugs given. If monitoring equipment for blood pressure, pulse and heart conditions are available, they should be used.

If breathing stops, insert a Guedel airway (Figure 14.4); give artificial respiration with a manual pulmonary resuscitator and oxygen, and check the pulse after every ten inflations. If there is no pulse, CPR is started and continued until expert medical assistance takes over.

In situations where a patient regains unassisted normal respiration and circulation, but remains unconscious, the patient is placed in the recovery position (Figure 14.8) and kept under continuous observation and monitoring to give immediate indication of any relapse.

Patients regaining consciousness after collapse are often anxious, confused and disorientated. It is particularly important to give immediate reassurance by telling them where they are and what has happened, and that they will be cared for until further help arrives or arrangements are made for them to return home.

A conscious patient who is breathless and distressed is sat upright in the dental chair and given oxygen.

If a patient is conscious, breathing normally and responds to questions, observation is maintained until medical assistance arrives or the patient has recovered sufficiently to return home.

The nurse's duty

Prompt treatment of collapse is essential for survival. Nurses play an important part in this by watching the patient closely for signs of impending collapse. The dentist can then be informed at once and valuable time gained. The dentist, or anaesthetist, decides the treatment and the nurse must assist efficiently. To do this the nurse must know how to clear an airway and perform CPR.

The emergency kit and any monitoring equipment must always be ready for instant use and the nurse must know what every item is for and how it is used. Nurses must also know how to obtain medical aid without delay. Telephone numbers of emergency services and the nearest doctor should be clearly listed by the telephone.

Whatever type of work is undertaken in a dental practice, the GDC requires all dentists and surgery staff to be adequately trained and equipped for basic life support and to practise it regularly, against the clock, so that everybody knows exactly what to do and no time is wasted. In addition to these requirements, practices administering GA or IV sedation must have the facilities for advanced life support.

Emergency kit

Practices using GA or IV sedation should have a sphygmomanometer, stethoscope and pulse oximeter; plus an ECG, capnograph and defibrillator for GA.

All practices should have:

1 Portable suction apparatus for clearing a blocked airway
2 Guedel airways to maintain a clear airway
3 A cricothyrotomy kit for opening a blocked airway
4 Manual pulmonary resuscitator and portable emergency oxygen supply
5 Syringes, needles and IV cannulas for injection of drugs
6 Some recommended drugs are:

- adrenaline: cardiac arrest; anaphylactic shock; asthma
- aspirin: heart attack
- aminophylline: asthma
- chlorpheniramine (*Piriton*): anaphylactic shock
- flumazenil (*Anexate*): overdose of IV sedation agent
- glucagon; glucose: hypoglycaemia
- glyceryl trinitrate: angina pectoris
- hydrocortisone: corticosteroid and anaphylactic shock; asthma
- midazolam: epileptic fits
- salbutamol (*Ventolin*): asthma; anaphylactic shock

Prevention

Collapse during dental treatment may be the result of existing illness, allergy or an adverse drug reaction. Such instances can often be prevented if adequate medical and dental records are taken. These must include details of past and present illness, allergies, drugs prescribed and the effects of previous dental treatment. Possible complications may then be foreseen and treatment modified accordingly. Chapter 30 gives more details on history-taking.

Written examination

Describe in detail the basic life support procedures to be carried out on a patient who has a suspected cardiac arrest in the dental surgery. (May 1995)

Write short notes on:
(a) fainting
(b) an epileptic fit (*grand mal*)
(c) cardiac arrest. (November 1990)

Summary

Fainting

Causes

- Fear
- Pain
- Injection of local anaesthetic
- Sight of blood
- Excessive heat

Effect

- Reduces blood supply to brain → Unconsciousness

Symptoms

- Feeling of faintness
- Thirst – dry mouth
- Hot

Signs

- Pallor
- Clammy skin
- Feeble pulse
- Shivering
- Sighing
- Unconsciousness

Treatment

- Lower head
- Keep under continuous observation

Prevention

- Reassure patient
- Remove excessive clothing
- Adequate ventilation
- Reasonable surgery temperature

Other causes of collapse

GA and sedation $\left\{\begin{array}{l}\text{Blockage of airway}\\ \text{Overdose of drug used}\\ \text{Fainting}\\ \text{Adverse drug reaction}\end{array}\right.$

Adverse drug reaction $\left\{\begin{array}{l}\text{Allergy – penicillin, amoxycillin}\\ \text{Corticosteroids}\\ \text{Depression; high blood pressure}\end{array}\right.$

Diabetes → hypoglycaemia → give sugar or glucose
Epileptic fit → prevent further injury

angina pectoris ← glyceryl trinitrate

Heart attack → chest pain

myocardial infarction → cardiac arrest ← CPR
Stroke

Treatment

ABC

AIRWAY   BREATHING   CIRCULATION

1 Summon medical assistance → 999
2 Clear airway
3 Check breathing and pulse
4 Pulse but no breathing → artificial respiration

2 operators → 1:5

5 No pulse → CPR → inflations:compressions

1 operator → 2:15

6 Monitor, time and record vital signs
7 Stimulant drug
8 Breathing and pulse restored → recovery position
9 Keep under continuous observation

Nurses's duty

- Observe patient.
- Monitor vital signs.
- Emergency kit ready.

- Summon medical assistance.
- Assist during resuscitation.

Prevention

Medical history $\left\{\begin{array}{l}\text{Illness}\\ \text{Allergy}\\ \text{Drugs}\end{array}\right.$

Dental history → Effects of past treatment

Emergency kit

- Portable suction
- Oro-pharyngeal (Guedel) airways
- Cricothyrotomy outfit
- Manual pulmonary resuscitator
- Portable emergency oxygen supply
- Syringes, needles, IV cannulas
  - Adrenaline
  - Aspirin
  - Chlorpheniramine (*Piriton*)
  - Flumazenil (*Anexate*)
  - Glucagon, glucose
  - Hydrocortisone
  - Midazolam
  - Salbutamol (*Ventolin*)

16 Extractions and Minor Oral Surgery

The removal or extraction of teeth is carried out under local or general anaesthesia. The decision on whether to extract or conserve teeth, and the choice of anaesthesia may depend on the patient's medical and dental history. These factors are discussed in Chapters 9, 14, 15 and 30. Teeth are extracted for various reasons but the commonest are as follows:

1 Pain which cannot be relieved by conservative measures
2 Alveolar abscess – acute or chronic
3 Caries – cases unsuitable for conservation
4 Periodontal disease – cases unsuitable for gum treatment
5 Prosthetics – teeth detrimental to the fit or appearance of dentures
6 Impaction
7 Orthodontics – misplaced teeth, or to create more space
8 Cosmetic – teeth of poor appearance, unsuitable for restoration

Extraction instruments

Instruments used for extractions are forceps and elevators.

Forceps

There are two basic types of forceps – roots and molars (Figure 16.1).
Root forceps have blades with rounded ends. There are many different patterns and they are named according to the angle which the blade makes with the handle, or the teeth for which they are designed; for example, lowers, straights, Read and bayonets. Every practitioner has particular forceps of choice for individual teeth but, generally speaking, they are used as follows:

- Lower roots – all lower teeth
- Straights – upper incisors and canine
- Read – upper premolars and molars
- Bayonets – upper premolars and molars

Some root forceps have narrow blades. These are used for small teeth such as lower incisors, and retained roots.
Molar forceps have pointed blades designed to fit the bifurcation (branching) of molar roots. There are three different patterns:

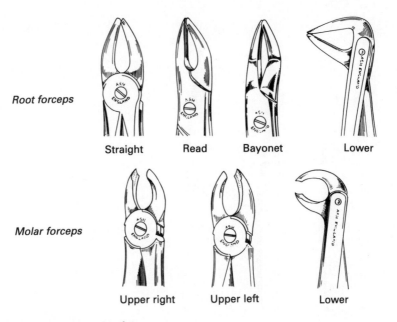

Figurer 16.1 *Extraction forceps.*

- Lower molars
- Upper right molars
- Upper left molars

Lower molar forceps have two identical blades which fit the buccal and lingual sides of the bifurcation. Left and right lower molars are extracted with the same pair of forceps.

Upper molar forceps have one pointed blade to fit the bifurcation of the buccal roots and a rounded blade which fits the single palatal root. Different forceps are needed for each side but nurses should have no difficulty identifying them correctly if they understand why the blades are different.

Elevators

These instruments are designed to elevate a retained root or impacted tooth out of its socket whence it can be easily removed. Many types of elevator are available but perhaps the most well known are Warwick James, Cryer and Coupland patterns (Figure 16.2).

Warwick James elevators are made in a set of three: straight, left and right curved. They are used for retained roots and impacted teeth.

Cryer elevators are for retained roots and impacted teeth. They have a triangular sharp end and are made in a set of two: left and right.

A **Coupland chisel** may be used as an elevator or for prising between the root and alveolar bone to dilate the socket and facilitate extraction.

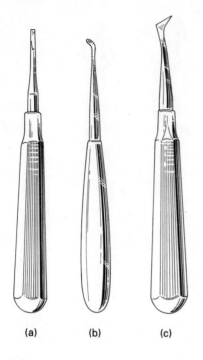

(a)   (b)   (c)

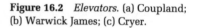

Figure 16.2   *Elevators.* (a) Coupland;
(b) Warwick James; (c) Cryer.

Preparation for extraction – the nurse's duty

The required instruments are sterilized and placed in a sterile dish ready for use. The patient is provided with a suitable bib, to prevent clothing being soiled; a disposable beaker of mouthwash; and a napkin for wiping the mouth after the extraction.

During an extraction the nurse may be required to hold the patient's head steady.

After extraction the forceps are carefully cleaned to remove all traces of blood, oiled if necessary, and then sterilized.

Care of the patient

Some patients require antibiotic cover to prevent infective endocarditis. This is described in Chapters 9 and 11. If any form of premedication is given to relieve nervousness, it is liable to make the patient quite drowsy. Such patients must be accompanied to the surgery by a responsible adult who stays in the waiting room and returns home with the patient afterwards. Patients are forbidden to drive a vehicle, operate machinery or take alcohol when premedicated.

Upon removal of the tooth, the dentist squeezes the socket walls together, places a gauze pad over the socket, and instructs the patient to bite on it for ten minutes. This helps to stop the bleeding. After treatment the patient is not dismissed until the bleeding has ceased. Advice is given, as follows, on the steps necessary to prevent bleeding and relieve soreness:

1 For the next 24 hours, *avoid*:

- Mouthwashing
- Very hot fluids
- Alcohol
- Strenuous exercise

2 Soreness can be relieved by taking some analgesic tablets such as aspirin or paracetamol.
3 After 24 hours, any further soreness may be relieved by taking hot saline mouthwashes – a teaspoon of salt in a glass of hot water.
4 If prolonged bleeding or severe pain occurs, return to the surgery.

Complications of extractions

Complications during extraction are fracture of the tooth; perforation of the maxillary sinus; loss of a tooth. Complications occurring after extraction are bleeding and dry socket.

Fracture

The crown of a tooth may fracture and come away with the forceps, leaving the root behind in its socket. This is most likely to occur when the crown is extensively decayed or heavily filled. Alternatively a root fracture may occur during extraction, leaving the apex behind. This is most likely to occur in teeth with curved or fine roots.

If a crown or root fracture occurs, the dentist may remove the retained part while the anaesthetic is still effective, or defer removal until the extraction wound has healed. If a retained root fragment is small and uninfected it may be decided to leave it alone, in which case the patient is informed and reassured.

The removal of retained roots is minor oral surgery and the technique is described later in this chapter. An X-ray film is necessary before removal is attempted.

Maxillary sinus

The roots of upper premolars and molars are very close to the floor of the maxillary sinus. Just how close this relationship can be is best seen by looking at X-ray films of upper teeth, where their roots may be seen forming bulges in the floor of the sinus; or the floor may dip down into the trifurcation of molar roots. In such cases there may only be a thin layer of compact bone separating a root from the sinus (Figure 29.1).

It is not surprising, therefore, that the floor of the sinus may be perforated during an extraction. In the majority of cases the perforation is small and no harm results as the perforation is protected by the blood clot which fills the socket. Usually, neither the dentist nor the patient is aware of what has happened. However, if the perforation is larger, it may be detected by the presence of air bubbles in the socket; or the patient may notice fluid entering the nose after drinking or rinsing the mouth. A perforation of this kind is called an **oro-antral fistula**, which means an unnatural communication between the oral cavity and the maxillary sinus (antrum). Closure of these perforations is necessary to prevent infection of the sinus and inconvenience to the patient. Small perforations are closed by stitching the socket, but larger ones require coverage by a flap of gum stitched across the perforation.

Attempted removal of a retained root sometimes results in the root being pushed into the sinus, and this again may cause infection of the sinus. X-ray films are necessary to locate a root which has disappeared upwards, as it may be loose inside the sinus or just trapped beneath the mucous membrane lining the floor of the sinus. Appropriate minor oral surgery can then be undertaken to remove the root.

Loss of a tooth

If an extracted tooth slips out of the forceps it may be swallowed or inhaled. The patient may be aware of swallowing it; or may cough, which suggests inhalation of the tooth. On the other hand, the patient may not be aware that anything untoward has happened.

When a tooth disappears it must be looked for inside and outside the mouth. If it cannot be found in the mouth, aspirator or vicinity of the dental chair, the patient must be referred to hospital for a chest X-ray. If it has been swallowed, no action is necessary as it normally passes through the alimentary canal without doing any harm. But if it has been inhaled an urgent operation is necessary to recover it from the airway or lung, before it causes serious complications such as pneumonia or a lung abscess.

Loss of a tooth is more likely to happen under GA as the patient's protective reflexes are ineffective and the operative field is obscured by a copious flow of blood. To help prevent such accidents it is the nurse's duty to account for every tooth as it is extracted, and place it in a kidney dish so that another check can be made afterwards.

Bleeding

This is covered later in the chapter.

Dry socket

Dry socket (also called septic socket) is a very painful condition which develops a few days after extraction. It is an acute inflammation of the bone lining the socket and is caused by bacterial invasion of a socket. The natural protective barrier against such invasion is the blood clot which fills the socket immediately after an extraction. Thus anything which prevents formation of an adequate blood clot can give rise to a dry socket. Such factors are infection of the blood clot, failure of formation of a blood clot and disturbance of the blood clot.

Infection of the blood clot may occur in neglected mouths where gingival (gum) infection is already present. Hordes of bacteria invade the socket, overwhelm the defending white cells, disintegrate the blood clot and set up an acute inflammation of the unprotected bare bone of the socket. Pre-extraction scaling of the teeth reduces gingival infection and may prevent a dry socket. Alternatively, or additionally, the application of iodine or chlorhexidine to the gingival crevice (Chapter 12) just before extraction helps to reduce infection.

Failure of formation of a blood clot may occur in difficult extractions. Pressure on the bone during such an extraction crushes the blood vessels and results in insufficient bleeding to produce a protective blood clot. It is more common in the mandible than maxilla as the former has a thicker layer of compact bone.

Disturbance of the blood clot is caused by too much mouthwashing soon after extraction. This breaks away the blood clot and leaves the socket bare.

Treatment of dry socket

Treatment is aimed at the relief of pain and protection of the socket during healing. It is achieved by syringing the socket to remove debris; inserting a sedative dressing to relieve pain and prevent ingress of food; and by taking an analgesic drug.

The socket may be syringed with hot saline or any other preferred antiseptic. A commonly used sedative dressing is gauze incorporated with a soft paste of zinc oxide and eugenol. However, there are many different dressings for treating dry socket and practitioners vary in their method of choice.

Patients are advised that relief of pain and quicker healing can be helped by frequent mouthwashing with hot saline. The blood clot has already been lost so no further harm can be done by mouthwashing. At this stage it is very helpful, as hot saline keeps the mouth clean and increases the blood flow to the area, thus aiding healing.

Accidental extraction

Accidental extraction can happen for a variety of reasons. One example is the removal of an unerupted premolar while extracting its deciduous predecessor. As a premolar crown is surrounded by the deciduous molar roots (Figure 12.12) it can be dislodged or completely extracted together with the deciduous tooth.

Fortunately the accidentally extracted premolar can be saved by immediately replanting it in its socket. The periodontal membrane and pulp retain their vitality and the tooth subsequently erupts normally. Success is accomplished by immediate replacement, which gives no time for the periodontal membrane to become infected or dried out.

The same procedure can be adopted if a child's tooth – usually an incisor – is knocked out by a fall or a blow. Such a tooth is said to be **avulsed**. As long as the periodontal membrane remains vital the tooth can be pushed back into its socket, with complete success in many cases. This type of accident constitutes a dental emergency and it is essential that correct first-aid treatment is applied before the child reaches a dental surgery. The following advice should be given to the person reporting the accident:

1 Reassure the child that successful treatment is possible.
2 Retrieve the tooth and, holding it by its crown, rinse it gently in warm water. Do not use a disinfectant.
3 Put the tooth back into its socket.
4 If that is not possible, let the tooth lie loose in the child's own mouth. This will keep it moist in saliva.
5 If that is impracticable, immerse the tooth in a container of milk. Do not wrap it in anything.
6 Come to the surgery immediately.

Once the tooth has been replanted in its socket and an X-ray taken, no further treatment may be necessary, but a splint (Chapter 21) is sometimes required to immobilize it for a week or so, followed by root filling. Other injuries to children's teeth are covered in Chapters 21 and 24.

Minor oral surgery

Minor oral surgery embraces such procedures as the removal of impacted lower wisdom teeth, unerupted teeth, retained roots, cysts, alveolectomy, frenectomy, apicectomy (Chapter 24), gingivectomy (Chapter 25) and biopsy (Chapter 9). All take longer than an ordinary extraction and require special instruments (Figures 16.4, 16.5 and

16.6) and preparation. Because of the time involved, these operations are not often done under GA in the dental chair. They are usually performed in the dental chair under LA or in a hospital operating theatre under GA.

Impacted teeth

An impacted tooth is prevented from erupting fully by being jammed beneath another tooth. It usually occurs in jaws which are too small to accommodate all the teeth in their normal position. The commonest example is an impacted lower third molar (Figure 16.3).

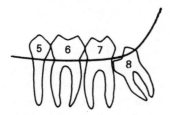

Figure 16.3 *Impacted lower third molar.*

Retained roots

A retained root is one which is left in the jaw following an incomplete extraction or total loss of the crown from caries.

Cysts

A cyst is a sac of fluid confined within a soft tissue lining. There are many different types found in various parts of the body. In dental practice they are most commonly seen as an abnormal cavity in the bone, at the apex of a dead tooth (**dental** or **apical cyst**); or surrounding and preventing eruption of an unerupted tooth (**dentigerous** or **follicular cyst**). If left untreated a cyst gradually enlarges, causing swelling of the jaw and displacement of other teeth. Whenever possible they are removed, complete with their lining.

Alveolectomy

Alveolectomy is just one of a variety of alveolar surgical procedures undertaken prior to making dentures. The bone surface is trimmed to make it smooth and even, so that dentures will fit better and feel more comfortable.

Frenectomy

This means the removal of a frenum. As mentioned in Chapter 12, a frenum is a band of fibrous tissue, covered with mucous membrane, which attaches the tongue and lips to the underlying bone. If the lingual frenum restricts the movement of the tongue, a lingual frenectomy is performed. If the upper labial frenum is too large it may allow a large gap to persist between the upper central incisors. It can also affect the fit of an upper denture. In such cases an upper labial frenectomy is often undertaken.

Apicectomy and gingivectomy are described in later chapters.

Technique

Although minor oral surgery covers many different procedures, the technique is virtually the same for all of them; and so is the order in which each stage of the operation is performed. The following description of the removal of a completely unerupted tooth may be used as a general example of minor oral surgery technique.

1   An incision is made in the gum overlying the unerupted tooth. This is done with a small razor-sharp knife called a **scalpel** (Figure 16.4). The area of gum outlined by this incision is called the *gum flap*.
2   The gum flap is prised away from the surface of the bone with a **periosteal elevator**, which resembles a cement spatula. The flap is then held aside with a **tissue retractor** or the periosteal elevator itself.
3   This exposes the bare bone covering the unerupted tooth. Some of this bone must now be removed to reveal the underlying tooth. A straight handpiece and surgical bur or a **mallet** and **chisel** (Figure 16.5) are used for bone removal.
4   Having removed sufficient bone in this way, the tooth can be loosened and eased out of its socket by gentle leverage with an elevator. It may then be grasped with forceps and removed.
5   Any sharp edges of bone on the socket are removed with **bone forceps** (*rongeurs*) and their margins smoothed with a **bone file** or bur. The socket is then cleared of all debris with a **curette** (Figures 24.2 and 28.6d), followed by irrigation with warm sterile saline in a **Hunt syringe** or a large disposable syringe.
6   Finally, the gum flap is **sutured** (stitched) back into place. The flap is held in position with toothed **dissecting forceps** (Figure 16.6) and the small curved needle (half circle) is held with special needle holders or **Spencer Wells forceps**. The loose ends of black silk thread are then cut off with fine scissors.

Instruments

- Aspirator tubes; saliva ejector
- Sterile towel and towel clip
- Mirror, probe and tweezers

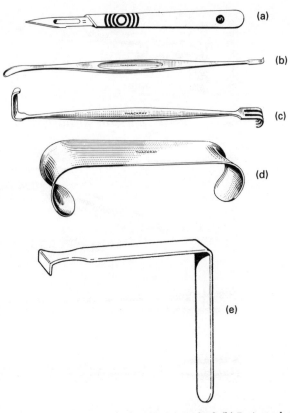

Figure 16.4 *Minor oral surgery instruments. (a) Scalpel; (b) Periosteal elevator; (c) Tissue retractor; (d) Kilner cheek retractor; (e) Austin retractor.*

- LA equipment
- Scalpel, periosteal elevator and swabs
- Retractors
- Straight handpiece and surgical burs; mallet and chisels
- Forceps and elevators
- Bone forceps (*rongeurs*); bone files
- Curettes
- Hunt syringe or disposable syringe and sterile saline
- Dissecting forceps, needle holder, needles and thread, scissors

Preparation and procedure

A sterile operative field is required. The necessary instruments are autoclaved and transferred, with sterile Cheatle's forceps, on to a sterile towel laid on a trolley or other convenient place. Also placed on the sterile towel are sterile swabs and a dish containing sterile hot saline, together with another sterile towel and towel clip. The

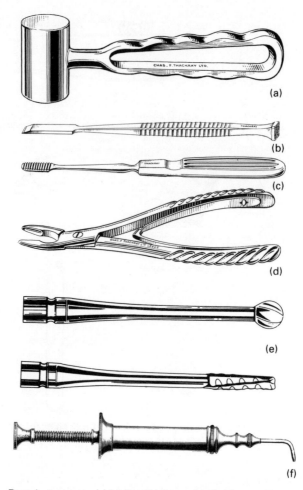

Figure 16.5   *Bone instruments.* (a) Mallet; (b) Bone chisel; (c) Bone file; (d) Bone forceps (rongeurs); (e) Surgical (bone) burs; (f) Hunt syringe.

patient's X-rays are mounted on a viewing screen and placed where the operator can see them.

A mouthwash is provided and a saliva ejector placed in the patient's mouth. A sterile towel is draped over the patient and fastened behind the neck with a towel clip. The patient is instructed not to touch the outside of the towel. LA is then given and the operation performed.

The nurse's duty during the operation is to provide the dental surgeon with a clear operative field. This is done by mopping up the blood with swabs or a sucker, and retracting the lip, cheek or tongue as required.

After the operation all instruments are scrubbed clean and

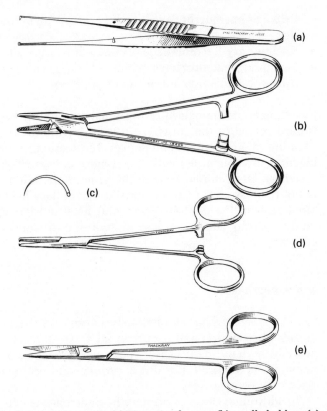

Figure 16.6 *Suture instruments.* (a) Dissecting forceps; (b) needle holders; (c) suture needle; (d) Spencer Wells forceps; (e) scissors.

sterilized; all traces of blood are removed from work surfaces; and all contaminated zones are disinfected.

Care of the patient

This is described in the previous section on extractions. Before and during the operation, the nurse applies a lubricant, such as petroleum jelly, to the patient's lips to prevent soreness caused by stretching or wide opening; and watches the patient's condition throughout. After operation the patient is given some analgesic tablets, or a prescription for them, and is instructed to return a few days later for the removal of stitches.

Haemorrhage

Haemorrhage means bleeding. It may be classified into three types: primary, reactionary and secondary.

- **Primary haemorrhage** is bleeding occurring at the time of operation.
- **Reactionary haemorrhage** occurs a few *hours* after operation.
- **Secondary haemorrhage** occurs a few *days* after operation and is caused by infection at the site of operation.

Reactionary haemorrhage is the most important. Patients suffering from it return to the surgery, up to a day after an extraction, complaining of a bleeding tooth socket. Most examination questions on bleeding are concerned with reactionary haemorrhage. Primary haemorrhage is, of course, seen at the time of operation and the patient is not dismissed until it has ceased. Secondary haemorrhage is not often seen in the dental surgery and need not be considered separately. Healthy adults can lose up to a pint of blood without any ill-effects.

Primary haemorrhage

Primary haemorrhage is obviously caused by the cutting of blood vessels at operation and occurs in all extractions and other surgical procedures. It normally ceases very quickly, as the blood clots, and no treatment is required. But if it is profuse and prolonged, other measures may be necessary.

An additional cause of primary haemorrhage is failure of the blood clotting process. This is an uncommon but very serious matter, occurring in patients taking anticoagulant drugs; in liver disease; or some rare blood diseases such as haemophilia. Patients with such conditions may carry a warning card for presentation to any practitioner they attend.

Reactionary haemorrhage

When primary haemorrhage has ceased, the patient leaves the surgery with the tooth socket completely sealed with clotted blood. If anything is done to disturb the blood clot, such as vigorous and frequent mouthwashing with hot fluids, reactionary haemorrhage may occur later. Similarly an increased blood flow to the part may put an extra strain on the clot and cause it to break away. Strenuous exercise, very hot fluids and alcohol can give rise to reactionary haemorrhage in this way.

Such bleeding is rarely serious, being just a steady ooze in most cases. However, this trivial loss of blood alarms patients because a small quantity of blood, mixed with a large pool of saliva, appears to them as a profuse and dangerous haemorrhage.

Treatment

The basic principle of treatment of haemorrhage anywhere in the body is application of pressure to the bleeding part. The various measures available for treatment of a bleeding tooth socket depend on this principle. Pressure closes cut vessels and allows blood to clot. Primary and reactionary haemorrhage are both treated in the same way, as detailed below. Each dentist has a preferential method of treatment from the following:

Pressure pad

A sterile mouthpack or pad of gauze is placed over the bleeding socket and the patient is instructed to bite on it firmly for ten minutes.

Pressure pad and haemostatic drug

As above but a haemostatic drug is also used. A haemostatic drug is one which stops bleeding; for example, adrenaline, absorbable packs.

Adrenaline is applied to the part of the pad in contact with the socket. Absorbable packs, such as oxidized cellulose (*Surgicel*), fibrin foam and gelatine sponge are inserted in the socket before placing the pressure pad.

Suture

LA is given and a suture inserted. This draws the socket edges together and compresses ruptured blood vessels. An absorbable pack is often inserted in the socket before suturing.

If these measures fail to arrest haemorrhage it may become necessary to admit the patient to hospital.

Prevention

An updated history must be available, with details of drugs taken by the patient and any previous experience of bleeding following medical or dental treatment. Information suggesting a risk of bleeding may require referral for blood tests or admission to hospital for treatment.

Primary haemorrhage

If tests show the risk to be slight and that hospital treatment is unnecessary, the precaution of suturing the socket immediately can be taken at the time of extraction. When there is no history of previous haemorrhage, liver disease or anticoagulant drugs, sutures may still be required if excessive bleeding occurs. In all cases, however, the patient must not be dismissed from the premises until bleeding has ceased.

Reactionary haemorrhage

As described earlier, reactionary haemorrhage is caused by increasing the blood flow to the part or disturbing the blood clot. Thus it can be prevented by instructing the patient to avoid mouthwashing, very hot fluids, alcohol and strenuous exercise for the next 24 hours.

The nurse's duty

Sometimes the dentist is away when a patient returns with post-extraction haemorrhage. In such a case it is the nurse's duty to reassure the patient that the condition is not serious and can be easily remedied. After obtaining full details about the patient and the extraction, the nurse must contact the dentist for instructions.

Meanwhile the patient is made more comfortable by the provision of a mouthwash to remove the unpleasant taste and clean the mouth. Then, unless instructed to the contrary, the nurse may give the patient a pressure pad to bite on until the dentist arrives.

While waiting, the nurse should switch on the sterilizer and prepare the surgery. Mouth mirror, tweezers, cotton wool, swabs, suction, haemostatic drugs, LA and suture equipment may be required. It should all be ready when the dentist returns.

If the nurse is unable to contact the dentist, and a pressure pad is ineffective, help may be sought from an emergency dental service, the patient's doctor or a local hospital.

Written examination

Describe briefly the main constituents of blood and their functions.

What is the role of the dental nurse in the treatment of post-extraction haemorrhage? (November 1995)

Why may a partially erupted wisdom tooth need extracting? How would the dental nurse assist the dentist during the surgical removal of an impacted lower wisdom tooth under local anaesthesia? (November 1995)

Summary

Reasons for extractions

- Pain
- Alveolar abscess
- Advanced caries
- Advanced periodontal disease
- Prosthetic purposes
- Impaction
- Orthodontic purposes
- Cosmetic purposes

The nurse's duty

- Sterilize instruments required and place in sterile dish
- Provide patient with bib, mouthwash and napkin
- Steady patient's head
- Account for every tooth extracted
- Clean and sterilize instruments after use
- Disinfect contaminated zones

Care of the patient

- Antibiotic cover?
- Must be accompanied by adult and forbidden to drive, operate machinery or take alcohol if premedicated
- Not dismissed until bleeding has ceased
- Advice on prevention of bleeding and relief of after-pain

Complications

1 Fracture of tooth
2 Perforation of maxillary sinus → risk of infection or oro-antral fistula. Small perforations closed naturally by blood clot. Larger ones sutured. Root displaced into sinus must be removed.
3 Loss of tooth

     swallowed → usually harmless

     inhaled → risk of serious lung infection

     X-ray chest   tooth must be retrieved
4 Bleeding
5 Dry socket
6 Accidental extraction – incisor or unerupted premolar

Dry socket

Painful inflammation of socket caused by:

- Neglected mouth → infected blood clot
- Difficult extraction → no blood clot
- Excessive mouthwashing → loss of blood clot

Treated by:

1 Syringing socket
2 Sedative dressing
3 Analgesic drug

Accidental extraction

- Removal of unerupted premolar during extraction of deciduous predecessor → replant immediately
- Child's incisor knocked out (avulsed). Give following advice:

1 Retrieve, hold by crown, rinse in warm water
2 Replant in socket
3 If replantation impossible, keep tooth in milk or patient's own mouth
4 Come to surgery immediately
5 Dentist replants tooth, takes X-ray, may fit splint. May do root filling

Minor oral surgery technique and instruments

1 Sterile towel used as bib for patient
2 Incision – scalpel
3 Raise gum flap – periosteal elevator
4 Remove overlying bone – straight handpiece and burs or mallet and chisels
5 Extraction – elevators and forceps
6 Trim bone edges – bone forceps (*rongeurs*); bone files
7 Remove debris with curette; syringe with saline – Hunt (or disposable) syringe and sterile saline
8 Suture gum flap – dissecting forceps, needle holder, curved needles, black silk thread and scissors

Preparation – the nurse's duty

- Patient's X-rays on viewing screen
- Instruments set out on sterile towel:
    - Aspirator tubes; saliva ejector
    - Sterile towel and towel clip

- Mirror, probe and tweezers
- LA equipment
- Scalpel, periosteal elevator and swabs
- Retractors
- Straight handpiece and burs or mallet and chisels
- Elevators and forceps
- Bone forceps; bone files
- Curettes
- Hunt (or disposable) syringe and sterile saline
- Dissecting forceps, needle holder, needles and thread, scissors

HAEMORRHAGE

PRIMARY

Immediate onset

1 Normal occurrence
2 Anticoagulant drugs
3 Liver disease
4 Rare blood diseases

REACTIONARY

Hours later

Mouthwashing
Strenuous exercise
Very hot fluids
Alcohol

Treatment

- Pressure pad – bite on it for ten minutes
- Pressure pad with haemostatic drug – adrenaline, absorbable pack
- Suture
- Hospital – if bleeding persists

Prevention

Patient advised to *avoid*:

- Mouthwashing
- Very hot fluids
- Alcohol
- Strenuous exercise

Nurse's duty

1 Reassure patient
2 Inform dentist
3 Give mouthwash
4 Apply pressure pad
5 Prepare surgery

17 Caries

Causes of caries

Tooth decay is called caries and is one of the commonest diseases affecting civilized communities. It is caused by acid, which forms on the tooth surface and dissolves away the enamel and dentine to produce a cavity. Acid is produced by the action of certain bacteria on sugar contained in the food we eat. These bacteria are normal residents of the mouth and are otherwise quite harmless.

Bacterial plaque

Millions of bacteria live in our mouths, flourishing on the food that we eat. Some of this food sticks to our teeth and attracts colonies of bacteria to the tooth surfaces concerned. This combination of bacteria and food debris on a tooth surface forms a thin, transparent, soft and sticky film called **plaque**. Some of the bacteria living in the plaque can turn sugar into acid, which in turn dissolves enamel to produce caries.

The micro-organism which initiates the process is **streptococcus mutans**. Large numbers of *lactobacilli* are then able to thrive in the acid environment, and this is put to practical use as a test for caries activity. By periodically counting the number of streptococci mutans or lactobacilli in a patient's saliva the level of caries activity and the effect of preventive measures can be assessed.

Sugar

As mentioned in Chapter 7 on digestion, all types of food are classi-fied into three distinct groups: protein, fat and carbohydrate. Of these, only carbohydrates can be turned into acid and thereby cause caries. The most important one of all is the refined carbohydrate called **sugar**. It can be instantaneously turned into acid by the bacteria concerned; and includes table sugar, sugar used in cooking, and sugar added to anything else taken by mouth, whether liquid or solid. Any food containing sugar can cause caries; and some obvious ones are cake, biscuits, jam, sweets, pastry, desserts, canned fruit, soft drinks, syrups and ice cream; together with hot beverages sweetened with sugar. Sugar is widely added to many savoury foods, too, in order to flavour or preserve them, but without making its taste apparent. Such foods can include soups, sauces, canned vegetables and breakfast cereals; and are accordingly sources of *hidden sugar*. Medicines may also contain hidden sugar and be a significant cause of caries in sick children (page 101).

Sugar occurring naturally in fruit, vegetables and milk does not cause caries. The prime cause is refined sugar (**sucrose**) processed from sugar beet and sugar cane, and commercial **glucose**, which together constitute such a large proportion of the manufactured and sweetened food in our diet.

Acid formation

Sugar enters the plaque as soon as it is eaten. Within a minute or two it is turned into acid by plaque bacteria and attacks the enamel surface below the plaque. Enough acid is produced to last for about 20 minutes; and in this initial acid attack a microscopic layer of enamel is dissolved away. This phase is called **demineralization**.

At the end of the meal or snack, when the intake of sugar is over, the acid persists for a period ranging from 20 minutes to two hours before it is neutralized by the buffer action (Chapter 7) of saliva. No further demineralization can then occur until such time as more sugar is consumed. In this phase where no more sugar is present in the plaque, some natural healing takes place; constituents naturally present in saliva enter demineralized enamel and restore the part lost by the initial acid attack. This healing phase is called **remineralization**.

What happens next is entirely dependent on the frequency of sugar intake. If it is confined to mealtimes only; for example, at breakfast, midday and early evening, there can only be three acid attacks a day on the teeth. The amount of time available for remineralization will greatly exceed that of demineralization and the initial phase of caries will be arrested. But if a series of snacks is eaten between meals the reverse will occur. Most snacks contain some sugar and the result is a rapid succession of acid attacks, with insufficient respite between them for saliva to neutralize the acid and allow the healing process of remineralization to become dominant. Caries can then spread rapidly through affected teeth as described in the section on the effects of caries.

The longer the sugar stays on the teeth, the longer the duration of acid production. Thus sweet fluids, such as tea or coffee with sugar, which are rapidly washed off the teeth by saliva, are not a major cause of caries; whereas the much more frequent consumption of very sweet soft drinks by children is far more serious. But, overall, the most dangerous sources of sugar are those which have a sticky consistency when chewed. The adherent nature of such foods allows them to cling to the teeth for a very long time, throughout which they are supplying plaque bacteria with the raw materials for prolonged acid formation and demineralization. Toffee and other sweets; cakes, biscuits, white bread and jam; and puddings with syrup or treacle are foremost among these sticky forms of sugar which cause caries.

Our modern diet is of such a nature that sugar is consumed nearly every time something is eaten; and the teeth are attacked by acid on each of these occasions. If snacks containing sugar are frequently taken between meals there will be a corresponding increase in the number of acid attacks on the teeth. The delicate balance between the forces of destruction (demineralization) and those of repair (remineralization) will then be completely upset in favour of tooth destruction and *irreversible* damage will ensue. Thus it is evident that the prime cause of caries is the frequent and unrestricted consumption of sweet snacks *between* meals. It is not the amount of sugar eaten but the *frequency* with which it is eaten that is all-important. This fundamental fact forms the basis of personal caries prevention and dental health education.

Sites of caries

The parts of a tooth most prone to caries are those where food tends to collect and plaque bacteria can flourish. Such sites are known as **stagnation areas**. Occlusal fissures and the spaces between the mesial and distal surfaces of adjoining teeth are the commonest stagnation areas. That is why caries occurs most often on occlusal and proximal surfaces. However, any other part where food debris can accumulate is a stagnation area where plaque will proliferate and caries is likely to occur. Such food traps are the necks of teeth covered by ill-fitting partial dentures; irregular teeth and unopposed teeth.

Minimal harm is caused by partial dentures which fit perfectly, but those which do not are a menace to dental health. They leave spaces between the necks of the teeth and plastic plate, or between clasps and teeth, which are dangerous stagnation areas.

During mastication, food which needs chewing actually helps to clean teeth which are in normal occlusion. It does not prevent plaque formation, but does reduce the amount of retained food debris which is responsible for the harmful effects of plaque. Teeth which are not in normal occlusion, such as irregularly positioned and unopposed teeth, are not exposed to this beneficial cleansing effect of mastication. Consequently food collects around these instanding or outstanding irregular teeth. It also covers the crown of any tooth which has lost its opposite number, and remains unopposed because the space has not been replaced artificially. To make the situation even worse, the sticky sweet food most likely to produce caries needs the minimum amount of mastication anyway, and therefore has a negligible cleansing effect – even on teeth in normal occlusion.

Effects of caries

Unrestricted consumption of sugar produces an abundance of acid-forming bacteria in the plaque which collects in stagnation areas. The resultant series of continual acid attacks prevents remineralization and allows acid to eat through the enamel until it reaches dentine. As enamel has no nerves the first stage is quite painless but once the dentine is breached, caries is then involving the sensitive part of a tooth and pain is liable to occur. Nevertheless pain is not usually felt until caries has extended a considerable way into dentine.

At first the pain only lasts for a short while and is brought on by contact with anything hot, cold or sweet. Later, however, as a cavity approaches the pulp, toothache becomes more severe and prolonged until eventually the pulp itself becomes inflamed. This condition of **pulpitis** is caused by the irritant action of bacteria and their acid products in the cavity. It is very painful and leads to death of the pulp, followed by formation of an **alveolar abscess**.

Although teeth are virtually defenceless against advancing caries the pulp does respond by forming secondary dentine (Chapter 12) as caries progresses. Unfortunately, however, caries advances too quickly to allow an effective barrier of secondary dentine to be formed.

Pulpitis

Pulpitis occurs when caries extends through the dentine to reach the pulp. The pulp is then said to be *exposed* and the sequence of events described under inflammation (Chapter 9) follows.

There is an increased blood flow through the apical foramen into the pulp. Swelling cannot occur, however, as the pulp is confined within the rigid walls of the root canal and pulp chamber. Pressure builds up instead and causes intense pain. A much more important result of this pressure, however, is the compression of blood vessels passing through the tiny apical foramen. This cuts off the blood supply and causes death of the pulp. When the pulp dies, its nerves die too, and the severe toothache stops abruptly. But the respite is short as pulp death leads to another very painful condition called alveolar abscess.

Pulpitis may be acute or chronic. It has many causes, apart from caries, but almost always ends in pulp death. Other causes of pulpitis are covered in Chapter 24.

Alveolar abscess

When pulpitis occurs, the pulp eventually dies as its blood supply is cut off by inflammatory pressure. The dead pulp decomposes and infected material passes through the apical foramen into the periodontal membrane and alveolar bone at the apex of the tooth. These irritant products give rise to another inflammatory reaction in the tissues surrounding the apex. Pus formation occurs and an acute alveolar abscess develops.

This is an extremely painful condition. The affected tooth becomes loose and very tender to the slightest pressure; there is a continual throbbing pain and the surrounding gum is red and swollen. Frequently the whole side of the face is involved in inflammatory swelling and the patient may have a raised temperature. Looseness is caused by swelling of the periodontal membrane. Pain is caused by the increased pressure of blood within the rigid confines of the periodontal membrane and alveolar bone. The tooth is so tender that it cannot be used for eating. Thus acute alveolar abscess may show all the cardinal signs of acute inflammation: pain, swelling, redness, heat, loss of function and raised body temperature.

Pulp death is sometimes followed by the development of a chronic alveolar abscess instead. This usually gives rise to very little pain and most patients are quite unaware of its presence. It may often be detected by the presence of a small hole in the gum called a **sinus**, which is a track leading from the abscess cavity in the alveolar bone to the surface of the gum. Pus drains from the abscess through the sinus into the mouth. This outlet prevents a build-up of pressure inside the bone and explains the lack of pain.

If an acute abscess is not treated it eventually turns into a chronic abscess by the drainage of pus through a sinus. This relieves the pain and the features of acute inflammation largely disappear. The relative freedom from pain does not last indefinitely, however, as a chronic alveolar abscess is liable to turn into an acute abscess at any time.

It should now be clear that pulpitis is followed by pulp death, and this eventually leads to an acute alveolar abscess, either directly or via a chronic abscess.

Treatment

If caries is allowed to progress untreated, it will cause toothache, followed by pulpitis and alveolar abscess. The object of treatment is to stop caries progressing further and thereby prevent or cure pain. Relief of pain and the replacement of damaged tissue will also restore function to decayed teeth.

The type of treatment given depends on the health of the pulp. If it is still vital, and not affected by pulpitis, the tooth can be **filled**. But if the pulp is inflamed, or already dead, treatment is by **extraction** or **root canal therapy**. The choice depends on the value of the tooth to the patient. If it is desirable, and technically feasible, conservative treatment is undertaken; otherwise it is extracted.

Filling

No drug can cure caries and nothing can make the lost tooth structure grow again. The best that can be achieved is the removal of all carious enamel and dentine and replacement by a filling. Patients with an excessive number of decayed teeth are obviously very susceptible to caries. In such cases, to prevent recurrence of caries on the surface being filled, the cavity may be extended to remove any other stagnation areas. Thus a tooth with a small occlusal cavity would have not only the carious part but all the occlusal fissures removed and filled. The occlusal surface should then be safe from further caries as there are no stagnation areas left for the lodgement of food. Similarly, teeth with mesial or distal caries may need the cavity preparation extended buccally and lingually to remove the entire stagnation area between the teeth (Figure 17.1).

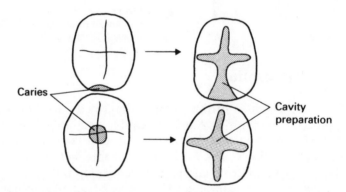

Figure 17.1 *Cavity preparation.*

Normally, however, for patients who exercise control over their sugar intake, attend regularly and maintain good oral hygiene, cavity preparation is restricted to the removal of carious tissue only. There is no need to remove sound fissures or to extend cavities in such patients.

Figure 17.1 shows the extent of cavity preparation for *susceptible* patients.

Diagnosis

Before caries is treated, it must first be detected. Large cavities are obvious to the naked eye but it is easier to treat caries before cavities reach such a size. Small occlusal cavities are found with a *blunt* pointed instrument called a **probe** (Figure 17.2). Mesial and distal cavities can be found with a special double-ended probe called a **Briault probe**.

By the time mesial or distal cavities are found with a Briault probe, caries is already far advanced. Detection at an earlier stage is achieved by taking X-ray films. A special film called a **bite-wing** (Figure 29.6) shows caries before it can be seen by any other method.

Another way of finding mesial and distal cavities at an early stage is **transillumination**. A bright fibre-optic light is placed against the crown and the cavity shows up as a dark shadow. This method is not as good as bite-wing X-rays but is quite useful on front teeth.

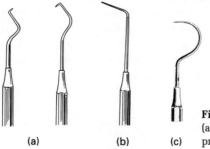

(a) (b) (c)

Figure 17.2 *Probes.*
(a) Ends of Briault probe; (b) Right angle probe; (c) Sickle probe.

Caries and civilization

The first sentence of this chapter described caries as a disease of civilized communities. Among primitive uncivilized people, caries is virtually non-existent but wherever civilization spreads, caries inevitably follows. The explanation of this fact is the difference in diet between civilized and uncivilized communities.

Civilized food, consisting to a large extent of non-fibrous sticky refined carbohydrate such as sugar and white flour, with little raw fruit and vegetables, requires hardly any mastication. The reverse is true of a primitive diet; refined carbohydrate is unknown and plenty of raw natural foods are eaten, needing the maximum amount of mastication. Mastication in itself cleans the teeth; so these uncivilized peoples, with a diet devoid of refined carbohydrates and requiring considerable mastication, have little food debris capable of acid formation left on their teeth after meals. Furthermore, the prolonged vigorous mastication necessary for this type of diet wears down cusps and eliminates fissures, thus removing the stagnation areas. This wear of the teeth, known as **attrition**, cannot possibly occur to such an extent on our civilized diet of soft cooked food which needs the bare minimum of chewing.

Prevention

Caries is a breakdown of tooth structure, caused by acid produced from dietary sugar trapped in plaque stagnation areas. Prevention of caries can therefore be achieved by:

1 Dietary discipline
2 Making teeth more resistant to acid attack
3 Elimination of stagnation areas

Dietary discipline

If all food debris containing sugar is cleaned off the teeth immediately after eating, the source of acid formation in plaque is lost and caries will not occur. Unfortunately this cannot be done completely as no method of cleaning can reach all the stagnation areas. Furthermore it is impracticable for most people to clean their teeth every time they consume sugar. The only sure way to prevent caries would be to eliminate sugar from our diet. But sugar is so widely used in the manufacture and cooking of food that its total withdrawal would be even more impractical.

However, a compromise can be made by confining sugar intake to mealtimes only, thereby reducing the frequency of acid attacks to a level where remineralization can predominate over demineralization. Eating sweets, cakes and biscuits, etc., between meals is the most important cause of caries; and if this habit can be overcome there will be a corresponding decrease in caries. Each time sugar is eaten acid is formed and attacks the teeth. Therefore the elimination of all such snacks between meals will reduce the number of acid attacks; and this, in fact, is the most effective dietary measure anybody can personally take to prevent caries.

The habit of eating snacks between meals is so widespread that many people are unwilling to give it up. However, the damage snacks cause can be minimized by substituting sugar-free alternatives such as fresh fruit, raw carrots, wholemeal bread, low-fat cheese, crisps and low-calorie drinks.

More education of the general public is still required to limit the disastrous dental effects of repeatedly eating sugar during school breaks, watching television, in cinemas, and last thing at night after the teeth have been cleaned.

Another way of cutting down on dietary sugar is to use artificial sweeteners, such as saccharin or aspartame, as a sugar substitute. Many products are now available which are sweetened in this way and their use will help prevent caries, as well as having other dietary advantages.

Acid resistance

The most important factor for making teeth more resistant to acid is **fluoride**. When present in the water supply it automatically forms part of the diet during the period of tooth formation and becomes a constituent of tooth structure. When these teeth erupt, the beneficial effect of fluoride continues as their crowns are then exposed to fluoride whenever water is drunk or food cooked in water is eaten.

The result is a reduction of about 50% in the number of carious teeth. In areas where fluoride occurs naturally in water, it is so effective that it is being added artificially to other public water supplies. This is known as **fluoridation**. It still has the same beneficial effect and causes no harm whatsoever to general health. Where fluoride is deliberately added to the public water supply it is in a concentration of **one part per million** (1 ppm). This gives maximum caries resistance and has no harmful effect on the teeth or the rest of the body. Some areas, however, have fluoride occurring naturally in much higher concentrations. While this is still caries-resistant and without harm to the rest of the body, it does have one great drawback: an unsightly mottling of the teeth. When added artificially though, at a concentration of 1 ppm, mottling (*fluorosis*) does *not* occur.

Where water fluoridation has not been instituted, an equally effective alternative is to take fluoride in the form of tablets or drops. But this is only applicable to a dedicated minority of parents as it must be administered to their children daily, from birth until adolescence, when the second permanent molars erupt. Such a degree of motivation and perseverance cannot be expected from the public at large.

Another way of making teeth more resistant to acid is to apply fluoride directly to the crowns of teeth; whereupon it promotes remineralization and the arrest of caries. This is known as **topical fluoridation** but it is not as simple or practical as the fluoridation of water supplies. Nevertheless it does produce a similar reduction in caries. The simplest and most convenient form of topical fluoridation is twice-daily brushing with **fluoride toothpaste**. Brushing with other toothpastes does not reduce caries to any extent as plaque in the stagnation areas where caries normally occurs is inaccessible to a toothbrush. But fluoride toothpaste allows the fluoride to penetrate plaque in the same way as dietary sugars.

An alternative form of topical fluoridation is the direct application of a fluoride solution, gel or varnish to the teeth by a dentist, hygienist or therapist. It is usually confined to children for whom dental treatment is potentially hazardous: for example, those with haemophilia or heart defects; those who are difficult to treat because of mental or physical handicaps; and those who are highly susceptible to caries. Three applications a year are sufficient and this is conveniently done during school holidays.

Saliva helps dissipate and neutralize the acid which is produced by plaque bacteria immediately after the consumption of sugar. It usually takes about 20 minutes for the acid attack to be overcome but, depending on individual variation, may take up to two hours. This helps to explain why, apart from dietary factors, people vary in their susceptibility to caries. The acid-resistant properties of saliva can be put to good use by promoting a greater flow of saliva. Fruit and sugar-free chewing gum are particularly effective at stimulating salivary flow and, taken at the end of a meal or between meals, can assist the antacid and remineralization functions of saliva.

Another form of acid attack, which is not dependent on sugar or plaque bacteria, is caused by the excessive consumption of acidic soft drinks and fruit juice. This is particularly common in children and gives rise to the loss of tooth substance by acid **erosion**. Teeth affected in this way become sensitive to very hot, cold or sweet fluids.

To summarize this section: a combination of strict dietary discipline to restrict the frequency and amount of intake of sugar and acidic drinks, together with twice-daily brushing with fluoride toothpaste, is the most effective way in which anybody can achieve almost complete self-protection against caries. The role of fluoride is covered again in Chapter 26.

Elimination of stagnation areas

As caries occurs in food stagnation areas, any means of reducing these can produce a corresponding reduction in caries. The methods available are directed against natural stagnation areas such as occlusal fissures, and acquired stagnation areas such as unopposed and irregular teeth, poorly fitting partial dentures and poor contact points.

Occlusal fissures are natural stagnation areas and these can be eliminated whenever a tooth is filled (Figure 17.1). However, they may also be eliminated by **fissure sealants** before caries occurs. These materials are used to fill the fissures without any cavity preparation and are described in Chapters 21 and 22. Moreover they can serve the dual role of filling material and fissure sealant in cases where only a small area is carious while the rest of the fissure system is sound; thereby limiting cavity preparation to the carious part and preserving the sound tissue.

Acquired stagnation areas include those associated with irregularly positioned or unopposed teeth, as these do not receive the normal self-cleansing effect of mastication. Additional food traps result from ill-fitting partial dentures, and teeth which have lost their contact point with a mesial or distal neighbour. This contact point is normally tight and prevents food packing between the teeth. But if it is lost through caries, or is inadequately restored by filling, the adjacent tooth can be affected by the food trap so formed.

Regular dental treatment plays a large part in preventing the onset of caries in acquired stagnation areas. By providing orthodontic or prosthetic treatment it can restore normal occlusion and the natural self-cleansing effect of mastication. Conservative treatment will maintain and restore tight contact points, and save teeth from extraction, thus avoiding the need for dentures. Existing partial dentures which permit food stagnation are replaced by new ones, correctly designed and well-fitting to prevent this.

Written examination

The prevention of caries is an obvious and frequent subject for examination questions, yet they are often poorly answered. In most cases, candidates know the methods but write them down in such a piecemeal and illogical order that the examiner remains unconvinced that the candidate has sufficient grasp of the subject to achieve a pass mark.

In order to demonstrate to an examiner that you do understand a subject, it is essential to give the most important points first and in their correct order of importance. This applies to any subject but in the case of individually attainable caries prevention a logical order would be:

1   dietary discipline by the reduction of frequency of sugar intake
2   twice-daily use of fluoride toothpaste
3   regular dental inspection

What causes dental caries and how can it be prevented in a young child?
Describe oral health instruction a dental nurse would give to a teenager. (November 1990)
Describe the progression of dental caries from the enamel surface to a dental abscess.
What symptoms may the patient complain of at each stage? (November 1996)

Summary

Stagnation areas

- Fissures ⎫
- Mesial and distal surfaces ⎪
- Irregular teeth ⎬ Plaque formation
- Unopposed teeth ⎪
- Ill-fitting partial dentures ⎪
- Loose contact points ⎭

Cause

- High frequency of sugar intake → demineralization predominant

- Sweets ⎫
- Cake ⎬ Sugar + plaque bacteria → acid
- Biscuits ⎭
- Acid dissolves enamel and dentine → cavity

Effects

1 Acid dissolves enamel → painless.
2 Acid dissolves dentine → slight pain.
3 Cavity approaches pulp → pain increases, lasts longer.
4 Pulpitis → severe prolonged pain.
5 Death of pulp → pain disappears.

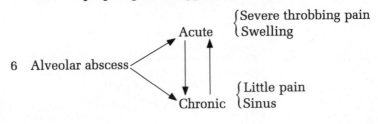

6 Alveolar abscess

Acute { Severe throbbing pain / Swelling

Chronic { Little pain / Sinus

Treatment

1 Pulp not involved → filling
2 Pulpitis ⎫ Extraction
3 Pulp dead ⎬ or
4 Alveolar abscess ⎭ root canal therapy

Prevention

1 Water fluoridation – 1 ppm
2 No snacks or acidic drinks between meals → remineralization predominant
3 Twice-daily brushing with fluoride toothpaste
4 Regular dental attendance
   - Conservation
   - Orthodontics
   - Prosthetics
   - Fissure sealing
   - Topical fluoridation
   - Oral health instruction

18   Fillings

The conservative treatment of caries, when the pulp is vital and unexposed, is by filling. If the pulp is exposed or dead, root canal therapy is usually necessary before the crown of the tooth is permanently filled.

Fillings are inserted in teeth to replace the part destroyed by caries. The normal function of the tooth is thereby restored, pain is prevented, and the vitality of the pulp is preserved. In front teeth, fillings restore normal appearance; in back teeth, stagnation areas can be eradicated and further caries prevented.

Temporary fillings

These are inserted as a temporary measure only. They are too soft or soluble to use as permanent fillings. The temporary fillings are:

- Zinc oxide and eugenol cement
- Zinc phosphate cement
- Polycarboxylate cement
- Gutta-percha

Permanent fillings

For premolars and molars, a metal filling such as **amalgam** or **gold** is used. In front teeth, where these fillings would show, non-metallic **composite** or **glass ionomer** fillings are used instead as their colour matches the tooth. As tooth-coloured materials are weaker than metal fillings their use is generally confined to front teeth.

Classification of cavities

Cavities are classified into five different types, depending on the site of the original caries attack. This is called **Black's classification**, after the American dentist who devised it. In general usage, his classification of cavities also applies to the fillings inserted in each class of cavity.

1   Class I cavities are those involving a single surface; in a pit or fissure. Thus a class I filling could be an occlusal filling; or a buccal or lingual filling.

2 Class II cavities involve at least two surfaces; the mesial or distal, and the occlusal surface of a molar or premolar. Thus a class II filling could be a mesial-occlusal (*mo*) filling in a premolar, for example; or a mesial-occlusal-distal (*mod*) filling in a molar.
3 Class III cavities involve the mesial or distal surface of an incisor or canine.
4 Class IV cavities are the same as class III but extend to involve the incisal edge on the affected side.
5 Class V cavities involve the cervical margin of any tooth. Thus a class V filling could be a labial cervical filling in an upper incisor; or a lingual cervical filling in a lower molar.

Cavity preparation

A permanent filling cannot be inserted directly into a carious cavity. Careful preparation of the cavity is required to ensure that all caries is removed; that the filling will be a permanent fixture; and caries will not recur at its margins. The general principles of cavity preparation are as follows:

1 Undermined enamel is chipped away with an **enamel chisel** (Figure 18.1).

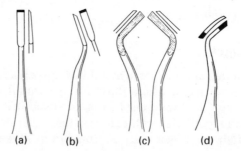

(a)   (b)   (c)   (d)

Figure 18.1   *Chisels* (a) Straight; (b) Bin-angle; (c) Hatchet; (d) Cervical margin trimmer.

2 Caries is removed with an excavator (Figure 18.2), or a large round **bur**.
3 The cavity is formed into a retentive shape and, in susceptible patients, is extended to remove the entire stagnation area; for example, occlusal fissures, on the carious surface. This is done with a **handpiece** and **burs**.
4 Burs, chisels, and **cervical margin trimmers** (Figure 18.1) are then used to finish off the cavity according to the type of filling necessary.

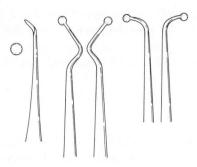

Figure 18.2 *Excavators.*

Retention of fillings

Permanent fillings are meant to stay put permanently and the cavity must be specially prepared to provide maximum retention. Before explaining how this is done, it is necessary to consider the types of fillings used. There are two types available: plastic and pre-constructed.

Plastic fillings are soft and plastic on insertion but set hard in the cavity. They include temporary cements, gutta-percha, amalgam, glass ionomer cement and composite fillings.

Pre-constructed restorations are **inlays**, **crowns** and **veneers**. These are made in the laboratory, after the teeth have been prepared, and are then cemented into place.

Retention for plastic fillings is obtained by simply **undercutting** the cavity to make the entrance smaller than its inside dimensions (Figure 18.3). Thus a plastic filling can be packed in when soft but cannot come out when hard. For fillings involving occlusal and mesial surfaces, or occlusal and distal, a **dovetail** is cut in the occlusal surface to prevent the filling coming out mesially or distally (Figure 18.3).

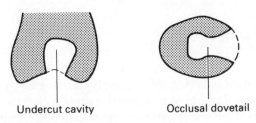

Undercut cavity   Occlusal dovetail

Figure 18.3 *Cavity preparation for plastic fillings.*

Sometimes it is not possible to prepare cavities which are sufficiently undercut to retain a plastic filling. In such cases they may be made retentive in other ways: by dentine pins for amalgam; acid etching for composites: and chemical bonding for glass ionomer cement. These methods are covered in the appropriate chapter.

Inlays and crowns are hard and rigid when inserted and cannot utilize undercuts for retention. To prevent them coming out occlusally, they rely on parallel cavity walls and adhesive cement. As with plastic fillings, an occlusal dovetail is used to prevent dislodgement mesially or distally.

Cavity lining

Before a permanent filling is inserted the cavity may need to be lined. A **lining** is an insulating layer of cement which protects the pulp against conduction of heat or cold through metal fillings; or against the chemical irritation of non-metallic fillings. Pain, and possibly death of the tooth, may occur through failure to insert an adequate lining.

The linings used are zinc oxide and eugenol cement, zinc phosphate cement, polycarboxylate cement and calcium hydroxide.

Insertion

The technique of inserting a filling varies with the type of cavity and filling material used. This matter is therefore discussed separately under the appropriate filling material.

Polishing

Permanent fillings may need trimming to remove any high spots or proud edges, followed by polishing to provide a clean, smooth, comfortable surface. Some fillings can be polished immediately after insertion but those with a long setting time are polished at a subsequent visit. The instruments and materials used depend on the type of filling and are detailed in the chapter concerned.

Control of saliva

Fillings inserted in wet cavities are always unsatisfactory. No matter what material is used a cavity must stay perfectly dry during insertion. Linings and cements cannot adhere to wet cavities; while amalgam and acid etching techniques are ruined by saliva contamination. The following methods are used to control saliva.

Suction

The patient holds a **saliva ejector** attached to the unit or **aspirator**. Many different types are used but those with a flange to keep the tongue away are particularly helpful. The nurse assists by holding a wide bore aspirator tube or using a retractor to keep the tongue or cheek away.

Absorbent materials

Cotton wool rolls or absorbent pads (*Dry Guards*) are placed in the buccal or lingual sulcus to absorb saliva and to keep the soft tissues away from the teeth. Napkins may also be used for the same purpose.

The cavity

The cavity itself is dried with cotton wool, followed by a short blast of compressed air from the warm air syringe on the unit.

Rubber dam

This is the best method of all. Rubber dam is a thin sheet of rubber which is placed over a tooth to isolate it from the rest of the mouth. A **rubber dam punch** (Figure 18.4) is used to punch a small hole in the rubber, which is then fitted on so that the tooth projects through the hole. The rubber dam is kept in place by a **rubber dam clamp** which is fixed on the tooth with **rubber dam clamp forceps**. Finally a **rubber dam frame** is used to support the sheet of rubber. A napkin is placed between the patient's chin and the rubber to make it more comfortable; and a saliva ejector is provided. **Dental floss** is used to work the rubber between the teeth.

Rubber dam may be applied to any number of teeth. It enables the operator to keep a tooth dry and maintain a sterile field; and prevents bits of filling material, debris or small instruments falling into the patient's mouth.

It is more comfortable for patients as it prevents water spray or irrigation fluids entering the mouth; and far better for the dentist, too, improving access and visibility by keeping the tongue, lips and cheek out of the way. It also helps prevent cross-infection of patients and chairside staff, by minimizing the cloud of infected debris spread by the use of compressed air and waterspray.

The two main uses of rubber dam are: in root canal therapy, to maintain a sterile field and prevent inhalation or swallowing of small instruments; and during the insertion of fillings to avoid failure caused by saliva contamination. Rubber dam clamps are often used alone to hold cotton wool rolls in place, especially when filling lower molars.

Ideally, rubber dam should be used for all fillings, but most operators consider it too time-consuming for routine use.

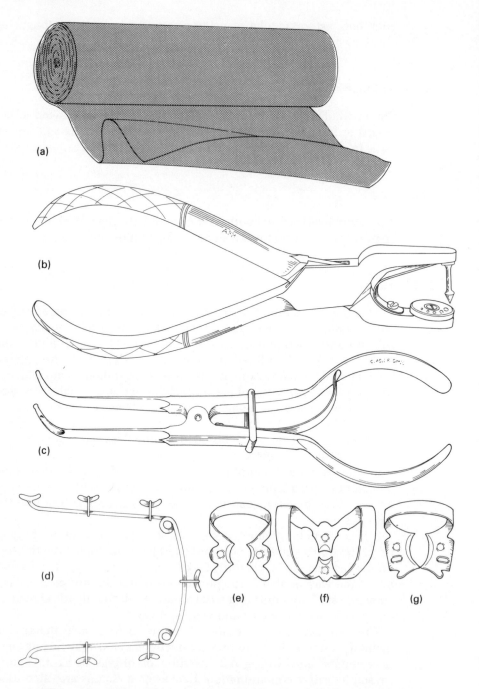

Figure 18.4 *Rubber dam instruments*. (a) Rubber dam; (b) Rubber dam punch; (c) Rubber dam clamp forceps; (d) Rubber dam frame; (e) Premolar clamp; (f) Incisor (butterfly) clamp; (g) Molar clamp.

Instruments

For each patient the instruments required are:

1 Mirror, probe, tweezers, napkins, waste receiver
2 Aspirator, saliva ejector, absorbent pads, cotton wool rolls and cotton wool for keeping the cavity dry
3 Enamel chisels and cervical margin trimmers for removing undermined enamel and smoothing the cavity margins
4 Excavators for removing caries
5 Handpiece and burs for drilling away hard tissue
6 **Plastic instruments** (Figure 18.5). These have blunt ends for manipulating, packing and trimming the filling or lining
7 Special instruments and drugs. Some fillings require the use of certain instruments or drugs which are not used for other fillings. These special requirements are dealt with under the appropriate filling materials.

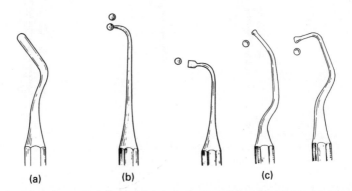

(a) (b) (c)

Figure 18.5 *Plastic instruments.* (a) Flat plastic; (b) Ball ended burnisher; (c) Pluggers.

Handpieces

Cavities are cut with burs fitted in a handpiece. The speed of cutting depends on the type of handpiece used.

Low-speed handpieces (up to 4000 revolutions a minute) are driven by a miniature compressed air or electric motor at the base of the handpiece. A **contra-angle** handpiece is used most often as it provides access to every tooth. For easily accessible teeth, and laboratory work, a **straight** handpiece is used (Figure 18.6).

Air turbine handpieces run at very high speeds of up to 400,000 revolutions a minute. There is a tiny air turbine motor in the head of the handpiece which is driven by compressed air. They are contra-angled and are used with a built-in water spray to counteract the heat generated by high-speed cutting. The advantages of air turbine

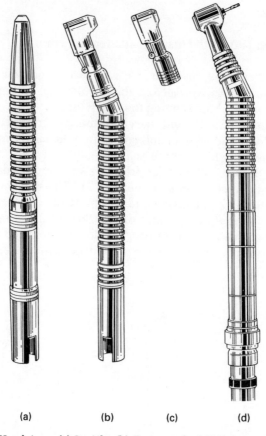

(a)   (b)   (c)   (d)

Figure 18.6 *Handpieces.* (a) Straight; (b) Contra-angle; (c) Miniature; (d) Air turbine.

handpieces are the ease and speed of cutting, and absence of vibration. Disadvantages are the difficulties caused by water spray, and the high-pitched whistling noise.

Burs

Burs for low-speed handpieces are made of steel. They are used for cutting dentine, the removal of caries, trimming dentures and other laboratory work.

Burs for air turbine handpieces have **diamond** or **tungsten carbide** cutting surfaces and are used for high-speed removal of enamel, dentine and old fillings.

Straight handpiece burs and mandrels (Figure 18.9) have a long plain shank. Burs and mandrels for low-speed contra-angle handpieces are short and have a notch in the shank which fits by a **latch grip**. Short burs are also used for air turbine handpieces but they have a plain shank which gives a **friction grip** (Figure 18.7).

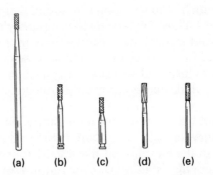

Figure 18.7 *Burs.* (a) Steel for straight handpiece; (b) Steel, latch grip, for low-speed contra-angle handpiece; (c) Steel, latch grip, for miniature contra-angle handpiece; (d) Tungsten carbide, friction grip, for air turbine handpiece; (e) Diamond, friction grip, for air turbine handpiece.

Contra-angled low-speed handpieces with smaller heads, and using even shorter burs, are used on children. They are called **miniature** handpieces and burs.

The cutting ends of burs are made in many different shapes (Figure 18.8) but those most commonly used are as follows:

1   Round – used for gaining access to cavities; and at low speed for removing caries
2   Pear – used for undercutting cavities
3   Fissure – used for shaping and outlining the cavity

Enamel chisels

Although enamel is the hardest tissue in the body it is a brittle material; and where caries has destroyed its underlying dentine, any remaining

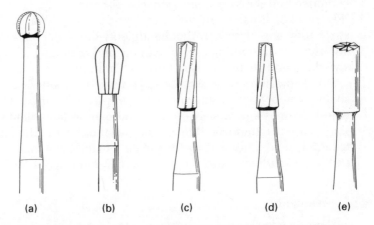

Figure 18.8 *Bur shapes.* (a) Round; (b) Pear; (c) Fissure; (d) Tapered fissure; (e) End-cutting.

enamel which is unsupported by sound dentine can break off during mastication. Thus it is essential during cavity preparation to remove all unsupported enamel. This can be done by chipping it away with an enamel chisel. These sharp hand instruments have a similar blade to a carpenter's chisel and are usually single-ended (Figure 18.1). They have tungsten carbide blades and are also used for smoothing cavity margins.

- **Straight** chisels resemble a miniature wood chisel
- **Bin-angle** chisels have their cutting edge at right angles to the plane of the handle, just like a garden hoe
- **Hatchet** chisels, as their name implies, have their cutting edge in the same plane as the handle
- **Cervical margin trimmers** are modified hatchet chisels with a curved blade for removing unsupported enamel from the cervical margins of class II cavities.

Excavators

Excavators are sharp double-ended hand instruments for the removal of carious dentine. Their spoon-like cutting edges may have a round or oval outline (Figure 18.2).

Plastic instruments

Plastic instruments are blunt double-ended instruments with round or flat ends for inserting and manipulating linings and plastic fillings (Figure 18.5).

Polishing instruments

There is a great variety of polishing instruments but they generally comprise fine abrasive stones, wheels, discs and strips, finishing burs (Figure 20.2), brushes and polishing pastes. Apart from hand abrasive strips they are all used with a handpiece. Finishing burs and stones are used for smoothing cavity margins and trimming fillings. Abrasive discs and strips are used for fine trimming and polishing.

Small abrasive stones, wheels and brushes are manufactured with a shank which fits the appropriate handpiece (Figure 18.7). Larger wheels, stones and abrasive discs require an independent mounting shank called a **mandrel**. Wheels and metal discs are fitted on a *Huey* mandrel; sandpaper discs with a metal centre use a *Moore* mandrel; and plain sandpaper discs a *pinhead* mandrel (Figure 18.9).

Care of instruments

All cutting instruments must be kept sharp. Blunt ones are inefficient and painful.

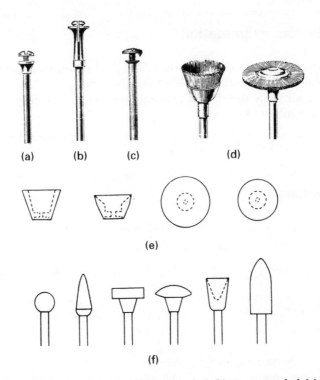

Figure 18.9 *Polishing instruments.* (a) Huey mandrel; (b) Moore mandrel; (c) pin-head mandrel; (d) polishing brushes; (e) abrasive rubber cups and discs for Huey mandrel; (f) mounted fine abrasives.

Hand instruments such as chisels and excavators must be sharpened regularly on a small flat oilstone (**Arkansas stone**), or with an abrasive disc in a straight handpiece. Burs are cleaned with a bur brush (Figure 18.10) or ultrasonic cleaner and discarded when blunt.

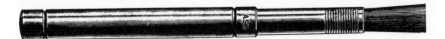

Figure 18.10 *Bur brush.*

All handpieces must be lubricated regularly according to manufacturers' instructions. If this is not done, wear takes place and causes excessive vibration and reduced speed. Low-speed handpieces should be stripped periodically to clean their internal mechanism; and worn bearings are replaced as necessary. The chuck on straight handpieces can be adjusted if the bur slips. Manufacturers' instructions must also be obeyed when sterilizing handpieces. The methods used are described in Chapter 10.

Written examination

Why is moisture control important during dental procedures?
What methods are available to achieve this?
Explain how the dental nurse can assist in moisture control.
(November 1993)

Summary

FILLINGS

Plastic

Pre-constructed

Inlays   Crowns   Veneers

Temporary

Permanent

Zinc oxide and eugenol
Zinc phosphate
Polycarboxylate
Gutta-percha

Amalgam
Composite
Glass ionomer cement

Functions of permanent fillings

- Restoration of part lost by caries
- Conservation of proper function of teeth
- Prevention of pain
- Prevention of further caries
- Restoration of appearance of front teeth

Black's classification

- Class I   Single surface → pit or fissure
- Class II   Mesial and/or distal, and occlusal → molars and pre-molars
- Class III   Mesial or distal → incisors and canines
- Class IV   Mesial or distal with involvement of incisal edge → incisors and canines
- Class V   Cervical margin of any tooth

Cavity preparation

1 Remove undermined enamel
2 Extend cavity to remove stagnation areas and prevent recurrence of caries in susceptible patients
3 Remove residual caries
4 Finish off according to type of filling

Retention of plastic fillings

- Undercut cavity
- Occlusal dovetail

Retention of inlays and crowns

Parallel cavity walls
Occlusal dovetail
Adhesive cement

Other methods of retention

- Dentine pins → amalgam
- Acid etching → composites
- Chemical bonding → glass ionomer cement

Cavity lining cements

- Zinc oxide and eugenol
- Zinc phosphate
- Polycarboxylate
- Calcium hydroxide

Functions of cavity lining

Protection of pulp and prevention of pain from:

1 Conduction of heat or cold through metal fillings
2 Chemical irritation of non-metallic fillings

Control of saliva

1 Suction – aspirator and saliva ejector
2 Compressed air syringe
3 Absorbent materials in sulcus – cotton wool rolls, pads, napkins

4   Rubber dam clamp and cotton wool rolls
5   Rubber dam

Use of rubber dam

1   Prevent moisture contamination of fillings
2   Prevent inhalation or swallowing of debris and small instruments
3   Prevent bacterial contamination during root treatment
4   Reduce cross-infection of patient and chairside staff

Rubber dam equipment

- Rubber dam punch
- Rubber dam clamps
- Rubber dam clamp forceps
- Rubber dam frame
- Floss

Instruments

All fillings

- Mirror, probe, tweezers, napkins, waste receiver
- Saliva ejector, aspirator tubes, absorbent pads, cotton wool rolls, cotton wool → keep cavity dry
- Chisels → remove undermined enamel; smooth cavity margins
- Excavators → remove caries
- Handpiece and burs → remove hard tissue
- Plastic instruments → manipulate, insert and trim plastic fillings

Handpieces

- Low-speed: straight, contra-angle, miniature
- High speed: air turbine

Burs

- Low-speed: steel; straight or latch grip
- High-speed: tungsten carbide or diamond; friction grip

Polishing

- Handpieces
- Finishing burs

- Unmounted coarse and fine abrasive stones, wheels and discs
- Mandrels: *Huey*, *Moore*, pinhead
- Mounted abrasives and polishing brushes
- Polishing paste

Care and maintenance

- Hand instruments → sharpen regularly
- Low-speed handpieces → lubricate regularly; strip and clean mechanism; replace worn bearings
- Air turbine handpieces → lubricate regularly

19 Temporary Fillings and Cavity Linings

The temporary filling materials are zinc oxide and eugenol cement, zinc phosphate cement, polycarboxylate cement and gutta-percha. They are not used as permanent fillings as they are too soft and soluble and would not remain intact for long periods. With the exception of gutta-percha they are also used as cavity linings. Although calcium hydroxide is not a temporary filling, it is an excellent cavity lining and is accordingly included in this chapter.

Uses of temporary fillings

1 As a first-aid measure to relieve pain
2 When there is insufficient time to complete the cavity and insert a permanent filling in one visit
3 For permanent fillings requiring more than one visit; for example, inlays and crowns, a temporary restoration is necessary between visits.

Purpose of cavity linings

1 Protection of pulp against thermal shock, such as conduction of heat or cold through metal fillings
2 Protection of pulp against the chemical irritation of non-metallic fillings

Zinc oxide and eugenol cement

Zinc oxide and eugenol cement (ZOE) is made by mixing *zinc oxide* powder and a drop of *eugenol* (oil of cloves) on a glass slab with a **spatula**. It can be thickened if necessary by squeezing in a napkin. Setting takes a few hours.

Uses

ZOE is used as a temporary filling; as a non-irritant lining for deep cavities; and as a sedative dressing for painful carious teeth and dry sockets. It also forms the main constituent of some impression pastes, periodontal packs, and root filling materials.

Advantages

ZOE is soothing and non-irritant to the pulp and can be safely used in deep cavities.

Disadvantages

It is too soft and slow-setting to use as a foundation for a permanent filling in one visit. But this can be overcome by using a strengthened quick-setting proprietary brand (e.g. *Kalzinol*). In this form it is generally regarded as a most satisfactory lining for metal fillings.

ZOE is not compatible with composite fillings. Manufacturers' instructions must always be followed in selecting a suitable lining for any non-metallic fillings.

Preparations containing eugenol may cause a burning sensation if they come in contact with the lips. This can be avoided by smearing the lips with petroleum jelly beforehand.

Zinc phosphate cement

Zinc phosphate cement (also called zinc oxyphosphate) is prepared by mixing a powder and liquid on a glass slab with a spatula. The powder consists mainly of *zinc oxide*; the liquid is *phosphoric acid.* Two different mixes are used: a thick mix of putty consistency and a thin creamy one. Setting takes a few minutes depending on various factors:

1 A warm slab accelerates the setting while a cold slab has the opposite effect.
2 A thick mix sets more quickly than a thin mix.
3 A dry slab must be used as moisture accelerates setting. It is most important to screw the cap on tightly, immediately after using the bottle of liquid, to prevent it absorbing moisture from the air. If this happens, the cement will set too quickly.
4 If a long setting time is required, when cementing a bridge, for example, a cold slab is necessary. A tiny quantity of powder is mixed with the liquid a minute or so before the cement is required. The rest of the powder is then added in small quantities at a time. This ability to prolong its setting time is the overriding advantage of zinc phosphate cement.

Experience soon teaches a nurse how much powder and liquid to set out, but occasionally too little or too much powder will be put on the slab. In the former case more powder can be added from the bottle, but the mixing end of the spatula must not be used for this purpose as it will contaminate and spoil the whole bottle. Excess unused powder may only be returned to the bottle if you are certain that it has not been contaminated by any liquid or mixed cement on the slab.

A cool *thick* glass slab should be used for mixing zinc phosphate cement. Thin slabs are warmed by the nurse's hand and can make the cement set too quickly.

Uses

A thick mix sets rapidly and is used as a temporary filling and cavity lining; and also to block out undercuts in crown or inlay preparations. As it is so adhesive, instruments used for inserting and manipulating it in a cavity are dipped in alcohol beforehand to prevent cement sticking to them.

A thin mix sets more slowly and is used to cement inlays, crowns, bridges and orthodontic bands into place.

Advantages

The advantage of this cement is that it sets very hard in a few minutes and therefore makes a sound lining for permanent fillings; and a durable temporary filling. Furthermore, its adhesive nature makes it satisfactory for cementing (*luting*) prefabricated restorations.

Disadvantages

In deep cavities it is irritant, and in these cases a sublining of calcium hydroxide is inserted before the zinc phosphate cement. Otherwise a different lining must be used. Zinc phosphate cement will not adhere to a damp cavity. Unless saliva can be kept away, the lining will fail.

Polycarboxylate cement

Polycarboxylate cement (for example *Durelon*) is prepared by mixing powder and liquid with a spatula on a glass slab or paper pad. The powder consists mainly of *zinc oxide*; the liquid is *polyacrylic acid*.

Many cements using polyacrylic acid have introduced replacement of the liquid by water. Polyacrylic acid, which is the normal liquid component, is dehydrated and included with the powder instead. The cement is then prepared by simply mixing the powder with water in the normal way (for example *Poly-F Plus*). The advantage of this *anhydrous* system is that only one bottle of material is needed; and there is no liquid to deteriorate, or to be used up too soon, or left over when the powder bottle is empty. Furthermore the normal liquid is rather viscous, difficult to dispense from the bottle and difficult to mix. Mixing with water is much easier and quicker.

Polycarboxylate cement may be prepared as a thin mix for cementing, or thick mix for lining. A measure is supplied by the manufacturer for dispensing correct amounts of powder. Instruments are dipped in alcohol or dry cement powder to prevent cement sticking to them; and are easier to clean afterwards if they are washed in water before the cement sets.

Uses

It is an alternative to zinc phosphate cement.

Advantages

It is less irritant than zinc phosphate cement and far more adhesive. For these reasons many operators prefer it to zinc phosphate for cementing inlays, crowns and orthodontic bands.

Disadvantages

It can be rather difficult to manipulate as it is so adhesive.

Calcium hydroxide

Proprietary products, such as *Dycal* or *Dropsin*, come in the form of a powder and liquid or as pastes which are mixed together on a pad or glass slab. If a non-setting application is required, it can be prepared by mixing calcium hydroxide powder and water into a paste on a glass slab or in a **Dappen's pot**.

Uses

As calcium hydroxide is non-irritant and compatible with all filling materials, it is used as a universal cavity lining. It promotes the formation of secondary dentine and the repair of hard tissue. It is also used for pulp capping, pulpotomy and other root treatment procedures (Chapter 24).

Advantages

Calcium hydroxide is the best lining material for non-metallic fillings as it has no deleterious effect on them or the pulp.

Disadvantages

In deep cavities, with metal fillings, it can only be used as a sub-lining as it forms too thin a layer to insulate the pulp against thermal irritation. Another lining must be inserted on top of the calcium hydroxide to provide a thicker layer of insulation against the conduction of heat or cold through metal fillings. In shallow cavities, calcium hydroxide alone is a satisfactory lining for metal fillings.

Gutta-percha

Gutta-percha (GP) is supplied as pink or white sticks which are softened over a flame and a portion is then inserted in the cavity. Once in the cavity it hardens very quickly and can be smoothed over with cotton wool soaked in a solvent such as *chloroform* or *Oil of Cajuput* (eucalyptus oil). Petroleum jelly smeared on the fingers will prevent GP sticking to them.

Uses

GP was once used as a temporary filling between visits for gold inlays but nowadays it is only used as an emergency temporary filling. Its main use in dentistry is in the form of ready-made points for permanent root canal fillings. Apart from fillings it is sometimes used to test the response of a tooth to heat, by placing some hot GP against the crown.

Black gutta-percha is used to form a soft lining for **Gunning splints** in the treatment of jaw fractures; and as a temporary plug or obturator for cleft palates and cyst cavities (Chapter 27). It is softened in the same way as the sticks by gentle heating.

Advantages

The advantage of GP is its simplicity. It requires no mixing; hardens immediately; and can be painlessly removed from a cavity with a warmed excavator, without any need for drilling.

Disadvantages

It is too soft to withstand a heavy bite, and decomposes if left in a cavity too long.

Practical examination

One of the two tests set in the practical examination often consists of mixing a cement, cavity lining or temporary filling material. For all these, observance of the following procedure is recommended:

1 Before starting your mix tell the examiner that you wish to wash your hands and wear a pair of operating gloves.
2 Select correct materials and mixing instrument.
3 Dispense correct amounts of powder and liquid.
Replace the bottle caps immediately.
Ask for the manufacturer's instructions if you are unfamiliar with the brand provided.
4 Dispense liquid on to centre of the mixing slab or pad. This confines the mixing area to the centre and avoids the embarrassment of losing some of your mix over the edge.
5 Cease mixing *immediately* the consistency is correct.
Collect the mix on to a clean area of the slab.
Wipe the mixing instrument and present your mix and the instrument to the examiner.
6 If you are dissatisfied with your mix, tell the examiner what is wrong with it and what its effect would be; for example, insufficient powder dispensed → mix too thin → would set too slowly → acidity may irritate pulp.
Offer to start again.

Special requirements are necessary for the following different materials:

Zinc oxide and eugenol cement

Test: Prepare a sedative lining for a deep cavity

- Select a clean, dry glass slab and spatula; and correct bottles of powder and liquid, e.g. *Kalzinol*
- Dispense and proportion powder neatly
- Dispense two or three drops of liquid. Replace bottle caps
- Mix to a putty consistency

Zinc phosphate cement

Test: Cementing a crown

- Select correct bottles of powder and liquid; and a clean, dry, cool, *thick* glass slab and spatula
- Dispense and divide powder into small portions. Replace cap
- Dispense two or three drops of liquid. Replace bottle cap immediately
- Mix sufficient portions of powder into the liquid to give a smooth creamy consistency

Test: Cementing a three-unit bridge

The differences between the requirements for this mix and the previous one are:

(a) A three-unit bridge contains two crowns and therefore requires more cement. Dispense double the quantity of powder and liquid.
(b) As bridges require more time for insertion, the cement must not set so quickly.

- Cool a *thick* glass slab under *cold* running water and dry it thoroughly
- Proportion the powder so that it can be mixed into the liquid in small increments
- Ensure slow setting by mixing one tiny portion of powder into the liquid first. Then wait a little before adding the rest of the powder by increments to achieve a smooth creamy consistency

Test: Lining a cavity

The difference between this test and the previous two is that a thick mix, almost of putty consistency, is required for a cavity lining. Thus more powder is required, but otherwise the test is performed in the same way as that for cementing a single crown.

Polycarboxylate cement

Test: Prepare polycarboxylate for cementing an orthodontic band

- Select correct bottles of powder and liquid, for example, *Poly-F Plus*
- Invert powder bottle to fluff powder before use
- Overfill powder scoop and remove excess with spatula to give flat surface level with edge of scoop. Do not press down on powder
- Dispense one scoop of powder to two drops of water on mixing pad
- Divide powder into two halves
- Add one half to liquid; as soon as wetted add other half
- Mix rapidly to creamy consistency – 15 seconds

Calcium hydroxide

Test: Prepare a calcium hydroxide dressing for a deep cavity

- Select correct materials, for example, *Dycal*
- Dispense equal lengths of base and catalyst paste on mixing pad
- Mix pastes immediately by stirring with applicator until a uniform streak-free colour. Take no longer than ten seconds
- Wipe the applicator and present mix and applicator to the examiner.

Summary

Uses of temporary fillings

- Relief of pain
- Inability to complete permanent filling in one visit
- Between visits for inlays or crowns

Cavity linings

Protect pulp against:

1 Thermal shock ← metal fillings
2 Chemical irritation ← other fillings

Zinc oxide and eugenol cement

- Powder: Zinc oxide
- Liquid: Eugenol (oil of cloves)
- Requirements: Glass slab and spatula

Uses

- Temporary filling
- Non-irritant lining
- Sedative dressing

Zinc phosphate cement

- Powder: Zinc oxide
- Liquid: Phosphoric acid
- Requirements: Thick glass slab and spatula
                 Alcohol

Uses

- Temporary filling
- Lining
- Cementing (luting) inlays, crowns, orthodontic bands

Polycarboxylate cement

- Powder   Zinc oxide
- Liquid: Polyacrylic acid
- Requirements: Glass slab or paper pad and spatula
                  Alcohol

Uses

- Alternative to zinc phosphate

Calcium hydroxide

- Powder: Calcium hydroxide
- Liquid: Water
- Requirements: Glass slab or Dappen's pot
                  Spatula

Uses

- Safest lining for non-metallic fillings
- Sublining for metal fillings
- Root filling, pulp capping, pulpotomy

Gutta-percha

- Pink or white sticks; softened over flame
- Requirements: Petroleum jelly
                  Chloroform or oil of Cajuput

Uses

- Root filling
- Pulp vitality tests

Comparison of temporary fillings

FILLING	USES	ADVANTAGES	DISADVANTAGES
Zinc oxide and eugenol cement	1 Temporary filling 2 Lining deep cavities 3 Sedative dressing for dry socket and gingivectomy	1 Non-irritant 2 Can be used in deep cavities	1 Soft 2 Slow-setting
Zinc phosphate cement	1 Thick mix: cavity lining; temporary filling 2 Thin mix: adhesive cement for inlays and crowns	1 Hard 2 Rapid set 3 Adhesive	Irritant in deep cavities
Polycarboxylate	1 Thick mix: cavity lining; temporary filling 2 Thin mix: adhesive cement for inlays, crowns and orthodontic bands	1 Less irritant 2 More adhesive	May be difficult to manipulate
Calcium hydroxide	1 Cavity lining 2 Endodontic treatment	1 Non-irritant 2 Can be used in deepest cavities 3 Compatible with all materials	Sublining only, in deep cavities under metal fillings
Gutta-percha	1 Emergency temporary filling for inlay cavities 2 Permanent filling for root canals 3 Vitality tests 4 Temporary obturator for cleft palates and cyst cavities 5 Lining for Gunning splints	No mixing	1 Too soft 2 Decomposes eventually

20 Amalgam

Amalgam is the most widely used permanent filling in dentistry and is prepared by mixing an **alloy** with **mercury**. The main constituents of amalgam alloy are silver (at least 60%), copper and tin. It is supplied in the form of powder or pellets, or together with mercury in prepacked disposable capsules.

Older brands of alloy contain zinc and this results in excessive expansion of amalgam if it is contaminated with saliva. Modern brands of alloy are zinc-free and have a higher copper content to improve their strength and durability.

As amalgam is a plastic filling and a good conductor, cavities are undercut for retention; lined to insulate the pulp against thermal shock; and the entire cavity varnished to give a good marginal seal before inserting amalgam.

Very large cavities may have too little crown structure left for retentive undercuts. Dentine pins (page 288) are used for retention in such cases.

Recommendations for best long-term results are:

1   In shallow cavities, three coats of cavity varnish suffice as a lining and marginal seal.
2   Medium cavities are lined with ZOE or glass ionomer cement (Chapter 22), and sealed with three coats of varnish.
3   Calcium hydroxide is used as a sublining in deep cavities.

Preparation

The alloy and mercury are mixed together in a mechanical amalgamator. Prepacked disposable capsules are best as they contain a correct ratio of alloy to mercury and avoid any danger of mercury spillage. Alternatively the alloy and mercury are dispensed separately into the amalgamator.

Precautions

Nurses must take great care with amalgam as mercury is poisonous. Correct preparation is also essential as an unsatisfactory mix may cause weakness and adverse dimensional changes in the filling. This will not be apparent on completion of the filling but results in early failure caused by leakage at the margins or fracture of the amalgam.

The adverse dimensional changes are excessive expansion or contraction, leading to food stagnation and recurrent caries at the margins. Manufacturers' instructions must be strictly followed to obtain satisfactory results.

The precautions necessary to avoid danger to the nurse and ensure a satisfactory filling are:

1 Correct proportions of alloy and mercury. Too much mercury causes expansion and weakness; too little causes contraction
2 Correct mixing time. Prolonged mixing causes contraction; inadequate mixing causes expansion and weakness
3 Gloves must be worn when handling mercury or amalgam. Any contact with bare fingers allows mercury to be absorbed through the skin and may give rise to mercury poisoning
4 No contamination with saliva during insertion. This causes expansion caused by gas production if alloys containing zinc are used

Insertion

The cavity must be thoroughly dried and saliva kept away from the tooth by means of cotton wool rolls, absorbent pads and a saliva ejector; or better still by using rubber dam. Amalgam is introduced into the cavity by means of an **amalgam carrier**, and packed into place with hand **amalgam pluggers** (Figure 20.1) or a mechanical condenser. A few minutes are then available before it sets for trimming away excess amalgam, carving it to the original anatomy of the tooth with plastic instruments, and checking the occlusion. Any

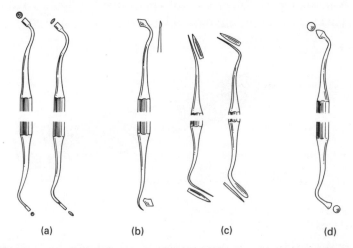

(a)   (b)   (c)   (d)

Figure 20.1 *Amalgam instruments.* (a) Serrated pluggers; (b) Carver; (c) Ward carvers; (d) Burnisher.

unused amalgam is kept in a sealed container, under old X-ray fixer, as it has considerable scrap value.

Although the initial set takes only a few minutes, it is not complete for several hours. The patient is therefore instructed to eat on the other side of the mouth for the rest of the day. At a subsequent visit the filling is polished with finishing burs, brushes and pumice paste. Amalgam finishing burs are made of steel for use in low-speed handpieces. They come in a variety of shapes but are recognized by having far more cutting blades than ordinary burs (Figure 20.2).

Blocked amalgam carriers cause much unnecessary trouble. To avoid blockage the nurse must always expel any residual amalgam from the nozzle before it sets.

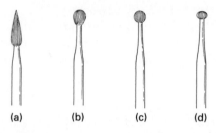

(a)   (b)   (c)   (d)

Figure 20.2   *Finishing burs.* (a) Flame; (b) Pear; (c) Round; (d) Oval.

Matrix outfits

Before amalgam can be inserted into a cavity involving two or more surfaces, such as mesial and occlusal, or mesial, occlusal and distal, a **matrix band** must be fitted round the tooth. This is to prevent amalgam escaping through the mesial or distal openings of the cavity during packing. The band is held tightly against the gum margin of the cavity by inserting a wooden or plastic wedge between the teeth. Various types of matrix outfit are available (Figure 20.3) and when packing is complete the band and wedge are removed.

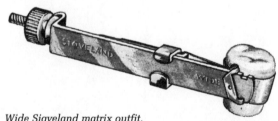

Figure 20.3   *Wide Siqveland matrix outfit.*

Advantages

The advantages of amalgam are its simplicity of use; great strength and durability.

Disadvantages

The colour of amalgam precludes its use in front teeth where it would show. As it is a good conductor, a lining is necessary in all but the shallowest cavities to prevent pain from sudden temperature changes, such as occur with very hot or cold drinks.

Mercury poisoning

It was formerly believed that mercury poisoning could only occur after several years of mishandling. However, it is now known that it can occur within a few months if a large quantity of mercury is spilled. Every nurse must accordingly understand the causes and prevention of hazards associated with the use of mercury and amalgam.

Poisoning can occur if the air contains mercury vapour. It will be breathed in and absorbed by the body. Similarly, if mercury or amalgam comes into contact with bare skin, it can be absorbed through the skin into the body. These are the two routes by which mercury poisoning could affect dental nurses: through skin contamination or the inhalation of mercury vapour.

Although the possibility of skin contamination is obvious when handling mercury or amalgam, the risk of inhaling mercury vapour is not. Both mercury and amalgam release mercury vapour at ordinary room temperature – and the higher the temperature, the more vapour is released. Mercury vapour is odourless and invisible, so it is of the utmost importance to keep all mercury and waste amalgam in sealed containers in a cool, well-ventilated place – not near a hot sterilizer or radiator.

Another source of mercury poisoning is the removal of old amalgam fillings. This releases a cloud of minute amalgam particles which can be inhaled or contaminate eyes and skin.

Apart from very rare cases of allergy, there is no evidence of danger to patients from their amalgam fillings.

Symptoms

The early symptoms of mercury poisoning may include headache, fatigue, irritability, nausea and diarrhoea. At this stage it is unlikely that mercury would be suspected. Later symptoms are tremor of the hands and visual defects such as double vision. The final stage is kidney failure.

Precautions

The routine use of gloves, mask and eye-wear for protection against cross-infection will also provide corresponding protection against amalgam hazards. Nurses are reassured that no danger exists if the following precautions are taken. However, they are so important that they are covered again, together with other occupational hazards, in Chapter 31.

To avoid absorption of mercury through the skin:

1 Always wear disposable gloves when handling mercury, mixing amalgam and cleaning amalgam instruments.
2 Do not wear open-toed shoes as the floor may be contaminated by spilled mercury or dropped amalgam.
3 Do not wear jewellery or a wrist watch as they may harbour particles of amalgam. Gold jewellery can be spoiled by contact with mercury or amalgam.

To avoid pollution of the air by mercury vapour:

1 Containers of mercury must be tightly sealed, and stored in a cool well-ventilated place.
2 When transferring mercury from a stock bottle, great care must be taken not to spill any. It is very difficult to find and recover mercury which has dropped on the floor or working surface.
3 Prepacked disposable capsules of mercury and alloy avoid any need to keep a stock of mercury.
4 For removal of old amalgam fillings, the use of a high-speed handpiece with diamond or tungsten carbide burs, water spray and efficient aspiration helps to reduce the aerosol of amalgam dust and mercury vapour; while the use of rubber dam will protect the patient. Surgery staff must wear masks, gloves and protective glasses throughout such procedures.
5 All traces of amalgam must be removed from instruments before sterilization, especially if a hot air oven is used.
6 Keep waste amalgam and mercury waste in a labelled, sealed, unbreakable container under old X-ray fixer solution.
7 Keep the surgery well ventilated.

Surgery hygiene

Much can be done to minimize any dangers of working with mercury by adopting the following recommendations:

1 Smoking, eating, drinking and the application of cosmetics should not take place in the surgery. Any of these actions could permit the absorption of mercury – from mercury vapour in the air or from contaminated hands.
2 The storage and handling of mercury should be confined to one particular part of the surgery, away from all sources of heat; or, better still, outside the surgery.

3 All handling of mercury and preparation of amalgam should be done over a drip tray (lined with kitchen foil) on a special work surface. A drip tray prevents the loss of spilled mercury and facilitates recovery. The work surface should not allow any spilled mercury to fall on the floor or roll into inaccessible places.
4 Any spillage of mercury must be reported to the dentist. Never be afraid to do this.
5 Special kits are available for the safe recovery of spilled mercury. Vacuum cleaners must never be used for this purpose as they vaporize any mercury they pick up and discharge it back into the surgery.
6 Floor coverings should not have any cracks or gaps in which mercury or amalgam can be trapped. Carpets should not be used.
7 Surgery equipment and plumbing should have easily accessible filter traps to collect particles of waste amalgam flushed through spittoons, aspirators or other suction apparatus. This waste should be collected and transferred to the surgery waste amalgam containers.
8 Waste amalgam should be saved for collection by authorized scrap-dealers for recycling. It must not be sent by post.
9 Efficient ventilation is essential at all times of the year. Avoid high surgery temperatures.
10 If, following a spillage of mercury or inadequate mercury hygiene, it is suspected that a risk of mercury poisoning exists, the public health authority should be notified so that tests can be carried out.

Mercury spillage

Accidental spillage of mercury or waste amalgam must always be reported to the dentist. If a spillage occurs, globules of mercury can be drawn up into a disposable intravenous syringe or bulb aspirator and transferred to a mercury container. Small globules can be absorbed by lead foil from X-ray film packets. Waste amalgam can be gathered with a damp paper towel.

Globules of mercury or particles of amalgam which are too small or too numerous to be recovered in this way can be rendered safe by smearing the contaminated area with a mercury absorbent paste. This consists of equal parts of *calcium oxide* and *flowers of sulphur* mixed into a paste with water. It should be left to dry and then removed with a wet disposable towel. Alternatively, a commercial mercury spillage kit may be used. Always wear disposable gloves for the recovery of mercury or amalgam.

Detection of mercury vapour

If a serious spillage occurs, or there are other reasons for suspecting mercury contamination in the surgery, tests are available for determining the amount of mercury vapour in the air. If such tests show an excessive concentration of mercury vapour, expert advice should be sought to trace and eradicate the cause. Hospital tests can also be arranged to check whether staff have absorbed dangerous amounts of mercury.

Practical examination

Prepare a matrix retainer (e.g. *Siqveland*) ready for an amalgam filling.

If you are unfamiliar with the matrix outfit provided, ask for the model you normally use. If it is not available, ask for the instructions on the outfit provided.

Select the correct width retainer and band for whichever tooth is specified. Choose a wide retainer and band if the test specifies a permanent molar; a narrow one for premolars and deciduous molars.

Fit the band on the retainer and adjust it to give a correct size loop for the tooth concerned.

Written examination

What are the uses of amalgam and what are its constituents? Describe the safe mixing and handling of this material.
Why might an amalgam restoration be lined and list the materials used for this purpose? (May 1995)

Describe the hazards associated with mercury in the surgery and the action to be taken in the event of a spillage. (May 1996)

Summary

Amalgam alloy

- Contains silver, tin, copper, zinc

Procedure

- Mechanical amalgamator
- Correct proportions of alloy and mercury
- Correct mixing time
- Adequate condensation
- No contact with skin → wear gloves
- No saliva contamination → expansion
- Keep waste amalgam and mercury waste in labelled, sealed, unbreakable container under old X-ray fixer solution
- Arrange collection of waste amalgam for recycling

Requirements

- Undercut cavity
- Lining
- Cavity varnish
- Mechanical amalgamator
- Disposable gloves
- Matrix outfit and wedges
- Amalgam carriers
- Amalgam pluggers and carvers
- Plastic instruments

Mercury poisoning

- Absorbed through skin or inhaled
- Keep mercury in a cool, well-ventilated place in tightly sealed containers
- Prepare amalgam over drip tray on special work surface
- Use prepacked disposable capsules of mercury and alloy
- Never permit contact of amalgam with bare skin; always wear disposable gloves
- Wear mask, gloves and glasses, and use aspirator, during removal of old amalgam fillings
- Wearing gloves, remove all traces of amalgam from instruments before sterilization

- Do not flush waste amalgam particles down surgery spittoons or sinks
- Store waste amalgam and mercury waste in unbreakable sealed and labelled container under old X-ray fixer
- Do not wear open-toed shoes, jewellery or wrist watch
- No carpets
- Keep surgery well ventilated
- Report mercury spillage to dentist

Mercury spillage

1 Must be reported
2 Collect mercury with disposable syringe, bulb aspirator or lead foil
3 Gather amalgam with damp paper towel
4 Remove remainder with mercury absorbent paste

21 Composite Fillings

Composite filling materials are tooth-coloured and are accordingly used for permanent fillings in front teeth. They can also be used for filling back teeth but do not wear as well as metal fillings. Consequently amalgam is still the most widely used material for back teeth.

Composite fillings consist of an inorganic filler in a resin binder. The inorganic filler, which acts as a strengthener, may consist of powdered glass, quartz, silica, or other ceramic particles. This is incorporated into the resin binder to produce a composite filling.

Composite filling materials

The composites used for permanent restorations contain a filler, resin binder and a catalyst. When the catalyst is activated it makes the filling set. The original composites, such as *Adaptic*, were supplied as two components: one containing a resin binder and filler; the other containing a catalyst. Mixing the two together activates the catalyst and makes the filling set. This method of mixing two components to produce setting is called a **chemical-cure** (self-curing) system. However, it has been almost superseded by materials containing a catalyst which is activated by exposure to light (e.g. *Tetric*). This setting method is called a **light-cure** system.

Apart from these two curing systems, composites also differ according to the teeth for which they are intended. Brands made specially for filling front teeth have a much finer grade of inorganic filler which improves their appearance and makes them easier to polish. These are called *microfine* composites. Brands intended for both front and back teeth contain a more durable filler, making them more resistant to masticatory wear. These are called *hybrid* composites and are more difficult to polish.

Chemical-cure system

Chemical-cure composites such as *Adaptic* and *Concise* are supplied as two pots of paste. One pot of paste is a mixture of resin binder and inorganic filler. The other contains a catalyst which acts on the resin to make the filling set. Different shades of paste are available and a shade guide may be provided.

A disposable plastic double-ended spatula is used to transfer the desired quantity of paste from one pot to a paper mixing pad. The other end of the spatula is then used to place an equal quantity of paste from the second pot on to the pad. It is essential to use different ends of the spatula for each pot; if the same end is used, the second pot will be ruined by contamination from the first. The two pastes are then mixed together with the same spatula to an even consistency. For mixing, it does not matter which end of the spatula is used but it must be discarded afterwards.

Light-cure system

Unlike chemical-cure composites, which cannot set until two components are mixed together, light-cure materials, such as *Durafill*, *Pekafill*, have introduced an ideal setting system to dentistry. All they need to make them set is exposure to bright light. A single component contains the resin binder, filler and a special catalyst which is only activated when a bright light shines on it. A special lamp is used to produce a spot of intensely bright light which activates the catalyst and makes the material set in about a minute. No mixing is required. The unique advantage of this system is that the dentist has complete control over setting. The dentist alone decides when it should set; and when ready, all that needs to be done is to shine a light on it.

The single component of light-cure composites enables manufacturers to supply their product in multidose dispensing syringes, or single dose capsules (compules) with an injector gun; thereby allowing a dentist to inject the filling directly into a prepared cavity. The dentist then has as much time as necessary to adapt, contour and trim the filling material before commanding it to set. In this way, the time-consuming removal of excess material which has set rock-hard can be avoided.

Just a thin layer of composite is needed to fill a shallow cavity and this only requires one application of the curing light. In larger cavities this would only cure the surface layer as the light cannot penetrate thick layers. In order to obtain full curing in such cases, the composite is inserted in a thin layer, then light-cured before adding another thin layer and light-curing again. This sequence is repeated incrementally until the cavity is completely filled with fully cured composite. One way of saving time in such cases is to partially fill a large cavity with a thick layer of lining material, followed by a surface layer of composite which can be cured in one application of the light. The best lining material for this purpose is glass ionomer cement which is described in Chapter 22.

Manufacturers provide special lamps to deliver a concentrated spot of bright blue light on the tooth concerned; together with special orange glasses or shields for patients or staff who find the light too bright for comfort. Light-cure materials are available for most uses of composites, and a new generation of cavity lining materials.

Rapid advances in dental materials technology are overcoming the limited penetration of curing lights. One solution is the use of **dual-cure** composites which utilize light and chemical-cure systems in one material. This allows the surface of a large restoration to be light-cured while the inner part undergoes a chemical cure. Another solution may be a **laser**-curing light which could penetrate the full thickness of a filling to produce an instantaneous complete set.

Technique

Composites are not adhesive and may irritate the pulp. An undercut cavity and lining are therefore required. Calcium hydroxide is a suitable lining for all these materials. The correct shade of composite is then selected.

For insertion of the filling it is best to use special composite filling instruments which have non-stick tips. As composite fillings are so hard, they can abrade ordinary metal instruments and result in a filling of poor appearance caused by the incorporation of metal particles. The filling is manipulated with a flat plastic instrument and contoured to the tooth with a clear polyester (*Mylar*) matrix strip, held in place with a crocodile clip matrix clamp (Figure 21.1). When set, it is trimmed and polished, but special finishing agents are needed as it is so hard. Tungsten carbide or diamond finishing burs or abrasive stones are used with waterspray for trimming excess material. White stones, fine abrasive discs, strips and rubber points are used for polishing (Figure 18.9). Manufacturers recommend the best polishing procedures for their own brands and these should be followed to give optimum results.

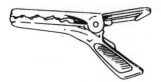

Figure 21.1   *Crocodile matrix clamp.*

In cavities which cannot be undercut sufficiently to provide adequate retention, most brands have their own particular systems for bonding composite directly to dentine by means of the special bonding agents described in Chapter 22.

Acid etching

Composite materials are far more versatile then their commonest use of filling a conventional undercut cavity in a front tooth. Their strength and durability allow them to be used for the restoration of fractured incisors and fissure sealing. Retention for these cases is obtained by using an **acid etch** technique, which bonds the composite directly to enamel.

Enamel is made retentive by applying phosphoric acid gel for up to a minute. This etches the surface by attacking the enamel prisms; and produces a retentive surface which is full of microscopic pits like a honeycomb. When the filling material is applied it flows into these pits and sets into hard tags, which effectively lock it to the enamel surface.

Surgery procedure for acid etching is as follows:

1   The tooth surface is cleaned with polishing paste in a rubber cup.
2   It is then washed with water and dried with compressed air. It is most important to check that the air is not contaminated with oil from the compressor. This can be done by holding a napkin over the syringe nozzle – whereupon any oil will show up on the napkin.
3   Any exposed dentine is protected from acid by coating with a calcium hydroxide lining material.
4   The acid gel is applied with a cotton wool bud, fine paintbrush or special dispensing syringe. The gel is distinctively coloured to ensure that it is confined to the required area.

Acid is caustic and must contact nothing but enamel. To achieve this, the tooth is isolated with cotton wool rolls and napkins, and full saliva control is essential. The best way is to use rubber dam. Protective glasses and a waterproof apron should be worn by supine patients. Spilt acid must be washed off with water.
5   After exposure to acid, the tooth is thoroughly washed with water and carefully dried with compressed air. It should now have a matt white frosted appearance. If so, the enamel has been successfully etched and is ready for application of the composite; but it must remain perfectly dry and free of saliva for successful bonding.

Restoration of fractured incisors

Before the acid etching technique was introduced, the most satisfactory way of restoring fractured incisors was by fitting a porcelain jacket crown. Unfortunately, this is unsuitable for children as the pulp chambers of immature teeth are too large and crown preparation may cause pulp damage. This, together with the fact that incisor fractures most commonly occur during childhood, meant that some other form of temporary crown had to be used – and these were of relatively poor appearance.

Composite filling materials and acid etching have transformed the treatment of fractured incisors. Small fractures in children and adults can be permanently restored in this way. Although porcelain jacket crowns remain the best treatment for extensive fractures, acid etched restorations provide children with a satisfactory alternative until such time as the tooth is ready for jacket crown preparation. Other injuries to children's teeth are covered in Chapters 16 and 24.

Cavity preparation for acid etched restorations is minimal and painless. After lining any exposed dentine with calcium hydroxide, the surface to be restored is outlined by cutting a tiny ledge in the surrounding enamel. It is then acid etched and a composite filling material is applied in a clear plastic crown form. When it has set, any excess is trimmed off and the restoration is polished where necessary.

The acid etch/composite filling technique is also used for building up malformed or misshapen teeth to improve their appearance; for the direct bonding of orthodontic brackets, porcelain veneers and small bridges (Chapters 23 and 28); and for the construction of temporary splints. The latter are mentioned on page 206, and are made by bonding a length of wire or fibreglass tape to the loose tooth and its neighbours with a light-cure composite.

Fissure sealing

As mentioned in Chapter 17, fissure sealing is a caries prevention measure. Occlusal fissures are natural stagnation areas where caries commonly occurs. If these fissures can be filled soon after eruption, the occlusal surface should then stay free of caries.

In the past, fissure filling was done by preparing an undercut cavity and using amalgam; but, as a preventive measure, this had the disadvantage of having to cut a cavity in sound enamel. The advent of new materials, such as composites and glass ionomer cement, allows fissure sealing to be done without any cavity preparation.

As composite materials are not adhesive, retention is obtained by acid etching the fissures. Whichever material is used, any existing caries is removed and the cavity is filled at the same time as the sound fissures. The sealant is introduced into the fissures and seals off these stagnation areas.

The application of fissure sealants should be done as soon as possible after eruption but requires a completely dry occlusal surface. This is difficult to achieve in young children but may be overcome by applying chlorhexidine varnish (Chapter 11), as a temporary seal, until a child is co-operative enough to permit the attainment of a dry field for sufficient time.

Unfilled resins

All the composite filling materials described so far consist of a resin binder incorporating an inert inorganic filler. They are accordingly called **filled resins**. A catalyst makes the resin set, while the filler remains unchanged throughout. This gives the unset material its paste consistency, and the set filling its hardness and durability.

Thus it is only the resin and catalyst which are actually involved in the setting process. Several brands of composite make use of this fact by providing a liquid base containing just the resin without a filler. This is called an **unfilled resin** and sets in the same way as all the others by using the same catalyst. These unfilled resins (e.g. *Delton*), are available in chemical or light-cure brands.

The advantage of an unfilled resin is its liquid consistency. Both resin and catalyst are liquids and the mixture can be easily flowed over acid etched enamel, into fissures, or mixed with a filled resin paste to give any desired consistency.

Unfilled resins are accordingly used as wetting agents, fissure sealants, and for surface glazing. As wetting agents they are flowed over acid etched enamel to ensure good penetration of the surface and a durable bond. A filled resin is then applied on top. It seems reasonable to assume that the use of a wetting agent would produce a better bond than direct application of a filled resin; but in practice it does not seem to make much difference.

Fissure sealants

Fissure sealants are unfilled resins, such as *Delton*, or filled resins which have been thinned by adding some unfilled resin (e.g. *Helioseal F*). Unfilled resins are flowed into the acid etched fissures, but filled resins are inserted with a packing instrument.

Surface glazing

As mentioned above, unfilled resins can be used as wetting agents to form the innermost layer of acid-etched composite restorations. However, they can also be applied as the outermost layer for glazing or 'varnishing' the surface of a restoration e.g. *Ketac Glaze*. They provide a smooth shiny surface and improve the appearance of older brands of material which are more difficult to polish than modern microfine brands. They can also be used to restore the appearance of a surface which has become stained. Another useful adoption of this property is mentioned on page 277.

Advantages of composite materials

They are stronger and more durable than any other tooth-coloured filling material. Their adhesion to acid etched enamel makes them suitable for the restoration of fractured incisors and for fissure sealing.

Chemical-cure composites are simple to mix as the amounts of each paste are not critical; while light-cure materials are easier still and give the dentist complete control over setting. Composites can also be used for building up the core of a crown preparation where too much of the original tooth structure has been lost; and for the direct bonding of small bridges and porcelain veneers (Chapter 23), and orthodontic brackets (Chapter 28).

Disadvantages

Although composites are hard enough for filling back teeth they are less resistant to wear than metal fillings. Furthermore their use for this purpose is, compared with amalgam, more difficult and time-consuming.

Written examination

Describe the procedure of, and the role of the dental nurse in, restoring an anterior tooth with a light-cured composite.

What precautions should be taken to avoid hazards to the patient and the dental team during this procedure? (November 1996)

Summary

Composite filling materials

1   Filled resins (*Pekafill, Adaptic*) consist of:

                          inorganic filler

  (a) base paste ⟨

                        resin binder

  (b) catalyst

2   Unfilled resins (*Delton, Ketac Glaze*) consist of:

  (a) base liquid ← resin
  (b) catalyst

Setting

- Chemical-cure → *Adaptic, Concise*
- Light-cure → *Pekafill, Durafill*
- Dual-cure → *ABC*

Types Microfine → front teeth e.g. *Silux Plus*

Hybrid → all teeth e.g. *Tetric*

Uses

- Permanent fillings
- Fractured incisors
- Enamel defects   } Filled resin
- Reshaping teeth
- Building up crown cores

- Fissure sealing
- Surface glazing } Unfilled resin
- Wetting agent

Bonding
- orthodontic brackets
- porcelain veneers
- direct bridges and splints

Conventional filling technique

1 Undercut cavity
2 Calcium hydroxide lining
3 Select correct shade
4 Insert with non-stick instruments
5 Apply transparent matrix band or strip
6 Trim excess under waterspray:
   tungsten carbide or diamond finishing burs
   abrasive stones
7 Polish under waterspray:
   white stones
   abrasive discs
   polishing wheels
   hand abrasive strips

Acid etching

Phosphoric acid → enamel → microscopic retentive honeycomb.

1 Polish tooth
2 Dry with oil-free air
3 Line exposed dentine with calcium hydroxide
4 Acid etch → white matt frosted surface
5 Wash with water
6 Dry thoroughly
7 Apply composite

Fissure sealing

Prevent occlusal caries:

1 Acid etch
2 Apply unfilled resin; or thinned filled resin

Advantages of composite fillings

- Strength
- Durability
- Difficult restorations possible ← acid etch technique
- Fissure sealing
- Surface glazing
- Bonding applications

Disadvantages

Less useful for permanent fillings in back teeth.

22   Glass Ionomer Cement

Glass ionomer cement (GIC), also known as glass polyalkenoate, consists of a powder and liquid which are mixed together on a paper pad. The powder is a glass-like mixture of **aluminosilicates**. The liquid contains **polyacrylic acid** (or polymaleic acid) and is similar to polycarboxylate cement liquid. Calcium hydroxide linings are unnecessary unless the cavity is very deep.

Uses

GIC has many different uses which depend on three outstanding properties:

1   It releases fluoride and thereby prevents the recurrence of caries in and around the cavity.
2   It bonds directly to enamel, dentine and cementum without acid etching. This chemical bond to tooth substance means that undercuts are not essential and makes it suitable for filling unretentive cavities; fissure sealing; a dentine substitute for restoring the excessive loss of tooth substance; and as an adhesive cement for inlays, crowns and orthodontic bands.
3   It can itself be acid etched. This allows it to be used as a retentive lining for composite fillings.

Permanent fillings

GIC is not strong enough for filling cavities which are exposed to the full force of mastication. Thus it is unsuitable for class I or II fillings (Chapter 18) in back teeth. Although GIC is tooth-coloured, its appearance is not as good as composite fillings as it is slightly darker and less translucent. Composites accordingly remain the material of choice for class III and IV fillings in front teeth.

The most useful application of GIC is for the permanent filling of class V (cervical) cavities anywhere in the mouth. Such cavities are naturally saucer-shaped, unretentive and not easy to undercut; and were accordingly very difficult to fill satisfactorily. GIC, such as *ChemFil*, *Ketac-Fil*, has provided the answer to this problem. Its darker colour is less important in cervical cavities in front teeth and does not matter in back teeth. Minimal cavity preparation is required and the filling provides its own retention by bonding directly to the cavity.

Cavities in deciduous teeth are also very suitable for filling with GIC as its natural retention allows minimal cavity preparation. Although it cannot withstand prolonged masticatory abrasion, the limited lifespan of deciduous teeth lessens the importance of this weakness.

Wherever and whenever it is used, its ability to release fluoride helps prevent further caries and, in that respect, it is superior to all other filling materials.

Cavity lining

As GIC is not very irritant to the pulp, and bonds naturally to dentine, it is suitable as a cavity lining beneath any permanent filling material. It is the strongest of all cavity linings and, together with calcium hydroxide, is superseding the traditional lining cements described in Chapter 19.

It is particularly useful for composite fillings. As shown in Chapter 21, composites can be bonded directly to enamel by etching it with phosphoric acid. This same procedure can also be applied to the surface of GIC. The entire area of exposed dentine is lined with a thick layer of GIC; then the lining and enamel cavity margins are etched to provide a bond for the top layer of composite. This completes the permanent filling and provides a surface with better strength and appearance than that of GIC alone. As the GIC is sandwiched between dentine and composite, such fillings are called sandwich restorations (Figure 22.1).

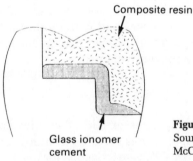

Composite resin

Glass ionomer cement

Figure 22.1 *Sandwich restoration.* Source: *Applied Dental Materials* (7th edn). J.F. McCabe, Blackwell Science Ltd, Oxford.

There is an alternative technique for bonding a layer of composite to GIC. Some of the dentine-bonding agents mentioned on page 278 can bond to unetched GIC as well as composites. After applying the bond to GIC, a layer of unfilled resin is applied on top of that, followed by the filled resin. Thus the dentine bonding agent adheres on one side to unetched GIC, and on the other to a layer of composite.

Dentine substitute

The restoration of teeth which have lost much of their natural crown poses a retention problem. One way in which this can be overcome is to replace most of the lost dentine with amalgam to form a core on which a gold veneer crown (Chapter 23) can be fitted. However, amalgam does not bond to tooth substance, so retention in such cases often requires the insertion of pins (page 288) into the remaining dentine prior to building up an amalgam core.

GIC avoids the need for a pinned amalgam core as it bonds directly to dentine and can therefore be used as a dentine substitute. The core is accordingly made entirely of GIC without pinning; and when set it is trimmed to shape ready for the crown impression.

Reinforced glass ionomer cement

GIC can be strengthened by adding powdered silver to the cement powder. This is done by the manufacturer and the silver/glass powder is then mixed with the liquid in the normal way. The resultant cement is stronger and is called a **cermet**, (e.g. *Ketac-Silver*). The silver component makes the cement too dark to use as an anterior filling, so cermets are mainly used as dentine substitutes for the preparation of crown cores, or as cavity linings in back teeth beneath a surface layer of composite or amalgam.

Adhesive cement

Inlays, crowns and orthodontic bands can be cemented into place with zinc phosphate or polycarboxylate cement. But GIC (e.g. *Aquacem*), is better as it forms a stronger bond with tooth substance. Furthermore it is the only luting cement which releases fluoride and thereby has a **cariostatic** (caries preventive) effect.

Fissure sealing

Fissures can be sealed with composites or GIC. The advantage of composites is that no cavity preparation is required as unfilled resins can penetrate acid etched fissures. GIC is too viscous for that and it is consequently necessary to widen the fissure slightly with a pointed diamond bur. It can then be flowed into the fissure.

The advantages of GIC for fissure sealing are its fluoride release which provides a cariostatic effect; and no need for acid etching. However, in practice, the two materials can be combined. If a part of the occlusal fissure system has already become carious, that part is filled with GIC. The remaining sound fissures and the GIC are acid etched and the entire fissure system is then sealed with composite.

Technique

Although GIC forms a direct *chemical* bond with tooth substance, it can only do so if the tooth surface is clean and free of cavity preparation debris. Cavities are accordingly *conditioned* with polyacrylic acid before inserting the cement. This must not be confused with the use of phosphoric acid for acid etching, which only provides a *mechanical* bond.

Complete saliva control is necessary at all stages and this is best achieved by the use of rubber dam. After preparing the cavity, the polyacrylic acid conditioner is applied for ten seconds, then thoroughly washed off and dried before insertion of the GIC.

Mixing

GIC may come in the form of powder and liquid which are mixed on a paper pad. The liquid constituent (polyacrylic acid) is usually dehydrated and included in the powder. This **anhydrous** version (e.g. *Legend*), only needs mixing with water. Alternatively it can come in the form of a capsule containing powder and liquid (e.g. *ChemFil Superior*), for use in a mechanical mixer. Manufacturers of hand-mixed brands supply measuring spoons to ensure that the correct proportions are used and proper consistency achieved – creamy for cementing and fissure sealing; thicker for fillings and linings. As GIC is so hard, an abrasion-resistant spatula, such as *agate* or stainless steel, should be used for hand-mixing.

Insertion

Very deep cavities are lined with calcium hydroxide before conditioning the cavity walls. Hand-mixed materials are inserted and manipulated with non-stick plastic instruments, whereas mechanically mixed brands are provided with a special injection gun. Permanent fillings are contoured to the tooth surface with a clear matrix strip which is held in place with a crocodile clip. Special shaped and contoured adhesive matrices are available for cervical cavities.

It is essential to avoid moisture contamination while setting, and to avoid dehydration through water loss after setting. Thus the cement must be covered with a waterproof varnish immediately the matrix is removed. A convenient varnish for this purpose is a light-cured unfilled composite, such as *Ketac Glaze*.

Finishing

Any removal of excess material, or polishing, should be deferred for at least one day as the heat produced during such instrumentation may dehydrate and weaken the filling. Ideally, trimming and polishing should be avoided altogether by inserting an exact amount of cement and relying on the matrix strip to give a polished surface. However, this cannot always be achieved and some finishing may be necessary. The cement manufacturers' recommended abrasive discs, strips and white stones should be used and dehydration avoided by lubricating the abrasives with petroleum jelly.

Advantages of glass ionomer cement

It forms a chemical bond with tooth tissue and releases fluoride. This natural adhesion and cariostatic effect makes it the best material for cervical fillings; lining unretentive cavities; and for cementing inlays, crowns and orthodontic bands. These same properties permit its use as a crown core without any need for pinning; and as a fissure sealant. As it can be acid-etched it forms a retentive lining for composite restorations.

Disadvantages

As it is darker and more opaque than composites, GIC is unsuitable for filling front teeth in young patients. It is not hard enough to withstand masticatory stress and is therefore unsuitable for permanent fillings involving the occlusal surface of back teeth.

Compomers

As the name implies, compomer is a term used to describe some of the new materials which combine the advantages of composites and GIC (e.g. *Dyract, Compoglass*). They are the latest generation of tooth-coloured filling and lining materials; and utilize the light-cure resin setting system, appearance and strength of composites; the fluoride release of GIC; and special bonding agents. Similar modified GIC materials, incorporating light-cure resins, also release fluoride but do not require bonding agents. These new developments combining various components of GIC, composites and bonding agents have not been in use long enough to assess their value.

Practical examination

Test: Filling

Mix the GIC (e.g. *ChemFil Superior*), for a class V filling:

1 Select correct bottles of powder and liquid
2 Invert the powder bottle to fluff the powder
3 Overfill the powder scoop and skim off excess with spatula to give a flat surface level with edge of scoop. Do not press powder into scoop
4 Dispense in ratio of one scoop of powder to one drop of water on the mixing pad or glass slab
5 Divide powder into two halves
6 Mix first half with the water in five seconds, using agate or stainless steel spatula
7 Add the second half and mix rapidly and thoroughly for ten seconds to a thick consistency, but retaining shine on surface
8 Complete mix should not take longer than 20 seconds

Test: Cementing

Mix the GIC (e.g. *AquaCem*), for cementing a jacket crown:

1–3 As for filling
4 Dispense in ratio of one scoop of powder to two drops of water, on the mixing pad or a glass slab
5 As for filling
6 Add one half to the water. As soon as it is wetted, add second half
7 Mix thoroughly and very quickly to smooth creamy consistency
8 Complete mix should not take longer than 15 seconds
9 A special spatula is not required

Written examination

Describe how the dental nurse would assist in the preparation, placement and finishing of a glass-ionomer restoration. (November 1994)

Summary

- Powder: aluminosilicate
- Liquid: polyacrylic or polymaleic acid

Uses

- Filling cervical cavities in all teeth
- Filling front teeth in older patients
- Filling deciduous teeth
- Cavity lining
- Crown core
- Cementing inlays, crowns and orthodontic bands
- Fissure sealing

Requirements

- Clean dry cavity
- Mixing pad and agate or stainless steel spatula; or mechanical mixer
- Cavity conditioner
- Non-stick plastic instruments for insertion
- Matrix strips
- Varnish

Advantages

- Direct bonding to tooth substance → fill and line unretentive cavities and act as dentine substitute
- Cariostatic ← releases fluoride
- Non-irritant to pulp – except in deepest cavities
- Suitable lining for all permanent fillings

Disadvantages

- Too dark and opaque for front teeth in young patients
- Cannot withstand heavy bite in posterior teeth

Compomers

Combination of composite and GIC.

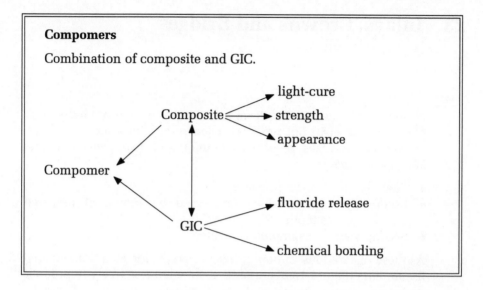

23 Inlays, Crowns and Bridges

Plastic fillings such as amalgam and composites are normally completed in one visit; but preconstructed restorations such as inlays, crowns and bridges require a minimum of two visits and one laboratory stage:

- First visit: tooth prepared
- Laboratory: restoration constructed on model of prepared tooth
- Second visit: restoration cemented

As these restorations cannot utilize undercuts for retention, tapered fissure burs (Figure 18.8) are used as they are less likely to produce undercuts. Any undercuts on the preparation are blocked out with the lining cement.

Gold inlays

Gold inlays are used as alternatives to amalgam fillings. They are generally confined to teeth which have lost cusps or are otherwise too weak to be satisfactorily restored with amalgam. Small uncomplicated cavities do not usually warrant the extra time and expense of gold inlays. The advantages of gold are that it does not tarnish and has great strength, which is far superior to that of any other material. Consequently much less tooth substance need be drilled away. Gold is also the material of choice for crowns where it does not show.

The disadvantages are the extra time and expense involved and, like amalgam, its unsuitability for front teeth where it would show.

First visit

The cavity is made retentive with parallel cavity walls and an impression is taken with an elastic material. This is sent to the laboratory, together with a recording of the occlusion. A temporary filling is then inserted and the patient is given an appointment for fitting the inlay. Gutta-percha is a convenient temporary filling as it can be removed in one piece without drilling, but most dentists prefer modern light-cure materials, such as *Fermit, Clip*.

Laboratory

A technician uses the impression to make a model of the prepared tooth and then constructs a wax inlay on the model. This is done by softening a stick of blue **inlay wax** over a flame and pressing it into the inlay cavity on the model. The wax is trimmed to the original shape of the tooth with a *Ward carver* (Figure 20.1) to make a **wax pattern** of the required restoration. The wax pattern is then cast in gold, polished, and returned to the surgery for fitting.

Second visit

The temporary filling is removed and the inlay fitted. Before cementing the inlay, the occlusion is checked and any high spots are removed with a carborundum stone. The edges are burnished to give a good marginal fit and the inlay is cemented with GIC, zinc phosphate or polycarboxylate.

This procedure, whereby the wax pattern is made in the laboratory from an impression, is called the **indirect method** of construction. The **direct method** is a procedure whereby a dentist makes the wax pattern in the surgery and the technician casts it directly in gold. For all but the simplest inlays, the direct method can be far more difficult and time-consuming for a dentist than taking an impression. For this reason it has been virtually superseded by the indirect method. All crowns and bridges are made by an indirect method.

Impressions

The elastic impression materials used for inlays, crowns and bridges are called **elastomers**, for example, *Aquasil, President, Optosil* and *Xantopren.* They consist of two components – base and catalyst – which are mixed together and loaded into an impression tray (Chapter 27). In the mouth they set into a solid rubbery consistency. There are many different types of elastomer, such as **silicones** and **polyethers**, but they are all used in much the same way.

Mixing

For hand-mixing the base and catalyst are supplied in tubes of different colour. They are mixed with a spatula on a pad, in the recommended proportions, to give a mix of uniform colour. Most makes are available in two different consistencies: *light-bodied* for syringing over a prepared tooth; and *heavy-bodied* for filling the impression tray.

Some brands use a putty for the heavy-bodied material. This is mixed with its catalyst by kneading in a gloved hand, but some of these materials cannot be used with every brand of glove.

Most elastomers are also supplied in cartridges which are inserted into a special gun and are extruded, ready-mixed, directly into the cavity or impression tray. This is obviously the most convenient, quickest and accurate procedure and is superseding traditional hand-mixing methods.

Technique

Before the impression is taken, the gum must be eased away from the cavity margin to keep it dry and permit a good impression. This is done by packing the gum margin with **gingival retraction cord** which consists of string or cord impregnated with an astringent, such as adrenaline or alum. It shrinks the gum away from the cavity margins, so that the impression material can reach every part of the preparation.

With such a wide range of these impression materials there is a corresponding range of techniques, but a typical procedure is as follows:

1 Pack gingival retraction cord into the gingival crevice
2 Mix light-bodied material and load into syringe
3 Mix heavy-bodied material and load into tray
4 Remove retraction cord
5 Syringe light-bodied material into cavity, ensuring that it covers the entire preparation and its margins
6 Insert impression tray of heavy-bodied material
7 Remove tray when material has set

For putty materials an impression is taken with the kneaded putty. Light-bodied material is then mixed and placed over the putty or syringed over the prepared tooth. The impression is then reinserted to provide the final impression. Alternatively both these stages may be combined into one by loading the tray with putty and covering it with a wash of light-bodied material before insertion.

As elastomers do not adhere to impression trays, it is necessary to use either a perforated tray, or apply a tray adhesive before loading, to ensure the safe withdrawal of the impression. It is then washed in running water, immersed in a disinfectant such as sodium hypo-chlorite, and rinsed in water again before despatch to the laboratory.

The advantages of elastomers are their combination of elasticity, strength and accuracy. This ensures an accurate undistorted impression of undercut areas and allows several cavities to be included in one impression. Their disadvantages are the elaborate technique required, long setting time and the sticky consistency before setting.

Occlusal records

Having obtained an impression of the prepared tooth, the next step is to record the occlusion between the prepared tooth and those which bite against it. An alginate (Chapter 27) or putty impression of the opposing teeth is taken and this provides the technician with a model of them as well as the prepared tooth. However, an additional record is needed to show the technician how the two models occlude together.

This is done by softening a sheet of pink or silver wax in a flame and placing it over the prepared tooth. The patient then closes into the wax to give an imprint of the opposing teeth on one side of the wax and the prepared tooth on the other. This wax **squash bite** allows the technician to fit the two models together in their natural occlusion and thereby produce a wax pattern in correct contact with its adjacent tooth and correct occlusion with its opposing teeth.

For a single inlay, a wax squash bite is usually sufficient; but for multiple-inlay preparations, crowns and bridges a more accurate recording than a squash bite is necessary. This is achieved by using an elastomer occlusal impression material instead of wax. Special trays are available which allow the opposing jaw impression and occlusal record impression to be taken at the same time.

Crowns

A crown is an artificial restoration which replaces at least three-quarters of the natural crown of the tooth. There are various types, made of various materials, and they require at least two visits.

At the first visit the tooth is prepared, using diamond discs, wheels and tapered fissure burs (Figure 18.8). An elastomer impression and occlusal records are then taken and, for front teeth, the shade is recorded. A temporary crown is then cemented and the patient is dismissed.

At the second visit, the temporary crown is removed and the permanent one positioned. It is then checked for appearance and occlusion before cementing with GIC, zinc phosphate or poly-carboxylate.

Temporary crowns

Temporary crowns are used to maintain appearance and prevent pain between visits. They also maintain the correct space and occlusion between adjacent or opposing teeth, and thus facilitate fitting of the permanent crown. Temporary crowns are made by fitting a **crown form** over the prepared tooth.

For front teeth a clear plastic crown form may be used. It is trimmed with **crown scissors** (Figure 23.1) and filled with a material which matches the teeth, such as composite or acrylic. Alternatively, tough

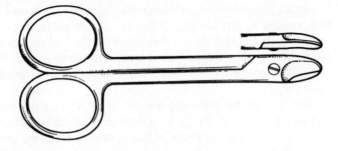

Figure 23.1   *Beebee crown scissors.*

tooth-coloured polycarbonate crown forms are used, and these only need trimming.

Metal crown forms made of aluminium or stainless steel are used on back teeth.

Trimmed temporary crowns are cemented with a material which is adhesive, but easily and cleanly removed for fitting the permanent crown; for example, a modified ZOE paste such as *Temp Bond.*

Stainless steel crown forms, cemented with GIC, are also used on badly broken deciduous molars instead of a permanent filling.

Jacket crown

A jacket crown is used for front teeth which are too mutilated to be restored by ordinary fillings. Such cases are very extensive caries, fracture of the crown, and severe pitting, discoloration, or deformation of the crown.

The outer coating of the natural crown is removed to leave a stump of dentine with a well-defined cervical shoulder, on which the artificial crown fits like a jacket (Figure 23.2).

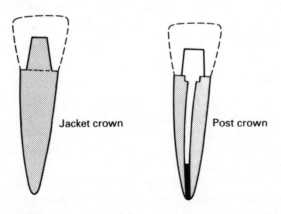

Jacket crown   Post crown

Figure 23.2   *Crowns.*

End-cutting burs (Figure 18.8) are often used for preparing the shoulder for such crowns. Jacket crowns are usually made entirely of **porcelain** (PJC). However, this is liable to fracture under a heavy bite, and such cases require a **porcelain bonded crown** (PBC). These have a porcelain facing bonded to a gold (or precious metal alloy) backing (Figure 23.3). Temporary or semi-permanent jacket crowns are made of acrylic.

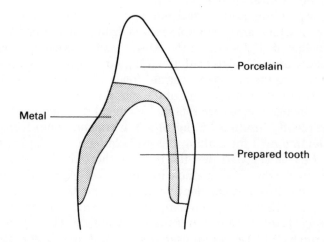

Figure 23.3 *Porcelain bonded crown.*
Source: *The Restoration of Teeth* (2nd edn). T.R. Pitt Ford, Blackwell Science Ltd, Oxford.

Post crown

When a crown is required on a tooth which has been root filled, a post crown is generally used. The natural crown is cut off and a post fitted down the root canal. The artificial crown is made on this post (Figure 23.2). Instead of cutting off the natural crown, it may be prepared as for a jacket crown and then strengthened by fitting a post.

The post may be a gold casting or a preformed stainless steel screw and stump, such as a *Kurer* post.

Whatever type of post is used, it is usually cemented into the root canal and an impression taken for a jacket crown to fit over the post stump. The stump may be part of a preformed post or built up with a composite material to resemble a jacket crown preparation.

Veneer crown

A veneer crown is a thin gold shell used in the construction of bridges (Figure 23.4). On back teeth it covers the entire crown and is called a

Figure 23.4   *Full veneer crown.*

full crown. On front teeth it covers all but the labial surface and is called a **three-quarter crown**.

Apart from bridges, full gold veneer crowns are also used to restore teeth which are unsuitable for amalgam, such as badly broken down teeth and split teeth. In the latter case the crown acts as a splint. On badly broken down teeth the full gold crown forms a protective shell covering the amalgam, cermet (page 276) or composite core which restores most of the bulk of the natural crown.

Amalgam cores are retained by metal dentine pins which are conveniently inserted by the *Stabilok* system, comprising a low-speed dentine drill for making the pinhole, and a matching threaded pin which is screwed into the hole by the same low-speed handpiece. Cermet cores are retained by their own chemical adhesion, while composite cores use dentine bonding agents (Chapters 21 and 22).

Full crowns on premolars are often made with a porcelain bonded buccal surface to improve their appearance. These porcelain bonded crowns (PBC) are often used instead of three-quarter crowns for front teeth.

Bridges

A bridge is a *fixed* replacement for one or a few missing teeth. The artificial tooth filling the gap has a gold backing or a gold base which is soldered to crowns on adjacent teeth. The artificial tooth is called a **pontic** and the supporting teeth are called **abutments**. The crowns or inlays on the abutment teeth are called **retainers**. Thus a bridge consists of one or more pontics soldered to gold retainers on the abutments, and is inserted by cementing the retainers on to the abutments (Figure 23.5). An elastomer impression is used when making a bridge, as all the teeth involved can be included in one impression. Full occlusal records are then taken and a temporary bridge is fitted between visits.

At the fitting stage, the occlusion must be correct before a bridge is cemented. Any high spots are found by closing the teeth together on **articulating paper** or a thin sheet of green wax called **occlusal indicator wax**. The paper or wax show the dentist which cusps are too high.

A bridge is an ideal replacement for a missing tooth as it is permanently fixed in place and functions as well as a natural tooth.

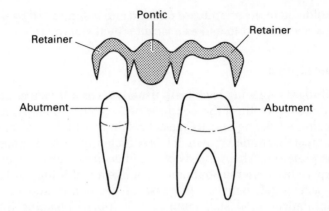

Figure 23.5 *Bridge components.*

Unfortunately it is very expensive and cannot be used to replace more than a few teeth.

Bridges can also be made by using **implants** as abutments. This saves having to make retainers on natural teeth and is described in Chapter 27.

Anterior bridges

Bridges replacing front teeth usually have a pontic consisting of a porcelain jacket crown on a gold stump. This permits easy replacement of the crown without having to remove the bridge. To prevent any gold showing, three-quarter or porcelain bonded crowns are used as retainers on the abutment teeth.

A bridge fixed at one end only is often preferred for the replacement of a single missing incisor. One variety of this type of bridge is called a **spring cantilever bridge** (Figure 23.6). The fixed end consists of three-quarter crowns on the premolars and the pontic is a porcelain jacket crown. The pontic and abutments are linked by a gold bar which is

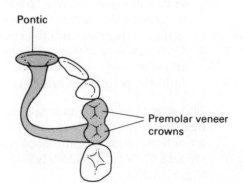

Figure 23.6 *Spring cantilever bridge.*

soldered to the retainers at one end and is supported by the palate as it passes forward to end as a jacket crown stump.

Posterior bridges

Bridges replacing back teeth usually have full veneer crowns on the abutment teeth. If the pontic is near enough to show, it has a tooth-coloured facing and its mesial retainer would be a three-quarter or porcelain bonded crown. If it is sufficiently far back, a **sanitary pontic** is preferred. This consists of a gold occlusal surface which spans the space between the abutments just like a real bridge. A large hygienic space is left between the base of the pontic and the gum which minimizes food stagnation and facilitates cleaning by the patient (Figure 23.7).

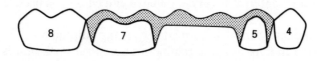

Figure 23.7   *Posterior bridge with sanitary pontic.*

Temporary bridges

A temporary bridge is necessary between visits to prevent pain, space closure, tipping or over-eruption of the abutment teeth. It may be made as follows:

1   Before the abutment teeth are prepared, the gap of the missing tooth is filled with a piece of cotton wool roll. A putty or heavy-bodied elastomer impression of the bridge area is then taken, the cotton wool discarded, and the impression put aside.
2   The abutments are then prepared and an impression for the permanent bridge is taken.
3   The first impression is now used to make a temporary bridge. A composite-type resin is placed in the part of the impression containing the abutment teeth and pontic area; and the impression is then reinserted until the resin sets.
4   On withdrawal of the impression, the temporary bridge is removed, trimmed, and cemented back into place with a temporary cement until the permanent bridge is cemented at another visit.

This direct method of making a temporary bridge is facilitated by new dual-cure materials (Chapter 21) utilizing cartridges and a special gun for automatic mixing and application into the impression (e.g. *Provipont DC*). Similar materials are also available as temporary cements (e.g. *Provilink*).

Surgery procedure

As bridges consist of one or more crowns, the surgery procedure is the same as that involved in the indirect method of inlay and crown construction. However, the following extra steps may be required:

1 Study models and X-ray films are first taken to decide the best design and plan the number and length of appointments needed.
2 A try-in visit for the crowns, to check their fit and occlusion; followed by an overall impression with crowns in place to facilitate soldering the pontic to the retainers.

Direct bonded restorations

Chapter 21 described composite filling materials and the technique of acid etching which allows composite materials to bond directly to enamel surfaces. This technique enables small anterior bridges to be made without having to crown the abutments. It also allows the use of porcelain veneers instead of jacket crowns in appropriate cases.

Maryland bridges

These bridges replace just one or two front teeth. The pontic has a porcelain bonded facing while the metal backing has wing-like flanges which rest against the palatal surface of the abutments, and are bonded directly to their acid etched enamel. The fitting surface of the flanges is made retentive by acid etching and sand blasting; and a chemical-cure adhesive resin, such as *Panavia Ex*, which bonds to both metal and enamel is used as a luting cement.

These Maryland bridges (Figure 23.8) conserve tooth tissue and are accordingly ideal for children. They are far quicker to make and can be replaced much more easily than conventional bridgework.

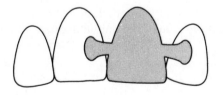

Figure 23.8 *Direct bonded bridge – palatal aspect.*

Porcelain veneers

Conventional jacket crown preparation requires the removal of a significant amount of dentine. While this may be harmless in fully developed adult teeth, it could result in pulpal damage in children and adolescents. In other cases it may be felt that labial enamel defects in incisors, which require a restoration to improve appearance, do not justify a full jacket crown preparation.

In such cases just the outermost layer of labial enamel may be removed and replaced by a porcelain veneer to restore normal appearance. After removal of the outer layer, the remaining labial enamel is acid etched and a laboratory made porcelain veneer is bonded to it with a light or dual-cure unfilled composite resin. The porcelain is etched with hydrofluoric acid to provide a retentive surface, but phosphoric acid is used for the enamel.

Practical examination

Mix sufficient material (for example, *Impregum*) for a crown impression and load it into a syringe
- Dispense equal, reasonable amounts from each tube, alongside one another, at the centre of the mixing pad
- Replace caps on the tubes
- Mix the catalyst and base with a spatula to give an even colour without any streaks of unmixed base or catalyst
- Strop the spatula blade on the edge of the mixing pad to remove streaks and collect mix on clean part of pad
- Wipe the spatula blade to remove any residual streaks and load the mix tidily into a suitable syringe for presentation to examiner

Written examination

A patient is to have porcelain veneers cemented on upper central incisors.
List the reasons these teeth may require porcelain veneers.
Describe the procedures and the role of the dental nurse in the placement and finishing of porcelain veneers. (November 1995)
How might the appearance of a discoloured central incisor be restored?
Describe the preparation of a vital incisor tooth for a porcelain jacket crown and list the instruments and materials you would lay out for this procedure. (May 1990)

How may a missing upper lateral incisor be replaced?
What impression materials may be required?
How should these materials be dealt with by the dental nurse
after removal from the mouth? (May 1991)

Summary

Inlay technique

First visit:

- Cavity prepared
- Undercuts blocked out with lining cement
- Elastomer impression
- Occlusal record
- Temporary filling inserted

Laboratory:

- Model made
- Wax pattern made on model
- Wax pattern cast in gold
- Inlay polished

Second visit:

- Temporary filling removed
- Inlay cemented with GIC, zinc phosphate or polycarboxylate

Elastomer impressions

1 Prepare tooth
2 Pack gingival crevice with retraction cord
3 Mix light-bodied material and load into syringe
4 Mix heavy-bodied material and load impression tray
5 Remove cord and inject into cavity
6 Apply impression tray

Crowns

First visit:

- Preparation
- Elastomer impression
- Occlusal records
- Shade taken
- Temporary crown fitted

Second visit:

- Cemented

Surgery requirements for inlays and crowns

- Tapered fissure and end-cutting burs
- Diamond discs, wheels and stones
- Lining cement
- Elastomer impression material, syringe, impression tray, tray adhesive and retraction cord
- Wax or elastomer for occlusal record
- Alginate or putty for impression of opposing teeth
- Shade guide
- Temporary filling or crown form
- Articulating paper, occlusal indicator wax Burnishers
- GIC, zinc phosphate or carboxylate cement

Bridges

- Replaced tooth: pontic
- Supporting teeth: abutments
- Abutment restorations: retainers

1 Study models and X-ray films
2 Prepare abutments; elastomer impression; occlusal records; fit temporary bridge
3 Try in retainers; overall locating impression; refit temporary bridge
4 Bridge cemented with GIC or zinc phosphate (for slower set)

Maryland bridge

- Small anterior bridge
- Retained by pontic flanges

- Flanges bonded directly to acid etched palatal enamel of abutments
- Easier and quicker to make and replace than conventional bridges
  Requires minimal preparation of abutment teeth
- Ideal for children

Porcelain veneers

- Outermost layer of labial enamel removed and surface acid etched
- Porcelain veneer bonded directly to labial surface
- Requires minimal loss of tooth tissue
- Ideal for children and cases with mild enamel defects

Comparison of permanent filling materials

FILLING	USES	ADVANTAGES	DISADVANTAGES
Amalgam	Permanent filling for back teeth	1 Simple technique 2 Rapid set 3 Strength	Lining usually required
Composite	1 Permanent filling for front teeth 2 Restoration of fractured incisors, misshapen and malformed teeth 3 Fissure sealant 4 Direct bonding of orthodontic brackets	1 Simple technique 2 Strength and permanence 3 Suitable for large and complicated restorations 4 Undercut or acid etch retention 5 Surface glazing	1 Not quite hard enough, and more difficult to use, for filling back teeth
Glass ionomer cement	1 Permanent filling in front teeth 2 Cervical cavities in all teeth 3 Deciduous teeth 4 Cavity lining 5 Dentine substitute 6 Adhesive cement 7 Fissure sealant	1 Chemical bond to tooth 2 Cariostatic 3 Non-irritant 4 Lining unnecessary	1 Too dark and opaque for front teeth in young patients 2 Too soft for back teeth
Gold	Permanent filling or crown for back teeth	Much stronger than amalgam	Involves far more time and expense than any other filling

24 Endodontics

Endodontics is the term used for all forms of root canal therapy. It includes root filling, pulpotomy, pulp capping and apicectomy.

Principles of endodontics

As explained in Chapter 17 on caries, pulpitis leads to pulp death. This in turn eventually leads to an acute alveolar abscess, which is a very painful condition. To prevent this chain of events, endodontic treatment or extraction is required whenever the pulp is inflamed or dead, or when an alveolar abscess is already present.

The basic object of endodontic treatment is to remove the inflamed or dead pulp and replace it with a permanent root filling. This seals each end of the root canal and removes the source of irritation which causes alveolar abscess. It will also allow the drainage and complete cure of an existing abscess. The root filled tooth will then function just as well as one with a normal pulp.

There are many causes of pulpitis and pulp death but the treatment is similar in each case: either extraction or endodontics.

Causes of pulpitis

The commonest cause of pulpitis is **exposure** of the pulp. This allows mouth bacteria to enter the pulp chamber and infect the pulp. Exposure of the pulp may be caused by:

1 Caries
2 Accidental exposure during cavity preparation
3 Fracture of the crown

Even when the pulp is not exposed, pulpitis can still occur. The causes are:

1 Irritation from unlined filling
2 Excessive heat during cavity preparation, such as the use of an air turbine handpiece without waterspray
3 Impact injury

Impact injuries are common in children with prominent front teeth.

The crown may fracture and expose the pulp. Alternatively the crown remains intact but the blow damages the apical blood vessels and pulp death ensues. Treatment of a tooth which is completely knocked out was described in Chapter 16.

Choice of treatment

In deciding whether to treat by extraction or endodontics, several factors are considered.

Extraction is the surest, quickest and simplest line of treatment, whereas endodontics may entail more than one long visit. Therefore, endodontic treatment is not undertaken unless the patient has a clean well-maintained mouth; prefers not to have an artificial replacement; is agreeable to lengthy treatment; and fully aware of the possibility of ultimate failure.

Many technical difficulties beset the endodontic treatment of multirooted teeth and for this reason they are often extracted instead. Endodontic treatment is most often done on front teeth as they are easily accessible and have only one root. It is consequently simpler and more likely to be successful than on back teeth. Furthermore, most patients would prefer to save a front tooth rather than have it extracted. Although premolars and molars are frequently extracted, they can be saved by endodontic treatment when necessary.

Vitality tests

The dentist's decision on whether to treat a decayed tooth by an ordinary filling, endodontics or extraction, depends on the state of the pulp. If it is dead, endodontics or extraction is necessary. If it is alive and unexposed, an ordinary filling will suffice.

The state of the pulp is not always apparent and vitality tests are often required to determine whether it is alive or dead. These tests depend on the painful response of the pulp to certain stimuli. If there is a response the pulp is vital; if not, it is probably dead. The following tests are used:

1 *Heat.* A stick of gutta-percha (GP) is heated in a flame and applied to the crown of the tooth. A film of petroleum jelly should be applied to the crown before the placement of GP to prevent it sticking to the tooth and causing excessive pain.
2 *Cold.* Cotton wool moistened with ethyl chloride, or an ice stick, is applied to the crown.
3 *Electricity.* An electronic pulp tester is applied to the crown.
4 *Drilling.* Cavity preparation without LA is painful when the pulp is vital.

5   *X-ray.* Alveolar abscess on a dead tooth will show on an X-ray film.

Root filling

The object of root filling is to remove the inflamed or dead pulp from a tooth and replace it with a sterile non-irritant, insoluble root canal filling. It is usually done in two stages: the first to prepare the canal; the second to insert the root filling. If no difficulties arise, both stages can be completed in one visit. However, many practitioners prefer a separate visit for each stage.

At the first visit:

1   The pulp is removed.
2   The root canal is enlarged and cleaned to prepare a dry, smooth, empty canal which tapers gradually from the pulp chamber towards the apex.
3   A temporary filling is inserted to cover the entrance to the empty root canal and prevent contamination of the canal between visits.

At the second visit:

1   The temporary filling is removed.
2   If the root canal is still clean and dry, it is filled with GP to seal off the entire canal to within a millimetre of the apex.

Root filling instruments

Special instruments used for root filling are barbed broaches, root reamers, root canal files, pluggers and rotary paste fillers (Figure 24.1).

Barbed broaches are disposable hand instruments for removing the pulp. They consist of a fine wire with multiple barbs. When the broach is inserted in a root canal and rotated, its barbs engage the pulp; whereupon the pulp can be withdrawn with the broach. Barbed broaches are always discarded after use.

Root reamers resemble wood drills and are used for enlarging root canals so that a filling can be inserted. They are made in standardized sets – all of the same length, but with an increasing range of widths. Each reamer is numbered or colour-coded to indicate its size. A small reamer is inserted in the canal and advanced to just short of the apex by hand rotation. This is repeated with successively wider reamers until the canal is large enough for filling.

Reamers are also available for use in low-speed handpieces.

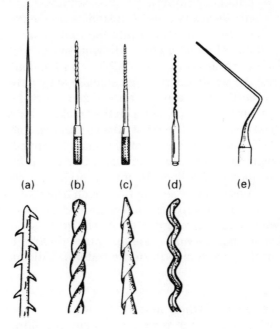

Figure 24.1 *Root canal instruments.* (a) Barbed broach; (b) Root canal reamer; (c) Root canal file; (d) Rotary paste-filler; (e) Root-canal plugger.

Special endodontic handpieces and ultrasonic instruments are also available which can ream and file root canals. They are particularly useful for the narrow, curved canals of multirooted teeth.

Root canal files are hand instruments which resemble reamers and are made in the same standardized range of sizes. Their function is to smooth and clean the walls of enlarged root canals and remove debris. They are inserted in the canal and used with an up-and-down filing action against the canal walls. Many practitioners use files exclusively instead of reamers, but in the same sequence of increasing sizes.

Root canal pluggers or **spreaders** have a long, tapered smooth point used to condense the GP filling against the canal walls and obliterate any gaps. They may have a long handle like a probe, or a small head like a root reamer or file.

Rotary paste fillers are engine instruments for inserting pastes into a root canal. They consist of a spiral wire which fits in a handpiece and propels the required material to the full length of the root canal.

Preparation

As the root canal must be disinfected before it is filled, all instruments and dressings must be sterile. A convenient arrangement is to keep a sealed container holding a complete sterilized root filling kit ready for immediate use at any time. Rubber dam is essential to prevent ingress of bacteria from the mouth into the root canal; and to prevent accidents such as inhalation or swallowing of tiny root canal instruments. It also improves access and visibility for the dentist.

Once the sterile instruments actually enter a root canal they are no longer sterile, and must be resterilized before being inserted again. This is most effectively done on the bracket table by an instantaneous dry heat method such as a **hot salt** or a **glass bead sterilizer**. This is kept at 225°C and root-canal instruments are dipped in it for up to ten seconds. An alternative method is to use a portable **hot air dental heater** such as the *Safe Air* model, originally designed to replace a naked flame when softening wax. Such heaters are based on domestic paint and paper strippers and emit a jet of very hot air. It has been shown that the *Safe Air* dental heater sterilizes root canal instruments in five seconds at a working temperature of 490°C. On removal from the hot air they are cooled in sterile water or a disinfectant.

Procedure

As mentioned earlier, more than one visit may be necessary. The following description is for a two-visit procedure:

1 LA is used if the pulp is still vital.
2 Rubber dam is applied. The tooth and rubber dam are then swabbed with a disinfectant such as chlorhexidine.
3 Access to the pulp is gained by drilling open the pulp chamber.
4 The pulp is removed with a barbed broach. Patients at risk of infective endocarditis require antibiotic cover for this stage.
5 The root canal is prepared with reamers or files. It is necessary to take an X-ray at the start of this stage, with a reamer in place, as a guide to the correct preparation of the canal.

   Once an X-ray shows the required length of canal preparation (1 mm short of the apex), all subsequent reaming and filing is kept to this length by fitting a stopper to each instrument before insertion. This prevents penetration of the apex or too short a preparation of the canal.
6 The walls of the root canal are smoothed and cleaned with files to produce a gradually tapering canal.
7 Throughout reaming and filing, the canal is irrigated with sodium hypochlorite to remove debris and disinfect the canal. A sterile disposable syringe is used for this purpose.
8 The canal is then dried with absorbent **paper points** and its entrance covered with dry sterile cotton wool.
9 The empty pulp chamber is sealed off with a temporary filling to prevent contamination of the empty, clean, dry root canal between visits.

10 At the next visit, if the root canal is still clean and dry, it is ready for insertion of the permanent filling. A **gutta-percha point**, matching the largest size file used, is selected. This is called the master point and has to be sealed to the apical end of the canal with cement.

11 Various proprietary brands of root canal sealers are available, many being based on a modified ZOE cement, for example, *Tubliseal*. The canal walls and the end of the master point are coated with sealer and the point inserted into the root canal.

12 The gap between the canal walls and the master point is filled by condensing successive GP points against the canal walls with a root canal spreader (plugger) until no space is left.

Warming the spreader softens GP and assists condensation against the canal walls. The use of self-locking tweezers facilitates handling of paper and GP points.

13 An X-ray is taken to ensure that the root filling is satisfactory and to check subsequent progress.

14 Having completely filled the root canal with GP, the access cavity is permanently filled with an appropriate material, such as composite or amalgam.

If, at step 10, the root canal is not dry, it means that apical infection is still present. In that case the canal is irrigated again with hypochlorite, dried with paper points and another temporary dressing is inserted in the access cavity. It should then be ready for a permanent root filling at the next visit. If not, a temporary root dressing of non-setting calcium hydroxide paste is inserted until the next visit. The paste can be made by mixing calcium hydroxide powder with sterile water or LA solution. The paste is inserted into the canal with a rotary paste filler.

Instruments

1 Mirror, probe and tweezers
2 LA equipment
3 Rubber dam equipment, aspirator and saliva ejector
4 Hot salt (or glass bead) sterilizer; hot air dental heater
5 Handpiece and burs
6 Barbed broaches, root reamers, files, spreaders and pluggers; rotary paste fillers
7 Locking tweezers, paper points and cotton wool
8 Syringe for irrigation with sodium hypochlorite
9 GP points and sealer cement
10 Ruler for measuring length of root canal

Sterilization

Endodontic kits are sterilized in a hot air oven or autoclave.

As GP points are destroyed by heat they are usually supplied in sterile packs. However, they can be disinfected in the surgery by immersion in sodium hypochlorite.

The hot salt sterilizer mentioned previously consists of an electrically heated container of ordinary table salt, or glass beads, whereas the alternative hot air dental heater produces an electrically heated jet of hot air. One of these is used at the chairside for instant sterilization of root canal instruments.

The operative area is disinfected by swabbing the tooth and rubber dam with chlorhexidine.

Pulpotomy

In adults, the conservative treatment of an exposed vital pulp is by root filling. But in children, growth of the root is not yet complete and an exposed tooth may still have a wide open apex, instead of the minute apical foramen. Root filling is unnecessary for these teeth as pulp death does not always occur. The wide open apex allows blood circulation through the pulp to continue, without being cut off by a build-up of inflammatory pressure. Instead of total removal of the pulp, followed by root filling, it is only necessary to remove the infected part of the pulp in the pulp chamber – a procedure known as **pulpotomy**. The very rich blood supply through an open apex allows healing to occur. The pulp survives and growth continues to its natural completion. In fully grown teeth, such healing is rarely possible and that is why the entire pulp must be removed and a root filling inserted.

The procedure in pulpotomy is similar to root filling in so far as a sterile technique is necessary. The pulp chamber is opened and the pulp tissue is removed from the pulp chamber only. The amputated pulp stump at the entrance to the root canal is then covered with a calcium hydroxide dressing. This stimulates the pulp in the root canal to form a layer of secondary dentine over itself. The pulp is thereby completely sealed off again, as it was before the exposure occurred, and normal growth continues until apical formation is complete. It may then be necessary to do a full root filling.

Procedure

The procedure is the same as root filling for steps 1–3.

4   The pulp in the pulp chamber is removed by the bur used to gain access.

5   The pulp at the entrance to the root canal is covered with calcium hydroxide paste and sealed with a temporary filling.

Instruments

1–5   As for root filling
6   Sterile cottonwool
7   Calcium hydroxide and sterile water
8   Temporary filling

Pulp capping

When a vital pulp is exposed, either root filling or pulpotomy is necessary to conserve the tooth. This cannot always be done immediately as pulp exposure often occurs unexpectedly, or presents as an emergency.

In such cases pulp capping is a valuable temporary measure. The exposure is covered with calcium hydroxide paste or *Ledermix* and the cavity is filled with a temporary cement. This prevents pain and protects the pulp from infection until root filling or pulpotomy are performed.

Apicectomy

Apicectomy is an operation for the removal of an infected apex and surrounding infected tissue. The purpose of apicectomy is to save the tooth in cases where root filling is either unsuccessful or impossible. It is the final alternative to extraction and is done for the following reasons:

1   Root filling unsuccessful
    (a)   Incomplete filling of inaccessible canal
    (b)   Escape of irritant cement through apex
2   Root filling impossible
    (a)   Canal blocked by broken instrument
    (b)   Alveolar abscess on tooth with post crown

Procedure

1   An incision is made in the gum and a flap raised off the bone with a periosteal elevator.
2   Using a straight handpiece and burs, a window is cut in the overlying bone to expose the infected apex.
3   The apex is cut off and infected tissue surrounding it is scraped away with a **curette** (Figure 24.2), which resembles a large excavator.

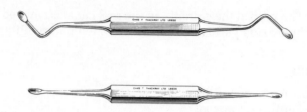

Figure 24.2   *Curettes.*

4   The cut end of the root is then examined to see if the remaining root filling is deficient. If so, a bit more filling is inserted in the cut end. Zinc-free amalgam or reinforced ZOE is usually chosen and the procedure is known as **retrograde root filling**.
5   Debris is removed by syringing with sterile saline and the gum flap is sutured back into place.
6   Sutures are removed a few days later and an X-ray is taken for record purposes. By comparing this X-ray with future ones, the progress of healing can be observed.

Instruments

Set out on sterile towel:

- Aspirator tubes or saliva ejector
- Sterile towel and towel clip
- Mirror, probe and tweezers
- LA equipment
- Scalpel, periosteal elevator and swabs
- Straight handpiece and burs
- Curettes
- Hunt or disposable syringe and sterile saline
- Dissecting forceps, needle-holder, needles and thread, scissors

---

Written examination

(a)   What are the reasons for root filling a tooth?

(b)   A patient asks the dental nurse what is involved in root canal treatment.
      What would you tell them?

(c)   Give a list of instruments and equipment which a dental nurse would lay out for the preparation stage of root canal treatment. (May 1996)

What is meant by the term apicectomy?

Why may it become necessary to perform this procedure on a tooth?

Describe the chairside role of the dental nurse during this procedure. (May 1995)

Summary

Conservative treatment of caries

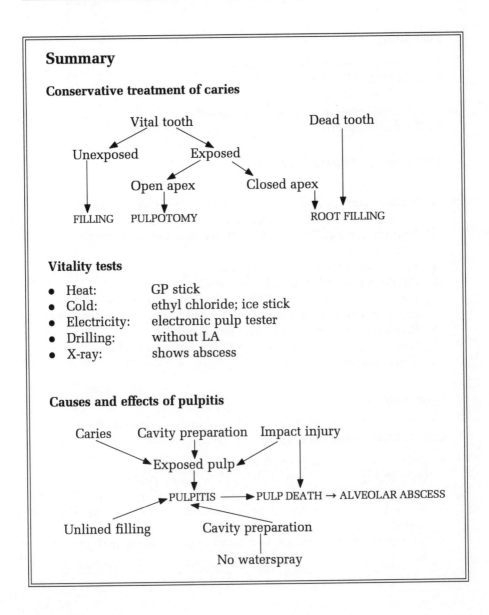

Vitality tests

- Heat: GP stick
- Cold: ethyl chloride; ice stick
- Electricity: electronic pulp tester
- Drilling: without LA
- X-ray: shows abscess

Causes and effects of pulpitis

Choice of treatment

CONSIDERATIONS	EXTRACTION	ROOT TREATMENT
Teeth treated	All	Mainly front
Success	Certain	Uncertain
Number of visits	One	One or more
Technique	Simple	Complicated
The patient	Will require partial denture or bridge	Must be aware of difficulties and keen to retain tooth

Root filling

1 Remove infected pulp ← antibiotic cover?
2 Enlarge and clean root canal
3 Disinfect root canal
4 Fill root canal → complete cure usually
5 If infection persists → apicectomy → complete cure

Technique and instruments

1 LA for vital tooth
2 Rubber dam applied. Tooth and dam swabbed with disinfectant
3 Gain access to pulp with handpiece and burs
4 Instruments sterilized by instant dry heat before reinsertion in root canal
5 Pulp removed with barbed broach
6 Root canal X-rayed with reamer in place
7 Root canal enlarged and cleaned with reamers and/or files; irrigated throughout instrumentation with sodium hypochlorite
8 Prepared root canal dried with paper points
9 Clean, dry, root canal filled with GP points and sealer
10 X-ray to show root filling

Pulpotomy

Children under 14 → growth not yet complete → exposed vital tooth may still have wide open apex.

1 Pulp removed from pulp chamber only
2 Pulp stump covered with calcium hydroxide paste
3 Good blood supply through open apex → healing occurs
4 Secondary dentine forms over remaining pulp → exposure sealed off
5 Normal growth continues → vital unexposed tooth with closed apex

Technique and instruments

1–3 As for root filling
4 Pulp in pulp chamber removed with bur
5 Dressing of calcium hydroxide and sterile water (or LA solution) placed over pulp stump and covered with temporary cement

Pulp capping

Temporary measure to protect exposed pulp. Calcium hydroxide or *Ledermix*.

Apicectomy

Surgical eradication of apical infection when root filling unsuccessful or impossible, for example:

- Infection persisting after root filling – inaccessible canal
- Alveolar abscess on tooth with post crown
- Canal blocked by broken instrument
- Escape of irritant sealer through apex

Procedure

1 LA (Antibiotic cover?)
2 Incision
3 Gum flap raised
4 Overlying bone removed
5 Infected apex cut off
6 Abscess cavity curetted
7 Retrograde root filling if necessary
8 Debris removed
9 Gum flap sutured
10 X-ray taken

Instruments

Set out on sterile towel:

- Aspirator tubes or saliva ejector
- Sterile towel and towel clip
- Mirror, probe and tweezers
- LA equipment
- Scalpel, periosteal elevator and swabs
- Straight handpiece and burs
- Curettes
- Hunt or disposable syringe and sterile saline
- Dissecting forceps, needle-holder, needles and thread, scissors

25 Periodontal Disease

Periodontal disease means disease of the supporting structures of the teeth. These are the gums, periodontal membrane and alveolar bone. The adjective relating to gums is *gingival*, and inflammation of the gum is accordingly called gingivitis.

Periodontal disease and caries are the commonest diseases of civilization. Caries is the major cause of tooth loss in children and young adults, while periodontal disease is the major cause in older people. This does not mean that periodontal disease starts much later in life – only that it takes so much longer than caries to cause tooth loss.

The earliest stage of periodontal disease is **chronic gingivitis** which is a chronic inflammation involving the gums alone. If allowed to continue, it spreads to the underlying periodontal membrane and alveolar bone. These are gradually destroyed and the teeth become very loose as their supporting tissues are lost. The name given to this late stage of the disease is **chronic periodontitis**. There is no obvious dividing line between the two stages, as untreated chronic gingivitis slowly progresses into chronic periodontitis.

Causes of periodontal disease

Periodontal disease is an infection caused by accumulation of **plaque** at the gum margin. Plaque is a tenacious transparent film of saliva, bacteria and oral debris on the tooth surface. Food debris adheres to plaque and the resultant paste of saliva and food remnants attracts far more bacteria which feed and multiply on it. It is the same plaque as that described in Chapter 17, on caries; but whereas caries can only occur when sugar is present in plaque, the presence of sugar is not necessary for periodontal disease to occur. Any sort of food debris will allow plaque bacteria to proliferate and cause periodontal disease.

Plaque can be removed by brushing; but in the absence of this counter-measure, it thickens as its bacterial population flourishes amid a permanent food supply. Toxic products of plaque bacteria then act as a continual source of bacterial irritation which causes chronic inflammation of the gum margin (chronic gingivitis). The plaque extends above and below the gum margin, and wherever it is present **calculus** (tartar) formation can occur.

Calculus is the hard rock-like deposit commonly seen on the

lingual surface of lower incisors. Two factors are necessary for its formation: plaque and saliva. Their interaction allows mineralization to occur within the plaque and produce a deposition of calculus. It is most easily seen opposite the orifices of salivary gland ducts – on the lingual surface of lower incisors and the buccal surface of upper molars. This visible calculus on the crowns of teeth has a yellowish colour and is called **supragingival calculus** as it forms above the gum margin. However, it also occurs in plaque beneath the gum margin on all teeth and in that situation it is known as **subgingival calculus**. This is harder and darker than supragingival calculus and its surface is covered with a layer of the soft bacterial plaque from which it was formed.

Calculus plays only a *passive* mechanical role in periodontal disease. Its rough surface and ledges create food traps which are inaccessible to a toothbrush and thus allow even more food debris to fertilize the plaque. The *active* role in periodontal disease belongs to plaque bacteria.

This description shows that supragingival plaque and calculus are associated with bad oral hygiene. If teeth are cleaned properly they do not accumulate. But if they are allowed to do so, they spread subgingivally and become inaccessible to toothbrushing.

Furthermore, there are some additional reasons for plaque formation which are not the patient's fault. These are caused by imperfect dentistry, such as fillings or crowns which have an overhanging edge at their cervical margin; fillings with loose contact points; and ill-fitting or badly designed partial dentures. All these defects are food traps which patients cannot keep clean. Plaque and calculus proliferate there and periodontal disease follows at these sites, even though the rest of the mouth may be perfectly healthy. As mentioned in Chapter 17, food stagnation also occurs on unopposed and irregular teeth, with consequent liability to periodontal disease as well as caries.

Chronic gingivitis

Normal healthy gums are attached to the teeth like a very tight cuff. At the edge of this cuff there is a minute space between gum margin and tooth surface called the **gingival crevice**. When food debris collects in this region, plaque accumulates inside the gingival crevice and subgingival calculus is produced (Figure 25.1).

The combined effect of plaque and subgingival calculus in the gingival crevice is to irritate the gum and produce a chronic gingivitis. In this condition the gum becomes swollen, thus loosening the tight cuff and greatly enlarging the gingival crevice. A vicious circle is now established: the enlarged crevice forms a **false pocket** around the

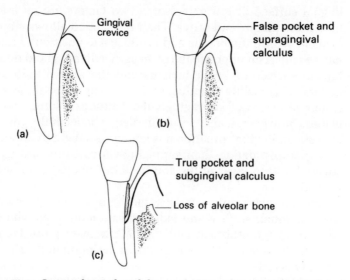

Figure 25.1 *Stages of periodontal disease.* (a) Normal appearance; (b) Chronic gingivitis; (c) Chronic periodontitis.

tooth, in which much more food debris can collect; further deposits of plaque and subgingival calculus are thereby formed; and these irritants keep up the inflammation. Bacterial poisons from the plaque ulcerate the floor of the gingival crevice and bleeding occurs on the slightest pressure.

An ulcer is any abnormal breach in the surface of the skin or mucous membrane. It has a raw base where the underlying tissues are exposed and may be very painful; for example, denture ulcer, herpetic ulcer. In chronic gingivitis the ulcers are painless and occur inside the enlarged gingival crevice. In any form of inflammation there is an increased flow of blood to the area and this explains why these subgingival ulcers bleed so readily when the slightest pressure is applied to the gums. Such bleeding is the earliest and most significant sign of periodontal disease, as opposed to caries where toothache is the first symptom.

Chronic periodontitis

If chronic gingivitis is not treated, bacterial poisons from the plaque soak through the ulcers in the gingival crevice and penetrate the deeper tissues. These poisons gradually destroy the periodontal membrane and alveolar bone; and while this is progressing, the gingival pocket deepens, thus further aggravating the condition. Whereas the false pockets of chronic gingivitis are caused by inflammatory swelling of the gum, in chronic periodontitis they are **true pockets** caused by destruction of the base of the gingival crevice and its attachment to the tooth. At the same time the gingival margin may recede, exposing the root to view. This **gingival recession** is commonly known as being *long in the tooth*. If no treatment is provided, so much bone is lost that the teeth eventually become too loose to be of any functional value (Figure 25.1).

This description of periodontal disease follows a slowly progressive but painless course of several years, but during that time pus and bacteria in the pockets cause bad breath (**halitosis**) and may affect the general health. Once periodontal disease is actually established it can be made worse by certain other factors, which do not in themselves cause the disease. Some of these aggravating factors are open lips, unbalanced or excessive masticatory stress, puberty and pregnancy. Certain medical conditions and drugs may also have the same effect, for example: diabetes, leukaemia, AIDS and other diseases where resistance to infection is poor; epilepsy treated with phenytoin (*Epanutin*); vitamin C deficiency; and treatment with immunosuppressant drugs such as cyclosporin and cytotoxic agents.

The rate of progress of periodontal disease depends on the balance between individual resistance and the toxic effects of plaque bacteria. Both these factors vary from time to time and in different parts of the mouth, and the predominant one determines whether the disease appears dormant or progressive.

Diagnosis

The diagnosis of periodontal disease is based on the medical history, appearance and recession of the gums, depth of gingival pockets, amount of bone loss, tooth mobility and the distribution of plaque.

Medical history

Periodontal disease affects the vast majority of the population, but most people are otherwise healthy and curable if they exercise adequate plaque control. However, patients with the following conditions are more at risk of severe periodontal disease and less likely to respond so favourably to treatment.

A regularly updated medical history is an essential feature of all patients' records, whatever their reason for attendance or the treatment required. As far as periodontal disease is concerned, the dentist will be particularly interested in illnesses, drugs prescribed, hormonal changes, such as pregnancy, and smoking habits.

Relevant illnesses are those where resistance is low, such as diabetes, leukaemia and other blood disorders; vitamin deficiencies; AIDS; and those requiring the use of immunosuppressant drugs, such as some cancer treatments and organ transplants. Some drugs such as phenytoin (*Epanutin*) used for epilepsy; Nifedipine (*Adalat*) used for angina pectoris and high blood pressure; and cyclosporin (*Sandimmun*), an immunosuppressant used to prevent rejection of transplants; can all cause severe overgrowth of the gums requiring surgical correction.

One of the most important diagnostic signs of early periodontal disease is gingival bleeding but this can be masked by heavy smoking as nicotine reduces bleeding. It also delays healing and upsets the delicate balance between disease resistance and the effect of bacterial toxins. There is far more awareness now of the significance of smoking as an adverse factor in periodontal disease; and as a cause of oral cancer (Chapter 9).

Periodontal examination

Normal healthy gums are firm and pink and do not bleed. They have a stippled surface, and the gingival crevice is less than 3 mm deep. In chronic gingivitis the gums have a soft, smooth surface, are darker in colour and swollen, bleed on pressure, and have a deeper gingival crevice which may contain subgingival calculus. In chronic period-ontitis these gingival changes may not be so obvious, as pockets are deeper and the active disease processes are occurring out of sight at that deeper level.

Tooth mobility and the appearance of the gums are easily checked; but detection of plaque and subgingival calculus, and assessment of pocket depth, gingival recession and bone loss, require examination with peridontal probes (Figure 25.2) and the use of special charts.

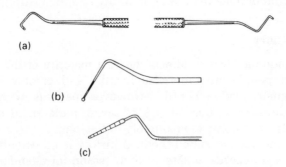

(a)

(b)

(c)

Figure 25.2 *Periodontal probes.* (a) Calculus probe; (b) WHO (CPITN) probe; (c) Pocket measuring probe.

A World Health Organization **(WHO) probe**, also known as a CPITN (community periodontal index of treatment needs) probe, is used for initial screening. This has a coloured band which assesses pocket depth by the amount of band showing (if any) after insertion into the gingival crevice; and a tiny ball on the end which detects subgingival calculus and prevents any bleeding caused by a sharp point.

A **pocket measuring probe** is used for charting. This has a blunt flat end (rather like that of a flat plastic instrument) with a millimetre scale marked on it. When inserted into the gingival crevice, pocket depth is read off from the scale.

Subgingival calculus is detected with a **calculus probe**. This resembles a Briault probe but has blunt ends which catch on the scales of calculus in the gingival crevice.

Bone loss can be assessed from pocket depth and X-ray films. As true pockets extend almost to the bone margin, a pocket measuring probe will indicate the amount of bone loss. X-rays show this as well, together with subgingival calculus and the cervical edges of restorations.

Plaque is normally invisible as it is a thin transparent film; but if a red dye is painted on the teeth, supragingival plaque is stained red and shows up clearly. Dyes used for this purpose are called **disclosing agents**. This part of the examination is left until last as dyes can mask gingival colour changes.

Charting

Whereas the mouth is divided into quarters (quadrants) for tooth charting (Figure 12.8), sixths (sextants) are used for periodontal charting. The sextants are upper and lower, left and right buccal segments (87654); and upper and lower labial segments (321 123). Each segment is subdivided into buccal (or labial) and lingual (or palatal) aspects.

A typical periodontal chart (Figure 25.3) has a 2 mm interval grid to record pocket depths; and boxes for the numerical scores of pocket depth, gingival recession, bone loss, tooth mobility, plaque distribution, and other factors such as imperfect fillings, dentures, or other sources of plaque accumulation.

The sextant system is also used by orthodontists for descriptive purposes.

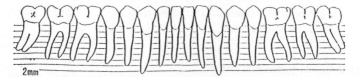

Figure 25.3 *Portion of periodontal chart.*

Treatment

Periodontal disease is caused by bacterial plaque. This occurs at the gum margins – on the surface of the teeth and on the surface of calculus. Therefore the fundamental aim of treatment is plaque control. Short-term success can be achieved by the combined efforts of the patient and the dental practice. But unless such teamwork is maintained on a permanent basis, the long-term result will be failure to control or cure the disease.

The patient's responsibilities are the removal of accessible supragingival plaque, giving up smoking, and attending regularly to check progress. The dental team are responsible for motivating and teaching patients how to do it, while the dentist and hygienist are responsible for the removal of plaque which is inaccessible to the patient's own efforts.

Accessible plaque is removed by **toothbrushing** and **flossing**. Subgingival plaque is inaccessible to patients and is removed by **scaling**. Once these aims have been achieved, and maintained, the causal sources of irritation which produce the disease are lost.

In chronic gingivitis, bleeding ceases, swollen gums return to their normal healthy condition and false pockets are thereby eliminated. The patient is then cured, but strict oral hygiene and regular dental checks are required thereafter to prevent recurrence of plaque and calculus formation.

In chronic periodontitis there is no regeneration of lost bone but mild cases can be cured in the same way as chronic gingivitis. In the advanced stages of the disease, scaling alone cannot eliminate true pockets if they are too deep to be accessible. In such cases they are removed surgically by recontouring the gum forming the pockets, and perhaps smoothing the bone. In this way, even advanced periodontal disease can be arrested, but a return of the condition is inevitable unless the patient follows the dentist's instructions on supragingival plaque control, and attends regularly to check progress and continue subgingival plaque control.

Apart from scaling and gingival surgery, appropriate treatment is given for any other conditions facilitating plaque retention: for example, unsatisfactory fillings, crowns and dentures; unopposed and irregular teeth.

As periodontal disease is an infection by plaque bacteria, an obvious approach to treatment is the application of antibacterial drugs directly into the gingival crevice and pockets. This approach is now one of considerable interest and research but it is too early to be certain of its future role.

Supragingival plaque control

Supragingival calculus and any overhanging cervical margins of restorations are removed in the surgery. At home, thorough, twice-daily toothbrushing by the patient will then keep accessible plaque under control. Appropriate instruction in the surgery, and the use of disclosing agents at home, will show patients how well they are performing, and indicate where improvement is required.

Parts which are inaccessible to an ordinary toothbrush are the interdental spaces below the contact points of adjacent teeth. They can be cleaned with dental floss, wood points and an interspace brush. The dentist or hygienist must give the patient special instruction in these methods as they can do more harm than good if used incorrectly or unnecessarily.

Dental floss is thread or tape which is worked between the teeth to keep their contact areas clean. Where recession of the gum has occurred, or gingival surgery has been performed, the resulting interdental spaces may be too large for flossing.

Wood points are used for these large spaces. They are soft wooden sticks which are passed through the spaces to keep them clear of food debris and reduce plaque formation.

An **interspace brush** (Figure 25.4) is a special type of toothbrush designed to clean interdental spaces in the same way as wood points. It has only one tuft of bristles.

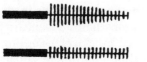

Figure 25.4 *Interspace brushes.*

Subgingival plaque control

This region is inaccessible to patients and is treated by regular scaling. This is done by a dentist or hygienist; and the patient's own efforts at supragingival plaque control are checked at the same time. Subgingival scaling removes plaque and calculus deposits from the gingival crevice and pockets.

Scaling instruments (Figure 25.5) are made in various designs appropriate for the removal of calculus from any part of a tooth. In general they are single-ended hand instruments with a very sharp end for planing away plaque and dislodging scales of calculus. Sharp instruments are essential and sharpening must be regularly undertaken. A calculus probe is used to detect subgingival calculus. When scaling is completed, which may take a few visits, the teeth are polished. This removes residual supragingival plaque and is done with a handpiece, small brushes or rubber cups, and polishing paste.

Subgingival scaling entails much instrumentation within the gingival crevice and pockets. This, in addition to the gingivitis

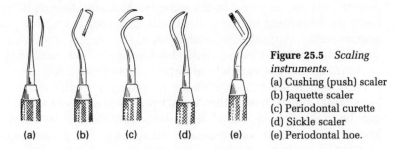

Figure 25.5 *Scaling instruments.*
(a) Cushing (push) scaler
(b) Jaquette scaler
(c) Periodontal curette
(d) Sickle scaler
(e) Periodontal hoe.

already present, produces considerable bleeding and requires the use of local anaesthesia. Antibiotic cover is also necessary for some patients before scaling and periodontal surgery (Chapters 9 and 11).

Patients are provided with a waterproof bib, eye protection and a saliva ejector. A supply of napkins is necessary for wiping the instruments during scaling, together with suction and water spray for keeping the area clear of blood. The nurse is often required to direct the spray for the operator and hold an aspirator tube. Full protective clothing for the prevention of cross-infection must be worn by chairside staff.

Scaling with hand instruments is a tedious procedure for operator and patient, but can be done much more easily and quickly with an **ultrasonic scaler**. This apparatus produces ultrasonic vibrations which are transmitted through a cable to a special scaling instrument. When it is applied to a tooth, the vibrations help loosen the plaque and calculus and they are flushed away by a water-cooling spray which is part of the apparatus. The scaling instrument consists of a special handpiece with a range of detachable scaling tips of various shapes. Use of a chlorhexidine mouthwash by the patient, before scaling, reduces any risk of cross-infection of staff.

Provided the patient achieves adequate supragingival plaque control; while the dentist deals with any restoration overhangs, imperfect partial dentures or other hindrances to plaque removal; and the hygienist or dentist can maintain subgingival plaque control; most cases of straightforward chronic periodontitis can be cured. However, cases will remain where this treatment alone cannot succeed. Patients with very deep pockets, especially those involving multi-rooted teeth, may present a problem of inaccessible subgingival plaque which can only be removed by surgical procedures to gain and maintain access to it.

Periodontal surgery

Periodontal conditions which do not respond to plaque control procedures such as meticulous oral hygiene by the patient, and subgingival scaling by a dental operator, may require treatment by minor oral surgery procedures. They are performed under local anaesthesia and may be undertaken by the patient's own dentist or by referral to a periodontal specialist.

Flap operations

Flap operations are similar to the technique described in Chapter 16 for the removal of an unerupted tooth. They cover a variety of procedures to remove inaccessible subgingival plaque and facilitate subsequent plaque control. Teeth with irregular gingival pocketing, a complex and uneven pattern of bone loss, or involvement of the **furcation** (the branching of roots of multi-rooted teeth), are those most likely to need such operations.

A gingival flap is reflected; alveolar bone surfaces are trimmed and contoured to eliminate bony pockets; all subgingival plaque and calculus is removed; and the gum is repositioned by suturing. There is no removal of gum but the gingival margin may be positioned more apically and thus expose more of the root.

Gingivectomy

Gingivectomy is the removal of a strip of gingival margin (Figure 25.6). It is mainly confined to cases with excessive overgrowth of gum caused by certain drugs used for medical conditions. The drugs involved are phenytoin, nifedipine and cyclosporin (page 312).

The excess gum is removed with a **gingivectomy knife**. There are many different types of gingivectomy knife available but probably the

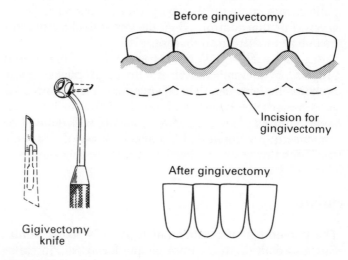

Gigivectomy
knife

Figure 25.6 *Gingivectomy.*

most convenient is a **Blake knife** (Figure 25.6), which uses disposable blades. The strip of incised gum is removed with tweezers and the raw area covered with a **periodontal pack** to protect the gum and promote rapid painless healing. The pack is removed about a week later and thorough scaling is then performed. A modified form of ZOE may be used as a pack but proprietary brands, (for example *Coe-Pak*, *Peripac*, *Barricaid*), are more popular and convenient. Packs are usually unnecessary for flap operations as the gum flap is sutured back into place and no raw areas are left exposed.

Following gingival surgery, patients are given or prescribed analgesic drugs to relieve after-pain; given an appointment for removal of sutures or pack a week later; and instructed to avoid smoking, eating hard food and using a toothbrush on the operative area meanwhile. A soft diet and chlorhexidine mouthwashes are advised instead.

After-care

After periodontal treatment is completed, whether by scaling and polishing alone or by surgery as well, it is then the patient's responsibility to keep teeth clean and free of plaque. They are accordingly shown how to do it, as already described, and encouraged to use disclosing agents at home to check their own performance.

It must be emphasized to patients that toothbrushing and inter-dental cleaning to remove supragingival plaque are of paramount importance following periodontal treatment. Failure to perform these essential tasks at least once daily will result in a reversion to the original condition of chronic periodontitis. Conservative treatment of periodontal disease by the dental team is a waste of time unless patients are prepared to co-operate by exercising rigorous supra-gingival plaque control. When neglect is likely, extraction is the best treatment for advanced disease.

Regular recall appointments are made to check and record the progress of plaque control and to chart pocket depth and tooth mobility. Patients can then be encouraged and motivated to maintain good periodontal health; and are given any further advice and treatment required. The frequency of recalls will depend on individual response to treatment and the effectiveness of home plaque control measures.

Prevention

The prevention of periodontal disease is rather similar to that of caries as both originate from plaque formation. In caries the plaque exerts its effect by acid formation, whereas in periodontal disease it is by bacterial irritation and calculus formation. Prevention consists of the parts played by the patient and the dental team.

It is the patients' responsibility to clean their teeth twice daily to remove supragingival plaque. They must also attend regularly for check-ups, and any required treatment, at the intervals determined by the dentist. These vary according to individual requirements but all patients should be seen at least once a year.

Preventive dental treatment involves many branches of dentistry: scaling, polishing and instruction in plaque control, to prevent gingivitis progressing to periodontitis; fillings, to restore contact points and prevent food packing between the teeth; orthodontics, to correct irregularities and encourage lip closure; prosthetics to restore function to unopposed teeth and evenly distribute the stress of mastication over all the teeth. As in the case of caries, ill-fitting partial dentures must be replaced by new ones, correctly designed to avoid accumulation of plaque at the gum margins.

Acute periodontitis

This chapter has only covered chronic periodontal disease so far. The reason for this is the universal prevalence of the condition and its responsibility for the major cause of tooth loss in adults. However, it can also occur as an acute inflammation of the gum or periodontal membrane in a healthy mouth, or as a complication of existing chronic disease.

Apart from some swelling and reddening of the gums, chronic gingivitis does not show the other cardinal signs of acute inflammation: pain, loss of function and a high temperature; but all these features are usually present in acute forms of periodontal disease.

Pericoronitis

This is an inflammation of the gum overlying an erupting tooth, and is probably the commonest type of acute periodontal disease. It can occur on any tooth but it soon resolves as the tooth erupts further. When it occurs in babies it is called *teething* and is generally regarded as a trivial normal condition.

However, a very serious and painful type of pericoronitis commonly occurs as the lower third molar erupts. This tooth often has insufficient space to erupt fully and becomes partially erupted and impacted against the second molar (Figure 16.3).

In such cases a gum flap over the partially erupted crown persists and this leads to food stagnation, plaque accumulation and secondary infection beneath the gum flap as it is inaccessible to a toothbrush. Acute inflammation supervenes and the gum becomes bright red, swollen, and too painful to eat on. The swelling usually results in the gum flap being continually bitten by the opposing upper third molar and this makes the pericoronitis even worse. The inflammation may spread to adjacent areas, resulting in more swelling, high temperature and trismus (page 130).

Treatment

The upper wisdom tooth is extracted if it is biting on the inflamed gum flap. The lower wisdom tooth is also extracted if it cannot erupt into good occlusion; but extraction is delayed until the acute inflammation has been successfully treated. This is achieved by giving metronidazole or an antibiotic and syringing beneath the gum flap with a disinfectant such as chlorhexidine to keep it clean. The patient is advised to help by taking hot saline mouthwashes after meals.

If the affected tooth can erupt into good occlusion it need not be extracted. A local gingivectomy is performed instead to remove the offending gum flap; but again this is delayed until the acute pericoronitis is cured.

Acute herpetic gingivitis

This condition is caused by the *herpes simplex* virus and most commonly affects infants. All the signs of acute inflammation (page 60) are present and the rest of the oral mucous membrane may be involved too in the form of tiny blisters which leave painful ulcers (*acute herpetic stomatitis*). The condition is short-lived but uncomfortable; the patient feels unwell and may be unable to eat solids, but it resolves without treatment and the gingival condition returns to normal.

However, the virus remains dormant in the body and can be reactivated later by a common cold to produce a *cold sore* on the lip. During the acute phase or presence of a cold sore, the condition is highly infectious and strict cross-infection control must be followed. The use of gloves is essential to protect dental staff against the very painful condition of herpetic whitlow which can occur from touching the infected area.

Acute necrotizing ulcerative gingivitis

This is abbreviated to ANUG and was formerly called acute ulcerative gingivitis (AUG) or Vincent's disease. It is an acute gingivitis characterized by pain and halitosis (bad breath). The affected gum appears bright red, with a covering layer of grey membrane where the gum margin has been destroyed by bacterial action. The bacteria involved are **bacillus fusiformis** and **borrelia vincenti** (Figure 8.1). All the features of acute inflammation are present: red, swollen, painful gums; loss of function, because it is too painful to chew hard food; and the patient often has a raised temperature.

It mainly affects young adults and usually occurs in areas already affected by chronic gingivitis. In many cases stress, heavy smoking and a lowered general resistance precipitates an attack; thus it is more common in winter when colds, influenza and other infections are rife.

Treatment

The principles of treatment are to kill the bacteria responsible for the painful acute inflammation, and follow this by plaque control to cure the preceding chronic gingivitis.

Metronidazole (*Flagyl*) or an antibiotic, such as penicillin, is given to kill the bacteria. Metronidazole is the drug of choice but penicillin is used for pregnant patients. Whichever drug is used to kill the bacteria, it is always necessary to scale the teeth afterwards to remove all plaque and calculus and prevent a recurrence. Throughout treatment, chlorhexidine mouthwashes are used to help keep the mouth clean.

Acute lateral periodontal abscess

This is an occasional complication of chronic periodontitis in which pus formation in a deep pocket is unable to drain through the gingival crevice. The pus accumulates instead at the base of the pocket to form an abscess. This condition must not be confused with an acute alveolar abscess (page 221), which follows pulp death and occurs at the root apex. Acute lateral periodontal abscess occurs on a *vital* tooth at the side of the root.

Treatment depends on the depth of the pocket and may entail extraction or surgical drainage in severe cases. Milder cases may be resolved with metronidazole or penicillin; but recurrence is probable unless the underlying periodontal disease is cured.

Practical examination

Mix sufficient periodontal pack (for example, *Coe-Pak*) to cover the lower incisor area.

1   Select correct tubes of material; large mixing pad or glass slab; spatula.

---

2   Dispense equal lengths from each tube, side by side at centre of mixing pad, ensuring that tubes do not contaminate each other. Replace caps.

3   Amount of material dispensed should be sufficient to provide a reasonable quantity without waste.

4   Mix rapidly until colour is uniform and no streaks remain.

5   Strop the spatula blade on the edge of the mixing pad to remove streaks and collect mix on clean part of pad. Wipe the spatula blade to remove any residual streaks, scoop some paste on to the spatula and offer it, handle first, to the examiner.

Written examination

Describe what the dentist may find when he carries out a periodontal examination of a patient with:
(a)   healthy gingiva
(b)   gingivitis
What advice should be given to a patient with gingivitis to improve their gingival health? (November 1995)

What is chronic gingivitis?
How does plaque contribute to this condition?
Describe the ways in which plaque is controlled. (May 1994)

Summary

Stages

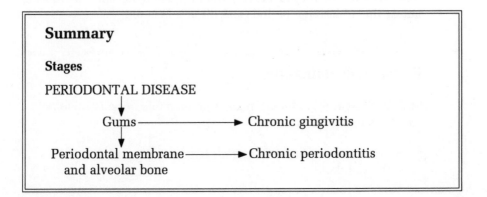

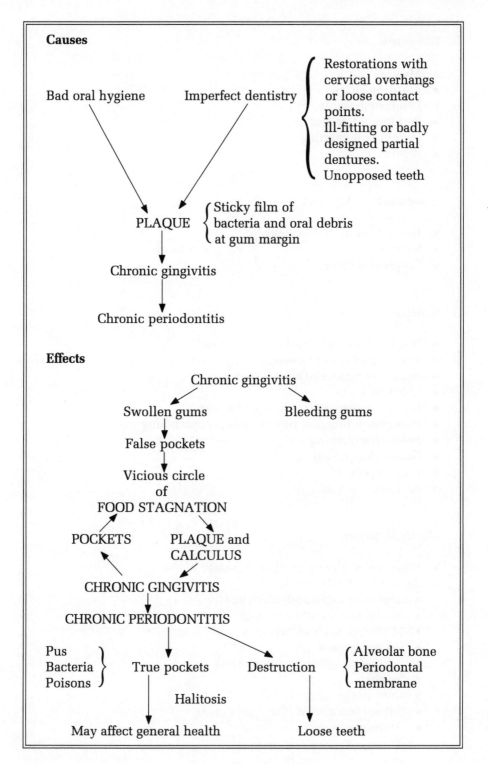

Causes

Bad oral hygiene   Imperfect dentistry { Restorations with cervical overhangs or loose contact points. Ill-fitting or badly designed partial dentures. Unopposed teeth

PLAQUE { Sticky film of bacteria and oral debris at gum margin

Chronic gingivitis

Chronic periodontitis

Effects

Chronic gingivitis

Swollen gums   Bleeding gums

False pockets

Vicious circle
of
FOOD STAGNATION

POCKETS   PLAQUE and CALCULUS

CHRONIC GINGIVITIS

CHRONIC PERIODONTITIS

Pus
Bacteria } True pockets   Destruction { Alveolar bone Periodontal membrane
Poisons

Halitosis

May affect general health   Loose teeth

Diagnosis

- Medical history
- Bleeding gums
- Disclosing agents
- Periodontal probes
- Periodontal charting
- X-rays

Treatment

- Instruction in oral hygiene ⎫
- Scaling   ⎬ Plaque control
- Gingival surgery   ⎭

Scaling

- Bib, napkins and chlorhexidine mouthwash
- Mirror, probe and tweezers
- Aspirator tubes and saliva ejector
- Calculus probe
- Scaling instruments; ultrasonic scaler
- Handpiece, brushes, rubber cups and polishing paste
- Protective clothing
- Glasses for patient
- LA equipment?
- Antibiotic cover?

Gingival surgery

- Wear gown, gloves, mask and glasses
- Set out on sterile towel:
  - Aspirator tubes and saliva ejector
  - Sterile towel and towel clip
  - Mirror, probe and tweezers
  - LA equipment
  - Scalpels or gingivectomy knives
  - Swabs
  - Gum packs (gingivectomy)
  - Suture equipment (flap operations)
  - Antibiotic cover?

After-care

Meticulous oral hygiene $\begin{cases} \text{Disclosing agents} \\ \text{Toothbrush} \\ \text{Dental floss} \\ \text{Wood points} \\ \text{Interspace brush} \end{cases}$

Regular inspection and treatment

Prevention

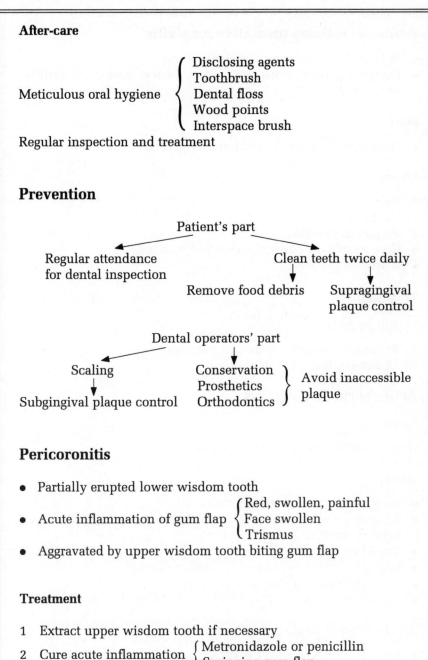

Patient's part

Regular attendance
for dental inspection

Clean teeth twice daily

Remove food debris

Supragingival
plaque control

Dental operators' part

Scaling

Subgingival plaque control

$\left. \begin{array}{l} \text{Conservation} \\ \text{Prosthetics} \\ \text{Orthodontics} \end{array} \right\}$ Avoid inaccessible plaque

Pericoronitis

- Partially erupted lower wisdom tooth
- Acute inflammation of gum flap $\begin{cases} \text{Red, swollen, painful} \\ \text{Face swollen} \\ \text{Trismus} \end{cases}$
- Aggravated by upper wisdom tooth biting gum flap

Treatment

1 Extract upper wisdom tooth if necessary
2 Cure acute inflammation $\begin{cases} \text{Metronidazole or penicillin} \\ \text{Syringing gum flap} \end{cases}$
3 Extract lower tooth if good occlusion impossible
4 Conserve tooth if good occlusion possible → gingivectomy to remove gum flap

Acute necrotizing ulcerative gingivitis

- Bacillus fusiformis and borrelia vincenti
- Lowered general resistance, stress, heavy smoking – mainly young adults

Sites

- Gum already affected by chronic gingivitis

Effects

- Pain
- Halitosis
- Bright red bleeding gums
- Grey membrane covering destroyed gum margin
- Raised temperature

Treatment

1 Kill bacteria $\begin{cases} \text{Metronidazole} \\ \text{Penicillin (pregnancy)} \end{cases}$
2 Scaling → remove plaque and calculus
3 Chlorhexidine mouthwashes

Acute herpetic gingivitis

Cause

Herpes simplex virus → mainly infants

Effects

- Bright red swollen bleeding gums
- Blistering and ulceration of oral mucous membrane (acute herpetic stomatitis)
- Raised temperature
- Highly infective → full cross-infection procedure
- Short duration and spontaneous cure
- Virus remains dormant → highly infective cold sores later

Acute lateral periodontal abscess

- Usually occurs in deep pocket at side of root of vital tooth
- Severe cases: treated by surgical drainage or extraction
- Mild cases: metronidazole or penicillin
- All cases: will recur unless underlying chronic periodontitis is treated

26 Prevention of Dental Disease

Most dental disorders arise directly or indirectly from two basic diseases of the teeth and their supporting tissues – caries and periodontal disease. The prevention of dental disease is therefore concerned with the control of plaque as this is the common factor in caries and periodontal disease. The methods of prevention are discussed in detail in this chapter, but first of all it is necessary to consider plaque itself.

Plaque

The full name is **bacterial dental plaque** but, in general usage and hereafter, it is simply referred to as plaque. As it plays such an all-important part in dental disease its origin and effects should be clearly understood by all whose work involves dental treatment or dental health education.

Plaque is a thin transparent layer of saliva, oral debris and normal mouth bacteria which sticks to the tooth surface and can only be removed by cleaning. It is then replaced within a few hours by a new deposit of plaque and may be regarded as a natural occurrence. The harm it causes comes from food debris which sticks to the plaque during meals and snacks and provides a plentiful supply of nourishment for its bacteria. They accordingly flourish, the plaque grows thicker, and caries and periodontal disease begin. Which of the two diseases predominates, depends on diet, the site of plaque and age of the patient; but the plaque is the same whichever disease occurs.

Caries is mainly a disease of children and young adults whereas periodontal disease predominates in later life. The difference is caused by the rate at which the two diseases progress. Caries can cause loss of teeth within a few years whereas periodontal disease may take decades. By the time periodontal disease has reached an advanced stage, the earlier onslaught of caries has already been overcome, and is no longer a problem; as the teeth which were susceptible to caries have already been treated, by extraction, filling, fissure sealing or exposure to fluoride.

Another reason for the difference is the diet of the two age groups. Consumption of sweets and sugary food and drinks is probably far greater, and far less controlled, in children; and their teeth are consequently much more vulnerable to caries. However, it must not be assumed that older people are immune to caries. It still occurs if childhood patterns of unrestricted, indiscriminate consumption of sweets persists. A typical example is the person who continually sucks mints after giving up smoking – and then develops rampant caries.

Plaque and caries

When food containing sugar is eaten, some of it sticks to the plaque and is turned into acid by plaque bacteria. The acid forms within the plaque and dissolves the underlying enamel to produce caries. Sites where this most commonly occurs are inaccessible to a toothbrush and are called stagnation areas. They comprise occlusal fissures and the contact areas between mesial and distal surfaces of adjoining teeth.

The most important thing to remember about the cause of caries is the unique role of sugar. Food which does not contain any cannot be turned into acid by plaque bacteria, and no matter how much plaque and food debris are present, caries will not occur unless sugar is present too. If there were no sugar for us to eat, there would be no caries.

Plaque and periodontal disease

Periodontal disease is caused by plaque at the gum margin. As in the case of caries, food debris sticks to the plaque and allows its bacteria to flourish. Bacterial poisons then irritate the gum margin and it becomes chronically inflamed – this, of course, being a natural reaction of the body to irritation.

If this plaque is not removed it spreads into the gingival crevice and the following sequence of events occurs: chronic gingivitis and sub-gingival calculus formation; causing inflammatory swelling, which transforms the gingival crevice into a false pocket (Figure 25.1), and permits more food stagnation and more plaque to form; thus establishing a vicious circle. The gingival crevice becomes ulcerated by bacterial poisons and they drain into the underlying tissues to begin destruction of the periodontal membrane fibres and alveolar bone; until, eventually, support for the teeth is lost and they become too loose to have any functional value.

The fundamental difference between periodontal disease and caries is that the latter is caused by dietary sugar; whereas *any* type of food can feed the plaque bacteria which cause periodontal disease.

Detection of plaque

Plaque is transparent and virtually invisible when it first forms. If oral hygiene is poor, it thickens and becomes more obvious as food debris adheres to its surface. Even then it may be difficult for dentists to make their patients understand its importance. Only when patients can clearly see it for themselves are they likely to take notice and realize the need for good oral hygiene.

Fortunately, the normally invisible plaque can be transformed into a dramatically convincing display by applying a red dye. It is painted on the teeth and then rinsed off with a mouthwash. Clean surfaces are unaffected but plaque is stained red and shows up vividly against clean white enamel.

Dyes used for revealing plaque are called disclosing agents. Originally, iodine was used but has been superseded by a red dye called *erythrosin*. It is applied as a solution or by chewing it in the form of tablets.

Prevention of dental disease

In the development of caries, the role of plaque is confined to acid formation; and this only happens in the presence of sugar. In periodontal disease there are no such limitations; it is the mere presence of plaque at the gum margin which causes the disease – no matter what kind of food is eaten.

The prevention of dental disease is therefore concerned with plaque control; but in the case of caries, additional measures such as dietary control and increasing the resistance of teeth to acid, are far more important. The methods of prevention are oral hygiene and dietary discipline, which are the patient's responsibility; preventive dentistry, which is the dental team's contribution; oral health education and increasing the resistance of teeth to caries, which are community health measures.

Oral hygiene

Oral hygiene consists simply of keeping the teeth clean and free of food debris, thus preventing the accumulation and persistence of plaque which leads to dental disease. It can be achieved by cleaning the teeth twice daily and not eating between meals. Cleaning is best performed by brushing as this is an effective way of removing plaque.

If brushing is not possible, loose food debris can be removed by finishing the meal with a detergent food. Such foods are raw, firm, fibrous fruits or vegetables, such as apples, pears, carrots, celery. By virtue of their tough fibrous consistency they require much chewing and stimulate salivary flow, thereby helping to scour the teeth clean of food remnants. Although plaque is unaffected by detergent foods they can remove some of the food debris which nourishes all plaque bacteria and enables some of them to produce acid.

Toothbrushing is the most effective way of cleaning teeth. When properly done it removes plaque, whereas detergent foods can only clean away loose food particles. Thus the role of detergent food is not that of a satisfactory alternative to brushing; but an additional measure at the end of a meal, or a substitute when brushing is not possible.

Toothbrushing

Brushing after meals can only be effective if it removes plaque. The object is to clean every accessible tooth surface after meals in order to remove food debris and plaque.

Toothbrushes with a small head and multitufted medium nylon bristles are probably the most effective. The brush is rinsed and a pea-sized portion of fluoride toothpaste added. Each dental arch is divided into three sections: left and right sides and front. Side sections are subdivided into buccal, lingual and occlusal surfaces; front into labial and lingual. This amounts to eight groups of surfaces in each jaw, and at least five seconds should be spent on each group. Each jaw is done in turn and the mouth is then cleared by spitting out. Brushes should be washed afterwards and allowed to dry. They only have a limited life and need replacement every few months as the bristles curl up and render the brush useless.

The actual method of brushing, whether by a scrubbing or rotary action, is immaterial. It is the end result – removal of plaque – that matters, not the method used. By using disclosing tablets, under guidance from their dentist or hygienist, individual patients can see for themselves which method suits them best.

Effective toothbrushing requires time, knowledge and skill. Many people lack these requirements and brushing is ineffective as a plaque control measure. The whole process can be made simpler for such people by using an electric toothbrush. It cleans effectively without effort, and is particularly valuable for children and the physically handicapped. Although no better than correct manual brushing, it is probably preferable as so many people find it difficult to achieve adequate plaque removal with an ordinary toothbrush.

Interdental cleaning

However good the toothbrushing technique, it is still impossible to clean interdental spaces perfectly with a toothbrush alone. Consequently these mesial and distal contact areas between adjoining teeth are more prone to caries and periodontal disease. To clean them adequately, dental floss, wood points and an interspace brush are used. These methods were described in Chapter 25.

Dietary discipline

It cannot be emphasized too strongly that even if teeth are thoroughly cleaned after meals, caries will still occur if sugary snacks are taken between meals. This is because plaque persists in the inaccessible parts of fissures and contact points. Acid forms in this residual plaque within minutes of eating sugar and caries will develop if frequent snacks are taken between meals. Then, as described in Chapter 17, a constant acid environment at the enamel surface allows demineralization to proceed unchecked, and leaves insufficient time between intakes of sugar for the natural defence mechanism of remineralization to occur. Although adequate toothbrushing and interdental cleaning twice daily may prevent periodontal disease, it cannot prevent caries unless accompanied by strict dietary discipline to eliminate sugary snacks between meals.

Preventive dentistry

Preventive dentistry includes instruction in oral hygiene; regular inspection for checking oral hygiene and to ensure early diagnosis of dental disease; any necessary treatment for the prevention and removal of areas inaccessible to plaque control; and specific caries-prevention measures such as fissure-sealing and topical fluoridation.

Instruction in oral hygiene

Dentists may delegate instruction in oral hygiene to their nurses providing they comply with the GDC requirements on page 10. Oral hygiene instruction is best given at the chairside, while posters and pamphlets in the waiting room serve as an extra reminder. Patients are told how dental disease arises and how it can be prevented. This entails an explanation of the all-important role of plaque and the effects it produces.

The most impressive way of demonstrating plaque on their own teeth is to give patients a disclosing tablet to suck. Patients can then see for themselves in a mirror whether they are cleaning their teeth properly. They are then shown how to use a toothbrush effectively, how to clean their interdental spaces, advised to clean their teeth twice daily, and warned against snacks between meals. They are also encouraged to use disclosing tablets at home to check their oral hygiene themselves.

However, they are not likely to heed such advice unless it is practicable. Patients must therefore be told how to care for their teeth when toothbrushing is not possible or convenient. The best substitute in such cases is to finish their meal with a detergent food such as fresh fruit, raw vegetable or sugar-free chewing gum. These increase salivary flow and will leave a minimum amount of food debris on the teeth; whereas a conventional sticky sweet dessert, such as jam roll and custard, will leave the maximum amount of acid-producing debris. A sweet drink of coffee or tea after meals will do no harm if patients are encouraged to use an artificial sweetener such as saccharin.

If plaque is thoroughly removed daily, by toothbrushing and interdental cleaning, periodontal disease can be prevented. But this is not sufficient for the prevention of caries. Acid production in residual or fresh plaque is so rapid that caries cannot be prevented if sugar is continually reintroduced by frequent snacks between meals. It must be impressed upon patients and parents that caries cannot be prevented by brushing alone. It must be combined with dietary discipline. Sweet snacks between meals should either be stopped altogether or replaced by sugar-free food such as fruit, nuts, low-fat cheese or crisps. Again, dietary advice must be practical if it is to be accepted. For example, parents who do not wish to deprive children of sweets can be advised to compromise by arranging for sweets to be eaten at meal times only, and not in between.

Expectant and nursing mothers are warned of the disastrous dental effects of using dummies or bottles with sweetened fruit juices. They can cause complete destruction of incisor crowns, by caries and erosion (Chapter 17); and colour photographs of such cases may help dissuade mothers from using them. Similar effects can arise from the long-term use of medicines sweetened with sugar, and these should be replaced by sugar-free alternatives.

Regular inspection and treatment

Prevention is better than cure. Patients should be encouraged to have a regular inspection every year. Oral hygiene could then be checked with disclosing agents and any deficiencies shown to the patient. Further instruction can then be given if necessary. Bite-wing X-rays may be taken at the same time for early diagnosis of caries.

These visits will detect incipient dental disease which can be treated far more easily in its earliest stages than later. Such treatment may involve all branches of dentistry:

1   Periodic scaling to remove inaccessible plaque and small deposits of calculus can prevent the onset of periodontal disease before it even reaches the stage of gingivitis.
2   Early treatment of caries enables affected teeth to be conserved rather than extracted.
3   If teeth have already been lost, carefully planned prosthetic treatment to restore normal occlusion and function will prevent food traps developing.

4 Any unsatisfactory dental treatment which itself promotes plaque formation (such as fillings with cervical overhangs, ill-fitting or badly designed partial dentures) is rectified.
5 For children, orthodontics can prevent or cure irregularities of the teeth which might otherwise form inaccessible stagnation areas.

Dental disease, arising as it does from the accumulation of plaque, can therefore be prevented to a large extent by patients' own efforts at supragingival plaque control and avoiding sugar between meals. Regular dental inspection and treatment can also prevent the vicious circle of dental disease developing, by providing treatment at the very earliest stages before caries and periodontal disease have time to cause serious damage to the dentition.

Topical fluoridation

Topical fluoridation means the direct application of fluorides to the teeth. It can produce a significant reduction in caries and consequently plays a valuable part in preventive dentistry for children.

The most economical way of applying fluoride is for patients to do it themselves by regular brushing, twice daily, with fluoride toothpaste. Even if their toothbrushing technique is not good enough to remove much plaque, it still allows fluoride to penetrate plaque and exert its beneficial effect of promoting remineralization. Together with dietary discipline, it forms the basis of effective and practicable caries prevention.

Topical application of fluoride may also be undertaken by the dentist, hygienist or therapist, but is usually confined to children with rampant caries; those with medical conditions such as haemophilia and heart defects which would make tooth extraction dangerous; and those who are too handicapped to achieve adequate oral hygiene. Fluoride applications are done three times a year, usually during each school holiday.

A popular method of application is an acidulated phosphate fluoride (APF) gel in a special applicator tray. Many such trays are available – some disposable – but they all provide full coverage of the entire arch; and some permit both arches to be treated at the same time. APF gels are pleasantly flavoured and well tolerated by children.

The technique has two stages: first a thorough polish to remove plaque, after which the teeth are washed and dried; and second, the APF gel is applied in the special tray for a few minutes. On removal of the tray, patients are instructed not to rinse, drink or eat for half-an-hour.

An alternative method is to paint the teeth with a fluoride varnish, such as *Duraphat*. As before, teeth must still be cleaned and dried first.

Roots exposed by gingival recession sometimes become very sensitive to hot or cold fluids. Fluoride varnish is applied to such areas to relieve this cause of pain.

Another method for this condition is the use of chlorhexidine varnish (Chapter 11). Apart from desensitizing such roots, its antibacterial action can arrest early caries of exposed roots. It can also be used as a temporary fissure sealant, as described in Chapter 21.

Fissure sealing

Topical fluorides exert most of their effect on mesial and distal (proximal) surfaces. Occlusal fissures are just as vulnerable to caries but they are less well protected by fluorides. Fortunately they can receive extra, and even better, protection by the application of fissure sealants. These materials are composite fillings or glass ionomer cement, and their use was described in Chapters 21 and 22. Successful fissure sealing should make an occlusal surface safe from caries. Like topical fluoridation, it can be done by hygienists and therapists; and is therefore of major importance in preventive dentistry as it can produce a significant reduction in the commonest disease of children.

Community health measures

Oral health education

Dental staff can explain the causes and prevention of dental disease to individual patients in the surgery, but this only benefits regular attenders. There still remains a need for greater effort by the public health service. Expectant and nursing mothers, parents of schoolchildren, and young teenagers are the groups most in need of advice on dental care. Publicity is still necessary to warn these groups of the damage done by dummies or bottles used with sweetened fruit juices; of acquiring the habit of unrestricted snacks between meals; and avoiding dental inspection until toothache develops. Doctors, midwives, health visitors, clinic staff and schoolteachers all have a part to play in helping the dental team to educate the public.

Nursing mothers should be encouraged to bring their babies when they have their own dental inspection. Toddlers will thereby accept the dental surgery as a place of interest and soon become regular and co-operative patients themselves, long before any treatment is necessary. The discipline of confining sweets to meal times and brushing after meals can be developed at an early age, and will establish good dental habits of lifelong value.

Parents should be warned of the danger of sugar and encouraged to restrict the consumption of sweets between meals. In school, steps should be taken to ensure that school dinners do not leave a film of sugary debris on the teeth; and the consumption of sugary snacks during breaks should be discouraged.

Young teenagers soon realize the importance of good appearance and this can be utilized in dental health education. Regular visits to the dentist for scaling and polishing, filling cavities in front teeth, orthodontics for straightening teeth, and the value of dietary discipline and oral hygiene; all these ways of improving appearance are freely available to them, but this powerful motivating factor could still be more widely communicated at national level.

Many excellent videos, films, posters and pamphlets are already available for display in clinics and schools, but these forms of dental health education are only reaching a small section of the population. To help reduce dental disease, the entire population needs to be shown how to maintain good oral health by dietary discipline, strict oral hygiene and regular dental inspection.

The message of dental health education can be condensed into three simple measures:

1 Reduce the frequency of consumption of food and drink containing sugar. Avoid acid drinks
2 Clean the teeth, twice daily, with *fluoride* toothpaste
3 *Regular* dental attendance at least once a year

Increasing resistance to caries

Increasing the resistance of teeth to acid attack has already been mentioned in Chapter 17. It can be done by fluoridation and fissure sealing.

Preventive dentistry provides dietary advice, topical fluoridation and fissure sealing for individual patients; but community health services can offer preventive measures to the whole population: at clinics where mothers can be advised on correct diet; and by the fluoridation of public water supplies. The community health measure of water fluoridation, mentioned in Chapter 17, is a subject of such importance to the dental profession that it is covered again here in more detail. Decisions to introduce fluoridation are made locally and all dental nurses should know its benefits so that, in any public debate, they may voice their opinion on the basis of knowledge rather than emotion.

Fluoridation

Fluoride is a natural constituent of most water supplies. It consequently forms part of the diet throughout the period of tooth formation and is incorporated into the full thickness of enamel. Thereafter its action continues by a surface (*topical*) effect on erupted teeth. Water containing one part per million (1 ppm) produces a 50% reduction in caries. Above 1 ppm the reduction is no greater but an unfortunate side-effect can occur: an ugly brown staining of enamel called *mottling*. Below 1 ppm there is no significant reduction in caries. Thus the ideal amount of fluoride in water is 1 ppm; at which level it has only one effect – a 50% reduction in caries.

Fluoride has no adverse effects on general health, even when it is in such high concentrations that mottling (fluorosis) is disfiguring. Public health surveys prove these benefits by comparing the number of decayed, missing and filled teeth (**DMF count**) in the populations of areas with differing amounts of fluoride in their water supplies.

Fluoridation of water supplies

A few places in the UK are lucky enough to have the right amount naturally present. This is known as **natural fluoridation**. Most places, however, are less fortunate as their water supplies are deficient in fluoride. But the same effect can be produced in these deficient areas by adding fluoride at the waterworks until it reaches the ideal concentration of 1 ppm. This is now being done on an increasing scale throughout the world and is called **artificial fluoridation**.

Fluoride only exerts its maximum effect if it is present in water until all the permanent teeth have erupted. Throughout this time, it is not only being incorporated into the structure of unerupted teeth, but is also exerting a topical effect on erupted teeth. This topical effect continues as long as fluoridated water is available. Fluoride makes enamel more resistant to acid attack and promotes remineralization; and these effects last throughout life. Fluoridation of water supplies is the simplest, cheapest, safest and most effective public health measure known for the prevention of caries. Without any personal effort, caries is reduced by 50% in the entire population, provided only that they use fluoridated water from birth until after eruption is complete.

Furthermore, this 50% reduction in caries can lead to a decrease in periodontal disease. It does this indirectly by reducing the number of teeth extracted or filled. This means fewer partial dentures, fewer unsatisfactory fillings, and consequently fewer acquired stagnation areas where plaque can accumulate. Thus it is untrue for opponents of fluoridation to say that it only benefits children. It benefits everybody and is of lifelong value.

Alternative forms of fluoridation

Until more health authorities are able to fluoridate their water supplies, some alternatives are available. These are fluoride supplements, toothpaste and topical fluoridation.

Fluoride supplements

If fluoride tablets or drops are taken daily throughout infancy, childhood and adolescence until every tooth has erupted, they produce similar results to water fluoridation. Only the keenest parents will keep this up until all teeth have erupted, so it is not a suitable method for the general public; but it is available free of charge for children by NHS prescription. The daily dosage depends on the fluoride content of local tap water; and supplements should not be used where the existing concentration is 0.7 ppm or more.

Fluoride toothpaste

Almost all toothpaste contains fluoride nowadays. When this is used regularly it is infinitely more effective for caries reduction than any other toothpaste. It has proved to be a major contributory factor in the control of caries as it exerts a topical fluoride action irrespective of individual toothbrushing efficiency. Only a pea-sized amount of toothpaste is used, but to produce its maximum effect the mouth should not be rinsed immediately after brushing. Residual paste should be spat out.

In the absence of mandatory fluoridation of water supplies, toothpaste is recognized as the most important and cost-effective fluoride delivery system.

Topical fluoridation

Topical fluoridation means applying fluoride directly to the crowns of teeth in the dental surgery, and was described in the section on preventive dentistry.

All these alternatives to fluoridation of water supplies are less effective. They require individual effort and only benefit the users. As a public health measure the case for water fluoridation is overwhelming. Until it is generally adopted, however, caries will continue to be, with periodontal disease, one of the commonest diseases of civilization.

Prevention of dental disease

To sum up the whole chapter: there is no single method of preventing dental disease. It can be reduced by a combination of all possible means. These are:

1   Fluoridation of water supplies
2   Dietary discipline
3   Plaque control and twice-daily fluoride toothbrushing

4 Regular dental attendance every year
5 Fissure sealing
6 Oral health education

If all these measures were applied, any individual could remain free of caries for life. But the prevention of periodontal disease is more difficult, as specific measures like fluoridation and fissure sealing only prevent caries and have no direct effect on periodontal disease. The only way of preventing the latter is by the control of plaque. At present this can only be achieved by a combination of perfect oral hygiene and regular dental attendance by the patient; and perfect preventive dentistry by the dental team. However, even the single measure of water fluoridation could reduce periodontal disease as well. It would do this indirectly by halving caries, thus reducing the number of plaque retention areas resulting from imperfect dentistry.

Written examination

What are the possible consequences of neglected oral hygiene?

What instructions and advice would you give to a teenager who presents at the surgery with poor oral hygiene? (November 1993)

Write notes on the following:

(a) dental plaque
(b) fissure sealants
(c) topical fluorides (May 1992)

Describe the uses and effects of the various types of fluoride in general use in dentistry. (November 1992)

Summary

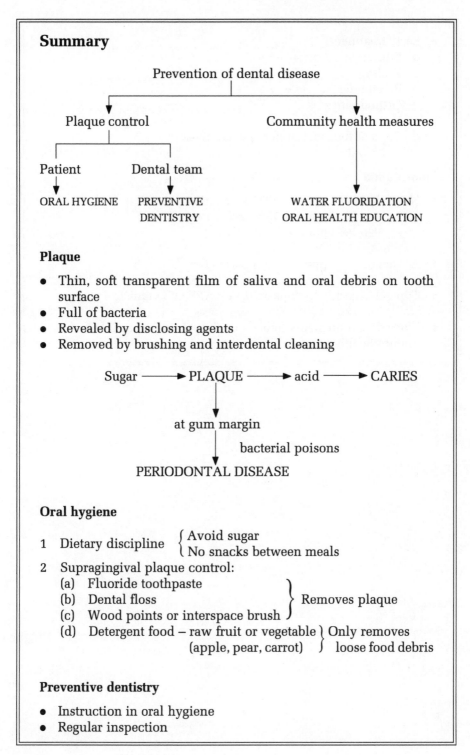

Prevention of dental disease

Plaque control — Community health measures

Patient — Dental team

ORAL HYGIENE — PREVENTIVE DENTISTRY — WATER FLUORIDATION ORAL HEALTH EDUCATION

Plaque

- Thin, soft transparent film of saliva and oral debris on tooth surface
- Full of bacteria
- Revealed by disclosing agents
- Removed by brushing and interdental cleaning

Sugar ⟶ PLAQUE ⟶ acid ⟶ CARIES

at gum margin

bacterial poisons

PERIODONTAL DISEASE

Oral hygiene

1 Dietary discipline { Avoid sugar / No snacks between meals
2 Supragingival plaque control:
    (a) Fluoride toothpaste
    (b) Dental floss   } Removes plaque
    (c) Wood points or interspace brush
    (d) Detergent food – raw fruit or vegetable } Only removes
           (apple, pear, carrot)   loose food debris

Preventive dentistry

- Instruction in oral hygiene
- Regular inspection

- Early treatment:
  - ○ Fillings
  - ○ Scaling
  - ○ Prosthetics
  - ○ Orthodontics
  - ○ Fissure sealing
  - ○ Topical fluoridation for special cases

Fluoridation

- Natural: Over 1 ppm → 50% less caries + mottling
            1 ppm → 50% less caries
  Under 1 ppm → Ineffective

- Artificial: 1 ppm → 50% less caries

- Topical: fluoride toothpaste (DIY); APF gel; varnish

- Fluoride supplements (tablets or drops): impracticable as community health measure

27　Prosthetics

Prosthetics is the branch of dentistry concerned with the replacement of missing teeth by dentures. Their purpose is the restoration of normal appearance, masticatory function and speech, as any of these may be adversely affected by loss of teeth. When there are no teeth left in a jaw, it is said to be **edentulous** and the artificial replacement is called a **full** or **complete denture**; if some teeth are still present the replacement is called a **partial denture**.

Effects of loss of teeth

If a tooth is extracted, and not replaced artificially, the opposing tooth has nothing to bite on and becomes functionless. Having no opposition, it overerupts and loses the beneficial cleansing effect of mastication. It consequently becomes a food trap and plaque retention area which produces localized gingivitis and caries. Furthermore, the two teeth on either side of the missing one may tilt towards each other and form similar food traps. Thus the loss of a single tooth can give rise to plaque accumulation resulting in caries and periodontal disease in at least six other teeth, as shown by the arrows in Figure 27.1.

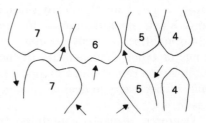

Figure 27.1 *Stagnation areas produced by loss of one tooth. Extraction of* 6̅| *results in overeruption of* |6̲ *and tilting of* 7̲5̲|*.*

If several teeth are missing, mastication cannot be performed efficiently and this could lead to malnutrition. People who lose all or most of their teeth tend to avoid foods which require much chewing, and change to a soft over-cooked diet which may be deficient in important nutrients. In addition the whole force of mastication is borne by the few remaining teeth; and if periodontal disease is already present it will be aggravated by this excessive stress.

It is therefore advisable to replace missing teeth as soon as possible, with a denture or bridge, in order to prevent these disorders arising.

Denture materials

Dentures are usually made of pink acrylic with acrylic teeth. Metal is often used for the framework of partial dentures, and for the palate of full dentures if there is a heavy bite. The metals used are stainless steel and chrome-cobalt.

Acrylic

Most dentures and orthodontic appliances are made of acrylic. This consists of powder called **polymer** and a liquid called **monomer**. When mixed together they form a plastic mass which has the consistency of dough. This sets into a hard acrylic by a process called curing. Curing is effected by heating the dough slowly in a special flask in an oven; or by adding a catalyst which allows it to cure at room temperature. These two methods of curing are known respectively as **heat-curing** and **cold-curing**.

Heat-cured acrylic is used for dentures and orthodontic appliances.

Cold-cured acrylic (also called self-cured or autopolymerized acrylic) is used for temporary crowns, denture repairs and impression trays.

Stages of full denture construction

Before any type of denture is made, a thorough history is taken of any previous experience of dentures, in order to assess the patient's co-operation and anticipate any difficulties. This is followed by clinical and X-ray examination of the mouth to detect any soft tissue abnormalities, excessive undercuts or alveolar resorption, retained roots or other abnormalities of the jaw bone. Surgical procedures, such as the removal of retained roots or alveolectomy (Chapter 16), may be necessary to deal with such problems before the dentures are made.

Dentures are made on models of the jaws in a dental laboratory. The technician makes these models by pouring **plaster of Paris** into an **impression** of the patient's jaw. The impression is taken by the dentist in an **impression tray** which is filled with impression material and held in the mouth until set.

Having obtained models of each jaw, they must be mounted in the same spatial relationship to each other as they are in the mouth; i.e. the upper and lower models are mounted in such a position that the distance between them, vertically and horizontally, is exactly the same as that between the jaws when the mouth is at rest. In order to achieve this, **occlusion rims** are constructed in the laboratory. They consists of a **baseplate** with a wax rim. A baseplate is a temporary plate made of acrylic, shellac or wax, which the technician moulds to the model and trims to the exact outline of the intended denture. The wax rim is attached to the baseplate in the same position as the teeth would be. These occlusion rims are then sent to the surgery, where they are worn by the patient while the dentist records the normal relationship of the jaws at rest. Although this stage is commonly referred to as *taking the bite*, more correct terms are **recording the jaw relationship** or **occlusal registration**.

The models and occlusion rims are then returned to the laboratory where the technician mounts them on an **articulator**. This is essentially a hinged mechanism for keeping models in their correct relationship as obtained at the occlusal registration stage. It can open and close to simulate some of the movements of the jaws. Once the models are mounted on an articulator, the wax rims are removed from the baseplates, and the false teeth fixed on, with wax, in their place. The baseplates with teeth attached are then fitted in the surgery to see that they occlude together correctly and are of satisfactory appearance. This is called the **trial insertion** stage or *try-in*. As the teeth are only embedded in wax, any alterations in arrangement or shade can easily be made at this stage.

These *waxed-up* **trial dentures** are now returned to the laboratory to be made into finished dentures, which are then fitted in the surgery.

The whole procedure is summarized as follows:

1 Surgery: dentist takes first impressions with stock trays
2 Laboratory: technician makes special trays on plaster models of jaws
3 Surgery: final impressions with special trays
4 Laboratory: occlusion rims made on final models (also known as working models)
5 Surgery: jaw relationship recorded with occlusion rims
6 Laboratory:
   (a) final models and occlusion rims mounted on articulator
   (b) wax rims replaced with acrylic teeth embedded in wax
7 Surgery: trial dentures checked in patient's mouth for appearance, fit and occlusion
8 Laboratory: wax replaced with acrylic for finished dentures
9 Surgery: finished dentures fitted; patient given appointment to return for any adjustments

Prevention of cross-infection

In order to prevent cross-infection of patients, surgery and laboratory staff, all work for a laboratory must be disinfected (and labelled as such) before despatch. Similarly, all work received from a laboratory must be disinfected before use. Immersion in sodium hypochlorite for ten minutes is suitable for most materials; but this cannot be used for aluminium impression trays; while chrome-cobalt can only withstand short periods of contact with hypochlorite. Alternatives in such cases are glutaraldehyde or chlorhexidine. Gloves should be worn by personnel handling laboratory work.

Impressions

Surgery procedure

The nurse sets out the patient's records, laboratory prescription pad, bowl of water for patient's existing dentures, mouth mirror and impression trays, and has the impression material ready for preparing and loading into a tray. A large kidney dish should also be available as some patients are liable to be sick. The patient is provided with a bib and mouthwash. After impressions have been taken, the nurse cleans off any impression material from the patient's lips. Patients who are prone to sickness during impressions can be helped by giving them a surface anaesthetic mouthwash, spray or lozenge beforehand (Chapter 11).

After removal from the mouth, impressions are first rinsed in cold running water to remove saliva and any blood, then disinfected by immersion in hypochlorite, and rinsed again in running water. Eye protection should be worn in case of splashing.

As the impression must reach the laboratory in perfect condition the nurse must take great care to handle it correctly. It should be very carefully packed if it is sent away to an outside laboratory; correctly labelled with the name of dentist and patient, and with full details on the prescription form of the work required and date for return.

Impression trays

Impression trays are of two kinds: edentulous and partial. Edentulous trays are used for taking impressions for full dentures and are semicircular in cross-section. Partial trays are used for impressions for partial dentures and have a box-shaped cross-section to accommodate the remaining teeth (Figure 27.2). For upper impressions both types of tray have a palatal section; which is, of course, absent in lower trays.

Those obtained from dental suppliers are called **stock trays**. They are made of metal for repeated use, or a weaker disposable material for single use. They may be perforated or unperforated, depending on the type of impression material to be used. Metal trays are sterilized in

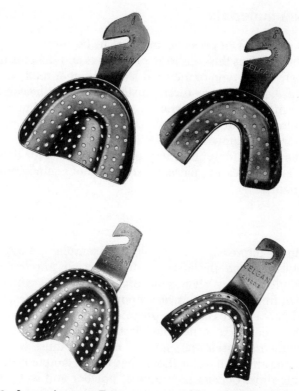

Figure 27.2 *Impression trays.* Top row: upper and lower perforated trays for partial denture impressions. Bottom row: edentulous impression trays.

an autoclave or hot air oven. Disposable trays are discarded after the model is made; and no time is lost on having to clean off the impression material. They should be used whenever possible.

Very often it is not possible to obtain an accurate impression with a stock tray. In such cases the model obtained from the first impression is used to make a **special tray**. With this *made to measure* individual tray a perfectly accurate final impression can be taken. Special trays are usually made of shellac baseplate or acrylic.

Laboratory procedure

The technician pours plaster into the impression to make a model of the patient's jaw. If required, this model is then used to construct a special tray. If so, the impression taken in this special tray is used for making the final (working) model; which is an exact reproduction of the required part of the patient's jaw.

Impression materials

The choice of impression material to be used depends on various factors, such as the condition of the jaws and the presence or absence of teeth. Each type of material has a different method of preparation and use, and manufacturers' instructions must be carefully followed if a satisfactory impression is to be obtained. Impressions for full dentures are called edentulous impressions while those for partial dentures are known as partial impressions.

The most widely used impression materials for dentures are alginate and impression paste. Elastomers and composition are used less frequently.

Alginate

Alginate impression materials; for example, *CA 37, Blueprint,* are elastic and can therefore be used for all impressions, partial or edentulous. They give an accurate impression which can be withdrawn from undercut areas without distortion or fracture.

Alginate impressions are prepared by mixing the powder and water with a spatula in a flexible plastic bowl. The tin is shaken before opening to loosen the powder but care must be taken to avoid inhaling any. The water should be at room temperature to give correct setting time. Correct measures of powder and water are mixed vigorously to a smooth consistency. This sets in a few minutes in the mouth and, on withdrawal, must be wrapped in a wet napkin until the model is made.

The advantage of alginate is its elasticity, which makes it the material of choice for most impressions; and also allows more than one model to be made from the same impression.

The disadvantages of alginate are:

1 If special care is not taken, alginate undergoes dimensional changes which would produce an inaccurate model. It may either absorb water and expand, or lose water and shrink. To prevent this happening the model must be made immediately. If this is not possible, dimensional changes can be delayed by wrapping the impression in a wet napkin and sealing it in a plastic bag; or by keeping it immersed in liquid paraffin. If an alginate impression must be sent away to an outside laboratory, the most convenient method is to wrap it carefully in wet napkins and seal it in an airtight plastic bag.

2 Because of these dimensional changes, the following procedure has been recommended for disinfecting alginate impressions:

   • Rinse in cold running water
   • Dip in sodium hypochlorite

- Rinse again
- Dip again in hypochlorite
- Cover with gauze dampened with hypochlorite for ten minutes
- Rinse well under running water

3 Alginate does not adhere to an ordinary tray so a perforated tray is preferable. An ordinary tray will do, however, if a special adhesive is applied. The only other materials requiring a tray adhesive are the elastomers.

Impression paste

Impression paste is a modified form of ZOE. Various other constituents are added to make it suitable as an impression material. It is supplied in two tubes: one containing the white zinc oxide mixture; the other containing the red eugenol mixture. Equal lengths from each tube are mixed together with a spatula on a paper pad, to give a uniform pink mix without any red or white streaks.

It is used for final *edentulous* impressions in a number of different ways:

1 First impressions are taken with composition or putty elastomer and well-fitting special trays made. Final impressions are taken in these trays using a wash of impression paste.
2 The specialized technique mentioned on page 348 utilizes a special tray with a perfect peripheral seal. A wash of impression paste is used to complete such impressions.
3 For relining loose dentures; the denture is used as an impression tray for the paste and is then sent to the laboratory for a new fitting surface to be processed in acrylic.
4 It is also used as a lining to improve the fit of baseplates in the occlusal registration and trial insertion stages.

The advantage of impression paste is the improved fit which can be obtained by its use in peripherally sealed special trays, baseplates or dentures. Furthermore, its accuracy can be checked or improved by reinsertion in the mouth and adding fresh paste where necessary.

A disadvantage is that it cannot reproduce undercuts and is therefore unsuitable for partial impressions. It also tends to stick to the lips and surrounding skin, but this can be avoided by smearing them beforehand with petroleum jelly.

Elastomers

The impression paste technique just described cannot be used where undercuts are present as it is not an elastic material. In such cases an acrylic special tray and a heavy-bodied elastomer (Chapter 23) are usually preferred. Light-bodied elastomer is used where the alveolar ridges are too soft and flabby to withstand distortion by more viscous impression materials. Silicone putty is replacing composition for first impressions for special trays, as it is just as easy to prepare and use.

The advantages of elastomers are their elasticity which makes them suitable for all types of denture. They are stronger than alginate; less liable to tear; more accurate; and easier to disinfect as they are not subject to significant dimensional changes.

The disadvantages of elastomers are their cost and longer setting time.

Composition

Composition (Impression compound) is a solid material which is softened by heat to a plastic consistency suitable for impression-taking. In the mouth it hardens rapidly on cooling and can then be removed. It is supplied in two forms: slabs which are softened in hot water; and sticks which are softened over a flame or hot-air jet. Whichever form is used, its temperature is always checked with the dentist's finger to reassure the patient. On removal from the mouth it is chilled with cold running water.

The slab form of composition is used mainly for first impressions for special trays. To avoid any adverse effect on composition the temperature of water used for softening it must not exceed that stated by the manufacturer. It varies from 55–70°C according to the particular brand, and should be checked with a thermometer; but in practices where it is used extensively it is more convenient to use a special thermostatically controlled hot water bath instead.

Composition sticks are called tracing sticks and may be green, brown or red according to the brand. As it is softened at a higher temperature than the slab form, it is quenched in hot water before insertion; otherwise it would burn the patient. It is used to form the periphery of acrylic special trays or baseplates. The periphery is built up bit by bit, repeatedly adding composition to it and retrying in the mouth until it forms a perfect peripheral seal with the soft tissues, thereby ensuring optimum retention for the final denture.

The advantage of composition is this ability to provide the best possible retention for a full denture by means of a perfect peripheral seal. When perfect accuracy is not essential, as in first impressions for special trays, composition has the advantages of requiring no mixing, and being so easy and quick to prepare and use.

The disadvantage of composition is that it cannot be withdrawn from undercut areas without distortion. Consequently it is unsuitable for final partial impressions.

Occlusal registration

Laboratory procedure

The technician makes occlusion rims on the final models obtained from the impression stage. They consist of wax rims on wax, shellac or acrylic baseplates. The rims represent the alveolar bone and teeth; and their purpose is to allow the dentist to record the patient's jaw relationship or *bite*.

Surgery procedure

The nurse sets out the patient's records, models, occlusion rims, sheets of pink wax, wax knife, shade and mould guides, a heat source (gas flame, spirit lamp or hot air jet) for trimming the wax rims, and a laboratory-prescription pad. The patient is provided with a bib and mouthwash and any existing dentures are placed in a bowl of water.

The occlusion rims are removed from their models, rinsed in disinfectant and washed in cold water before insertion in the patient's mouth. The sides of the wax rims are trimmed with a **wax knife** (Figure 27.3) until they represent the correct position of the teeth and give proper support for the lips. A **Le Cron carver** is used for fine

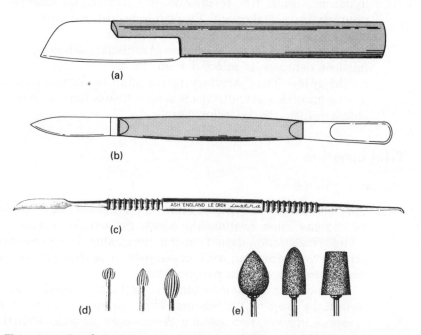

Figure 27.3 *Prosthetic instruments.* (a) plaster knife; (b) wax knife; (c) Le Cron carver; (d) acrylic burs; (e) acrylic stones.

trimming. The wax rims are then reduced or increased in height until the jaws are the correct distance apart when the rims are in contact. A hot flat metal surface, such as an electric iron, is useful for providing a flat, even occlusal surface on the wax rims. Some operators use a **Willis bite gauge** to determine the correct height of occlusion rims. This is based on the assumption that rim heights are correct when the distance between nose and chin equals that between eyes and mouth. The bite gauge facilitates comparison and measurement of these distances. Dividers can also be used for this purpose.

Once the wax rims are trimmed correctly they must be fixed together to register the correct jaw relationship. This can be done by cutting grooves in the rims and placing some recording material, such as a softened wax wafer, impression paste or a quick-setting light-bodied elastomer between them. When the patient closes together it is squeezed into the grooves and permanently records the correct relationship of the jaws at rest. Marks are also made on the upper rim to indicate the midline of the face and rest position of the upper lip.

Best results are obtained if dentures are made on an **anatomical articulator** but it entails extra surgery time at this stage, and in the laboratory. The extra steps required when such an articulator is used are for indicating the movements of the jaws during mastication; and consist of the **face bow** and protrusive bite registrations. A face bow is an accessory part of the articulator for recording the position of the upper occlusion rim relative to the mandibular condyles. The protrusive bite is taken with the mandible postured forward to obtain an occlusal record in the protruded position.

Finally the shade, shape and size of artificial teeth to be used in the finished dentures is selected from the manufacturer's shade and mould guide. The laboratory prescription is then written by the dentist and the nurse disinfects the occlusion rims in hypochlorite before despatch to the technician.

Trial insertion

Laboratory procedure

The technician seals the models and occlusion rims together in exactly the same relationship which the dentist recorded at the occlusal registration stage. Then they are mounted on an articulator to provide the technician with an accurate three-dimensional copy of the required parts of the patient's jaws.

The wax rims can now be removed and are replaced by the actual teeth to be used on the denture. They are mounted in wax on the baseplate in normal occlusion with the opposing teeth. Then the wax is moulded, trimmed and polished to produce a perfect copy of the final denture. This waxed-up denture is called a **trial denture**.

Surgery procedure

The nurse sets out the patient's records, articulator with models and trial dentures, wax knife, Le Cron carver, pink wax, heat source, and a large hand mirror. After the dentist has checked the occlusion of the trial dentures on the articulator, the nurse rinses them in disinfectant and washes them in cold water. She fits a bib on the patient, places any existing dentures in a bowl of water, and the dentist then fits the trial dentures in the patient's mouth. They are checked for comfort, stability and occlusion; and the patient is given a mirror to see the shade, shape and arrangement of the teeth. If the patient is dissatisfied with them, they are replaced on the articulator, and any necessary adjustments can then be made in the surgery. It is emphasized to the patient that such adjustments can only be done at this stage while the teeth are still embedded in wax; alterations cannot be carried out once the dentures are finished.

Finally the junction of hard and soft palate is marked on the upper model together with the extent of the pad of softer tissue in this region. This enables the technician to make a retentive posterior border (*post-dam*) for the final denture. The trial dentures are then disinfected again, remounted on the articulator and the laboratory prescription is written up for the technician.

Final insertion

Laboratory procedure

The technician invests the trial dentures in a plaster mould and eliminates all the wax by flushing with boiling water. The space formerly occupied by wax is now filled with acrylic dough and heat-cured in a warm oven. The acrylic dentures are then trimmed and polished ready for fitting. They are disinfected and kept in a bowl of water until the patient attends.

Surgery procedure

The finished dentures are kept in a bowl of water until ready for insertion. The nurse sets out articulating paper, occlusal indicator wax, straight handpiece, acrylic burs and stones, and a large hand mirror. She fits a bib on the patient, scrubs the dentures in disinfectant and rinses them in water when the dentist is ready to fit them.

Each denture is fitted in turn to check its retention and stability. Any necessary adjustments to the occlusion are made by biting on a piece of **articulating paper** or **occlusal indicator wax** (Chapter 23). These mark any high spots on the teeth which can be ground down with a carborundum stone in a straight handpiece. High spots on the fitting surface or overextension of the periphery can be localized by painting **pressure indicating paste** on the fitting surfaces. The offending parts are then removed with an acrylic bur or stone (Figure 27.3).

The patient is given a mirror to see the appearance of the new dentures and is shown how to insert and remove them. Instructions are given, as follows, on the care of new dentures:

1   They should be cleaned after meals with a scrubbing brush, soap and cold water; and handled with care as they can break if dropped. When cleaning, put water in wash basin to act as a cushion and prevent breakage.
2   Hot water should not be used as it may damage the acrylic.
3   Partial dentures should not be worn at night. Unless a patient practises perfect oral hygiene, night wear can only aggravate the effects of plaque.
4   At night, or any other time when the dentures are not worn, they must be kept in a glass of water. If allowed to dry out, acrylic is liable to warp and may not fit properly.

After care

An appointment is given for a few days later to see how the patient is managing the new dentures. Patients are advised to stop wearing a denture if it is hurting the soft tissues; but wear it again for 24 hours before their appointment so that the dentist can see the sore area and be able to deal with it. Articulating paper or occlusal indicator wax is used again to find any high spots on the teeth; and pressure indicating paste for detecting the causes of soreness or ulceration. A straight handpiece, acrylic burs and stones, polishing paste and brushes are used to trim offending surfaces and leave them smooth and polished. The dentures are then scrubbed with disinfectant, rinsed in water and returned to the patient.

Patients are also told that new dentures do not last for ever, and are advised to have them checked every year. Alveolar bone gradually changes its shape following the loss of teeth and the denture will eventually become too loose. By that time most patients will have learned how to control a loose denture; but the alveolar bone changes can adversely affect appearance as the loose denture may no longer provide adequate support for the lips and cheeks. It is consequently necessary to reline the fitting surface of a denture from time to time and perhaps make other adjustments. Relining is usually done with impression paste.

As already mentioned, patients are advised to clean their new dentures by scrubbing with soap and cold water, and to keep them immersed in water overnight. If such advice is followed the mouth should remain healthy and the use of proprietary denture cleansers should be unnecessary.

If this advice is not followed, the soft tissues covered by a denture may become inflamed. This condition is called *denture stomatitis* and is treated with antifungal drugs (Chapter 11) and oral-hygiene instruction. Similarly, the dentures may become stained and calculus may form on them. Patients with such dentures are advised to clean them by soaking in hypochlorite (e.g. *Milton*) for 20 minutes, rinse thoroughly and immerse them in water overnight. Dentures with metallic components should only be soaked in hypochlorite for ten minutes.

Partial dentures

There are two types of partial denture. One is made entirely of acrylic; the other consists of a metal skeleton with the artificial teeth embedded in acrylic. Both are made from alginate or elastomer impressions followed by the stages of denture construction already described. If only a few teeth are missing, the occlusal registration stage may be omitted. A wax squash bite (Chapter 23) is taken instead, at the final impression stage. In the laboratory, the squash bite shows the technician how the remaining teeth occlude. The models can then be mounted correctly on an articulator and the trial denture made. This is followed by a trial insertion in the surgery.

Acrylic partial dentures may have wire clips to improve retention. These clips, which are known as **clasps**, spring into the undercut areas of the teeth and prevent vertical dislodgement of the denture. They are made of stainless steel wire or chrome-cobalt.

Skeleton dentures are made of chrome-cobalt castings. They are much better dentures, as the metal skeleton is far stronger than acrylic. This allows construction of a less bulky denture, specially designed to avoid food traps and plaque retention round the gums and teeth. The remaining teeth are used for support and retention of the skeleton. Clasps are used for retention and **occlusal rests** for support. Occlusal rests are tiny lugs which fit on the occlusal surface of the enamel or in a groove cut into a filling. If there are no suitable fillings or surfaces, seats for occlusal rests may be made by bonding some composite filling material to the enamel.

Skeleton dentures take longer to make and are far more expensive than acrylic ones. Special tray elastomer impressions are necessary to ensure accuracy as it is difficult to make adjustments to metal castings. Extra visits may also be required: before the final impression stage, to prepare seats for occlusal rests; and after the occlusal registration stage, to try in the metal skeleton before waxing-up the teeth for the trial denture.

The after-care instructions for full dentures also apply to partial dentures but, because of their potential for plaque retention, patients are emphatically advised not to wear them at night, and to have a check-up twice a year.

Immediate dentures

Dentures are usually made some months after the teeth have been extracted, as this allows time for completion of the initial alveolar bone changes and gum healing. Many patients, however, are not prepared to wait that long for the replacement of missing front teeth. In such cases they can be provided with **immediate dentures** which are made *before* their front teeth are extracted, and are fitted immediately afterwards. But patients should understand that the rapid remodelling of alveolar bone which follows extractions necessitates relining or replacement of immediate dentures within a year.

Procedure

The dentist provides the technician with final impressions, an occlusal registration and shade of artificial teeth. The teeth to be extracted are cut off the model by the technician and the artificial ones fitted in their place. The denture is then waxed-up and processed in acrylic; disinfected and kept in water until ready for fitting.

In the surgery the teeth are extracted and the denture is fitted at the same visit. The patient is given an appointment to attend for check-up the next day and instructed not to remove the denture before then. After that it should only be removed for cleaning, and worn full-time until the dentist decides that it can be left out at night.

Overdentures

An overdenture is one which is fitted on top of standing teeth or retained roots. The advantage of an overdenture is the presence of natural roots remaining in the alveolar bone. These have the effect of greatly reducing the shrinkage of alveolar ridges which normally occurs after extraction of teeth. When teeth are extracted, the alveolar bone becomes redundant, as it has lost its natural function of providing support for the teeth. It consequently diminishes in size as the bone resorbs and this loss of bone may be so great that it becomes very difficult to make a denture which is not perpetually loose. Lower dentures pose the most awkward problems in this respect.

As long as any roots remain, there is hardly any loss of alveolar bone and these problems of difficult lower dentures are far less common. But dentures cannot be fitted directly on top of retained roots or teeth. In most cases a certain amount of preparation of the abutment teeth is required to remove undercuts and prevent caries. Retained roots are root-filled and ground to a dome shape level with the gum. If the root surface is irregular because of previous caries, the dome shape can be restored by fitting an appropriately shaped post crown. Teeth which still have intact crowns are usually treated by reducing the crown to a small tapered stump and fitting a full gold veneer thimble. Having prepared the remaining teeth or roots, the overdenture is then made in the usual way.

Overdentures are usually made as full dentures but they can be used as partial dentures in cases where some of the remaining teeth are unsuitable for the partial denture design. They are also used for patients with cleft palates and for those who have undergone surgical removal of part of their jaw. In such cases the alveolar ridges may be so misshapen that properly fitting conventional dentures cannot be made.

Where there are no remaining roots, **implants** can be used to support an overdenture. This is explained later in the chapter.

Obturators

An **obturator** is an appliance for plugging an abnormal cavity, such as a cleft palate; the space left after surgical removal of part of the jaw; or a cyst cavity. It usually consists of an ordinary acrylic denture bearing a plug which seals the cavity. This prevents the ingress of food and improves speech. If the cavity is very large, a hollow plug is used to lighten the obturator.

An obturator can be made in the usual way, using an elastic impression material. Alternatively the denture part is made first in acrylic and a temporary plug, made of black gutta-percha, is added. When this has been worn for a while, and moulded itself to the shape of the cavity, it is remade in acrylic.

Soft linings

The section on impression paste described its use for relining loose dentures: those which have been worn for many years; or immediate dentures which have lost their fit after a few months. Impression paste, as with all other conventional impression materials, sets in a few minutes and reproduces a totally artificial situation where the mouth is wide open and immobile throughout. The real and natural situation in the mouth is one of continual movement and change. Recording this real situation in an impression requires a material which takes hours to set while the denture is being worn and used. Such an impression is called a **functional impression** and it provides a much better fit.

The oldest functional impression material is black gutta-percha but this has been replaced by modern materials called **soft linings** which are a type of slow curing acrylic resin, such as *Visco-gel, Coe Comfort*. They usually consist of a powder and liquid which are mixed together and applied to the fitting surface of the denture for up to a fortnight. They are also used as a modern alternative to composition sticks for producing a perfect peripheral seal for full dentures. When set, the denture can be reconstructed in the normal way with heat-cured acrylic or it can be worn temporarily with the set material forming the new lining or peripheral seal.

Soft linings can also be used as **tissue conditioners**. These are required when the soft tissues become too sore, swollen or otherwise distorted, to withstand pressure from a denture. A soft lining accommodates any changes in the soft tissues and allows the denture to be worn without discomfort until the tissues have healed or a new denture can be made. Tissue conditioners may also be used when immediate dentures are first fitted, and for relining them during the first few months when the most rapid changes in alveolar shape take place.

Implants

Overdentures and bridges rely on teeth for retention. If there are no available tooth roots for an overdenture, or suitable teeth for bridge abutments (Chapter 23), artificial tooth roots implanted into the alveolar bone can be used instead. These implants are made of titanium and generally consist of threaded cylinders which are screwed into holes drilled in the bone. The cylinders also have an internal thread for a screw which attaches the artificial abutment to the implant (Figure 27.4). Up to six implants may be needed to retain a denture or extensive bridgework.

Construction

1   A team of oral or periodontal surgeon, prosthetic specialist, and hygienist examine and assess the patient, helped by study models and X-rays. They can then plan the preparation, construction and maintenance of an implant procedure.

2   LA or GA is used for the oral surgery procedure of inserting implants into alveolar bone. A gum flap is raised to expose the bone and special low-speed drills are used to prepare holes for the implants. They are screwed into these holes and the gum flap is then sutured back into place to completely bury the implants.

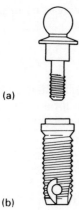

(a)

(b)

Figure 27.4 *Implant components.*
(a) Ball abutment for overdenture;
(b) Implant fixture.

3 After a period of up to six months, the implants become firmly embedded in the bone. This process is called **osseointegration**. Under LA a small incision is made in the overlying gum to expose the top of each implant, and the artificial abutments are then screwed on to the implants. Abutments may be in the form of stumps for fitting bridge pontics, or a bar for clipping on a removable overdenture (Fig. 27.5).

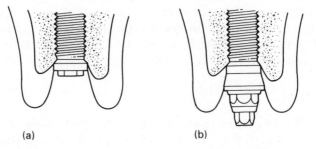

(a)   (b)

Figure 27.5 *Implant procedure.* (a) Stage 1: implant fixture; (b) Stage 2: crown or bridge abutment fitted.

Procedure

Patients are very carefully selected as implants can only succeed if meticulous oral hygiene and plaque control is maintained before and after the implants are inserted. A thorough medical history, and comprehensive clinical and X-ray examinations, are essential to confirm the feasibility of implants, and to exclude patients who are unsuitable for reasons of general or dental health, motivation or ability to attend for regular checks.

Implants and their abutment components are intended to act as natural teeth and it is essential that their supra- and subgingival parts are kept clean and regularly checked in the same way as natural teeth, as described in Chapter 25 on periodontal disease.

Advantages of implants

They allow full dentures to be worn in cases where there is insufficient alveolar bone to provide adequate retention for a conventional denture. They also permit the construction of bridges without having to crown adjacent abutment teeth.

Disadvantages

They require a specialist team and a highly motivated patient. They are accordingly very expensive.

Practical examination

One of the most commonly set tests in the practical examination is to mix an impression material such as alginate or impression paste, and load it into a tray. It requires correct mixing of the correct amount of material, and correct selection of the tray: perforated for alginate, unperforated for impression paste; edentulous for a full denture, box-shaped for a partial denture, and upper or lower depending on the specified jaw. The amount of material mixed should be sufficient to provide an adequate quantity without waste.

Alginate

1 Select a correct perforated tray. Do not choose a box-shaped partial tray if the test specifies a full denture. If you choose an unperforated tray, ask for tray adhesive.
2 If you choose a disposable tray you will have to fit the handle the correct way up. If you are unsure how to do this, choose the correct metal tray instead.
3 Shake the alginate container to loosen the powder.
4 Scoop up a heaped measure of powder and level it with the mixing spatula so that all the excess powder falls back into the container. Empty the powder measure into the mixing bowl and replace the lid on the alginate container.
5 Dispense a measure of water from the bottle of water provided. This will be at room temperature, whereas tap water will be too cold. Two measures of powder and a full one of water are usually required for an upper impression.

---

6 Pour the water on to the powder in the bowl and mix vigorously to a smooth, even consistency without any bubbles.
7 Fill the tray adequately and smooth the alginate with the
spatula.
8 Present the tray, handle first, to the examiner.

Impression paste

1 Dispense equal lengths of paste from each tube, side by side
at the centre of mixing pad, ensuring that the tubes do not
contaminate each other. Replace the caps.
2 Mix rapidly until the colour is uniform and no streaks
remain.
3 Paste should be controlled in one mass at the centre of the
pad to avoid any mess on the table top.
4 Strop the spatula blade on the edge of the mixing pad to
remove the streaks and collect the mix on a clean part of the
pad. Wipe the spatula blade to remove any residual streaks,
scoop some paste on to the spatula and offer it, handle first,
to the examiner.

Written examination

Describe the preparation, and different uses, of the following
impression materials:
(a) rubber base or silicone
(b) alginate
(c) zinc oxide and eugenol impression paste
(November 1996)

What information and advice would be given to a patient by
the dentist and the dental nurse following the provision of an
immediate full upper denture? (November 1992)

What dental procedures may be required before the dentist
constructs a partial chrome-cobalt denture?
List the surgery stages in the construction of such a denture.
(November 1991)

Summary

IMPRESSION MATERIAL	USES	ADVANTAGES	DISADVANTAGES
Alginate	Edentulous and partial impressions	Accuracy	Dimensional changes
Impression paste	Edentulous special tray impressions Lining baseplates Relining dentures	Accuracy Can be tried in mouth and additions made	Unsuitable for partial impressions Sticks to lips and skin
Elastomers	Putty: impressions for special trays Heavy-bodied: special tray edentulous impressions where undercuts are present Light-bodied: soft flabby ridges	Accuracy Stronger than alginate	More expensive than alginate Longer setting time
Composition	Impressions for special trays	Rapid and simple No mixing required	Unsuitable for final partial impressions
	Peripheral seal for special tray edentulous impressions	Best possible retention	Time-consuming

Possible effects of loss of teeth

1   Overeruption of functionless teeth ⎫ Food traps
    Tilting of teeth on each side of gap ⎭

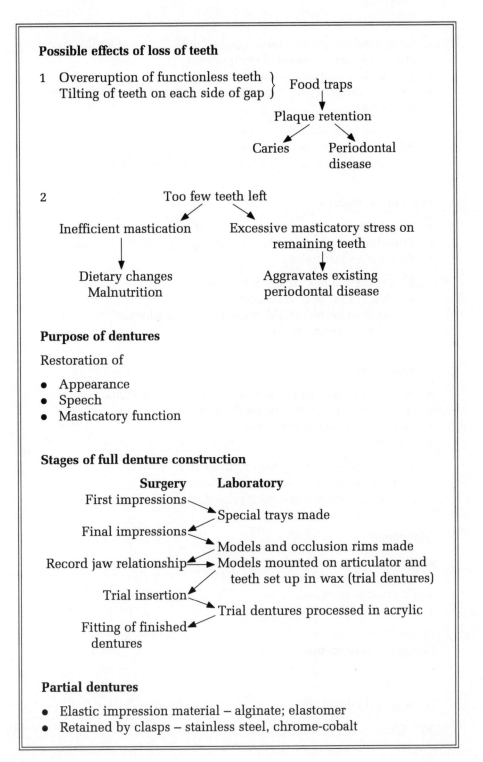

Plaque retention

Caries   Periodontal
                disease

2   Too few teeth left

Inefficient mastication   Excessive masticatory stress on
                                    remaining teeth

Dietary changes   Aggravates existing
Malnutrition   periodontal disease

Purpose of dentures

Restoration of

- Appearance
- Speech
- Masticatory function

Stages of full denture construction

Surgery	Laboratory

First impressions
                    Special trays made
Final impressions
                    Models and occlusion rims made
Record jaw relationship ⟷ Models mounted on articulator and
                                teeth set up in wax (trial dentures)
Trial insertion
                    Trial dentures processed in acrylic
Fitting of finished
dentures

Partial dentures

- Elastic impression material – alginate; elastomer
- Retained by clasps – stainless steel, chrome-cobalt

- Supported by occlusal rests – on occlusal surface of tooth, groove cut into filling, or bonded composite ledge
- Acrylic base or metal skeleton
- Skeleton more hygienic but expensive. May require extra surgery stages for:

  (a) preparing seats for occlusal rests
  (b) special tray impression
  (c) trying-in metal skeleton before teeth are added

Immediate dentures

- Fitted immediately after extraction of front teeth
- Provides immediate restoration of appearance and function
- Stages of construction:

  1 Impression and occlusal registration
  2 Denture made in laboratory
  3 Teeth extracted and denture fitted immediately
  4 Reline required before long

Overdentures

- Fitted over retained roots, standing teeth or implants
- Roots root-filled; standing teeth crowned
- Minimizes alveolar bone loss
- Used for:

  1 Potentially difficult lower full dentures
  2 Cases unsuitable for partial dentures
  3 Cleft palate and jaw surgery patients

Obturators

- Plug for abnormal cavity: cleft palate, cyst, jaw surgery
- Plug attached to denture
- Functional impression used – black gutta-percha or soft lining material

Surgery requirements

All stages

Disinfect all laboratory work on receipt and before despatch.

(a) Rinse in cold running water

(b)   Immerse in hypochlorite
(c)   Rinse again

Provide patient's records, bib, mouthwash and denture bowl

Impressions

- Mouth mirror, impression trays, laboratory prescription pad
- Prepare impression material
- Clean patient's face afterwards if necessary

Occlusal registration

- Mouth mirror, wax knife, Le Cron carver and heat source
- Models and occlusion rims
- Willis bite gauge, dividers, face bow
- Pink wax
- Shade and mould guides
- Laboratory prescription pad

Trial insertion

- Articulator with models and trial dentures
- Large mirror and mouth mirror
- Pink wax, wax knife, Le Cron carver and heat source

Fitting

- Finished dentures kept in water
- Articulating paper; occlusal indicator wax; pressure indicating paste
- Straight handpiece, acrylic burs and stones
- Large mirror and mouth mirror

Care of dentures

- Scrub with soap and cold water after meals
- Always keep dentures in water when not worn
- Do not wear dentures at night
- Check-up required at least once a year
- Clean old stained dentures with hypochlorite

Denture materials

- Full dentures: Acrylic
                   Metal palate – stainless steel, chrome-cobalt
- Partial dentures: Acrylic – wire clasps
                      Skeleton – chrome-cobalt casting
- Teeth: Acrylic

Uses of acrylic

Powder + Liquid → Dough
(Polymer) (Monomer)

Heat cured { Dentures
              Orthodontic appliances

Cold cured { Temporary crowns
              Denture repairs
              Impression trays

Soft linings

Slow-curing acrylic

1   Functional impressions
2   Tissue conditioners → sore or swollen soft tissues
3   Lining immediate dentures

Implants

- Artificial roots embedded in alveolar bone
- Made of titanium
- Abutments for overdentures or bridges are screwed on to top of implant
- Used when alveolar bone inadequate for retention of denture
- No need to prepare bridge abutments on existing teeth

28 Orthodontics

Orthodontics is the branch of dentistry concerned with the correction of irregular teeth. When the permanent teeth erupt, parents may notice that the front teeth are crooked or protruding. The condition is known as a **malocclusion** and treatment is sought to improve the child's appearance.

Aims of treatment

The aims of orthodontic treatment are to reposition the teeth so that appearance is improved and a good functional occlusion obtained. By correcting badly positioned teeth it may also eliminate some plaque retention areas and help to prevent caries and periodontal disease. Children in need of orthodontic treatment are often teased at school and become very anxious about their appearance. Successful treatment is of great psychological benefit in these cases.

Normal occlusion

Before learning the types and causes of malocclusion, nurses must understand what is meant by normal occlusion, and should refer back to Chapter 12. In normal occlusion all the teeth are well aligned and there is no crowding. Upper incisors slightly overlap the lowers vertically and horizontally and special names are given to this overlap. Vertical overlap is called **overbite** and horizontal overlap is called **overjet** (Figure 28.1).

For teeth to erupt into normal occlusion, the jaws must be in correct horizontal and vertical relationship to each other, and of sufficient

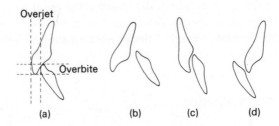

Figure 28.1 *Overbite and overjet.* (a) Class 1 occlusion; (b) Class 2 division 1 occlusion; (c) Class 2 division 2 occlusion; (d) Class 3 occlusion.

size to accommodate their full complement of teeth. The teeth can then erupt into a normal position of balance between the pressures exerted by the lips and cheeks on their outer side, and the tongue on the inner.

Types of malocclusion

The basic types of malocclusion are crowding, protruding upper incisors and a prominent lower jaw.

Crowding

Crowding is caused by insufficient room for all the teeth. It occurs in jaws which are too small to accommodate 32 permanent teeth. The teeth become crooked and overlapping, while those which normally erupt late cannot take up their proper position as there is insufficient room left. Thus the canines are usually displaced buccally, second premolars lingually and the lower third molars are impacted.

Early extraction of carious deciduous molars may also contribute to the crowding in these cases. The gap left by an extraction soon closes, as the back tooth drifts forward and takes up some of the space required for the permanent successor.

Protruding upper incisors

Many children attend for orthodontic treatment because their upper front teeth protrude between their lips. This condition usually arises from a jaw relationship in which the upper teeth are too far forward relative to the lowers. It is commonly associated with an open lip posture and is called a class 2 division 1 occlusion (Figures 28.1 and 28.2).

Prominent lower jaw

This condition, in which the chin is unduly prominent, is caused by a jaw relationship in which the lower teeth are too far forward relative to the uppers. It usually results in the incisors biting edge to edge; or with the lowers in front of the uppers, instead of behind them; and is called a class 3 occlusion (Figures 28.1 and 28.2).

Causes of malocclusion

Almost all kinds of malocclusion are genetic in origin; very few are acquired. The most common are inheritance of an abnormal jaw

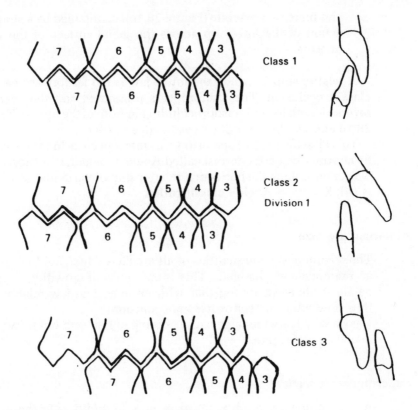

Figure 28.2 *Classification of occlusion.*

relationship or jaw size. Other genetic factors include supernumerary teeth and missing teeth. The most common acquired cause is a sucking habit.

Abnormal jaw relationship

With a normal jaw relationship the teeth should occlude in a class 1 relationship as shown in Figures 28.1 and 28.2. This is the most attractive type of occlusion and is accordingly regarded as normal. Abnormal jaw relationships give rise to either a class 2 or class 3 occlusion.

A jaw relationship in which the upper jaw is too far forward causes two different types of class 2 occlusion:

(a) **class 2 division 1** in which the upper incisors protrude, the overjet is increased (Figures 28.1b and 28.2), and the lower lip is trapped inside the overjet
(b) **class 2 division 2** in which the upper central incisors tilt back-wards into contact with the lowers, giving a decreased overjet

and increased overbite (Figure 28.1c), maintained by a strap-like action of the lower lip across the labial surface of the upper incisors

A relationship in which the lower jaw is too far forward causes a **class 3** occlusion. The chin appears prominent and the overjet is reversed, with lower incisors occluding in front of the uppers (Figures 28.1d and 28.2); or in milder cases, edge to edge.

This classification of occlusion was introduced as long ago as 1899 by an American orthodontist called Angle. It remains the most useful way of describing the horizontal relationship of the dental arches and is still known as **Angle's classification**.

Abnormal jaw size

The commonest abnormalities of all are jaws which are too small to accommodate all the teeth. This is the cause of crowding. Unfortunately it often occurs together with an abnormal jaw relationship, thus producing an even worse malocclusion.

Jaws which are too large cause spacing of the teeth but this type of malocclusion is rare.

Supernumerary teeth

A supernumerary tooth is an extra one, in addition to the normal complement of 32 teeth. It occurs most commonly in the upper incisor region and may either prevent a central incisor erupting or cause it to erupt in an abnormal position.

Missing teeth

Missing teeth is the opposite condition to supernumerary teeth. Upper lateral incisors are often missing and orthodontic treatment may be necessary to close the resultant gaps. Sometimes, instead of being absent, upper lateral incisors are tiny conical teeth. Again the appearance is unsightly and treatment may be necessary. The other teeth which are most commonly missing are third molars and second premolars. If several teeth are missing, the condition is called **partial anodontia** but this is a rare occurrence.

Sucking habits

Habits such as finger or thumb sucking can cause displacement of front teeth resulting in a decreased overbite and increased overjet. This may correct itself when the habit ceases.

Treatment of malocclusion

Orthodontic treatment may involve extractions and the use of removable or fixed appliances.

Extractions

When the jaw is too small to accommodate all the teeth properly they become crowded and irregular; often resulting in overlapping of the incisors, labially displaced canines and/or impacted lower third molars. Such malocclusions are treated by extractions. The commonest teeth to be extracted for this purpose are first premolars and the resultant space provides room for straightening the front teeth. If there is an abnormal jaw relationship, such as class 2 division 1, there may be no apparent crowding; but extractions are still necessary to provide space for moving protruding incisors backwards and thereby improve appearance.

Crowded teeth often straighten themselves after extractions, but appliances are usually required to reposition them in good alignment.

Appliances

Orthodontic appliances may be removable or fixed. They all require a great deal of co-operation from the patient and parents as treatment may last up to two years, and necessitates wearing the appliance all the time, and maintenance of a high standard of oral hygiene throughout.

Appliances work by applying pressure to the teeth. This results in a remodelling of the alveolar bone surrounding the teeth concerned, allowing them to be guided by the appliance into the desired position. However, appliances cannot be discarded as soon as the teeth have been aligned. A period of retention with an appliance is then required to hold them in their new position until the alveolar bone changes become stabilized. Relapse towards the original condition is likely if the patient fails to co-operate in this final stage.

Care of appliances

Most orthodontic appliances contain delicate wire springs, designed to fit precisely against the teeth to be moved. Patients and parents are accordingly advised to take the greatest care of their appliances and not to miss their monthly adjustment appointment. Failure to keep appointments prolongs the overall treatment time.

Removable appliances must only be removed and inserted as directed by the dentist. Careless handling may distort the springs and produce discomfort or undesirable tooth movements. They should be removed and cleaned with brush, soap and cold water after meals; and patients are warned that failure to do this can result in rapid caries and a sore palate (denture stomatitis).

Fixed appliances are less robust than removable ones and even greater care must be taken over oral hygiene.

Whichever type of appliance is used, patients are instructed to contact the surgery at once if any difficulties arise, without waiting until their next appointment. If attending a different dentist for orthodontic treatment, they must still visit their own general practitioner for routine dental inspection and treatment.

Removable appliances

A removable appliance resembles an acrylic partial denture but instead of teeth it contains springs made of stainless steel wire. The springs press against the teeth to be moved and guide them in the required direction. The appliance is held in place by stainless steel clasps. It is made in the same way as a denture, on a model of the jaw obtained from an alginate impression, but special trays, occlusal registration and trial insertion stages are unnecessary. Most appliances are retained at the back by clasps called **Adams cribs** on the first molars (Figure 28.3). Retention for the front varies according to the tooth movement required.

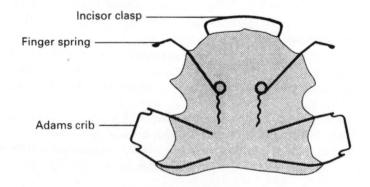

Incisor clasp

Finger spring

Adams crib

Figure 28.3 *Removable upper orthodontic appliance.*

Canines are moved back into the first premolar extraction spaces by palatal *finger springs* or *buccal retractors*. It usually takes about six months and leaves sufficient space to align the incisors. This takes another six months or so and is most commonly achieved with a wire *labial bow* which rests against the labial surfaces of the incisors. Apart from the springs and bows already mentioned, screws and elastic bands may be used as alternative or additional means of tooth movement. When the incisors are aligned, a new appliance with a labial bow is made to retain them in their new corrected position for about six months. This appliance is called a **retainer**.

Instruments required to adjust removable appliances are **Adams universal pliers, Adams spring forming pliers** (Figure 28.4) and **wire cutters**. A black marking pencil or eyebrow pencil is used to mark the acrylic where trimming is required or to indicate spring positions.

The advantages of removable appliances are ease of cleaning, simplicity of construction and repair, and the short amount of surgery time needed for fitting and adjustment. The main disadvantage is their limited range of tooth movement. They only achieve tilting, and while this is sufficient for many cases, it is unsuitable for more severe types of malocclusion where bodily tooth movement or rotation is required.

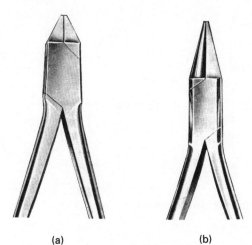

(a) (b)

Figure 28.4 *Orthodontic pliers.* (a) Adams universal pliers; (b) Adams spring forming pliers.

Fixed appliances

Fixed appliances (Figure 28.5) consist of an **archwire** made of springy stainless steel or special alloy which is bent or preformed into the desired ideal shape of the dental arch. When all the teeth are bound to the archwire it forms them into its own ideal shape. It rests in **orthodontic brackets** which are attached to the labial or buccal surfaces of incisors, canines and premolars. These brackets are made of stainless steel or tooth-coloured materials (Figure 28.5) and are fixed to the teeth by acid etching and direct bonding with a composite or GIC material. The ends of the archwire fit into **buccal tubes** welded to stainless steel **orthodontic bands** on the first molars. The bands are cemented with zinc phosphate, polycarboxylate or GIC.

The archwire is attached to the brackets with fine **ligature wire**,

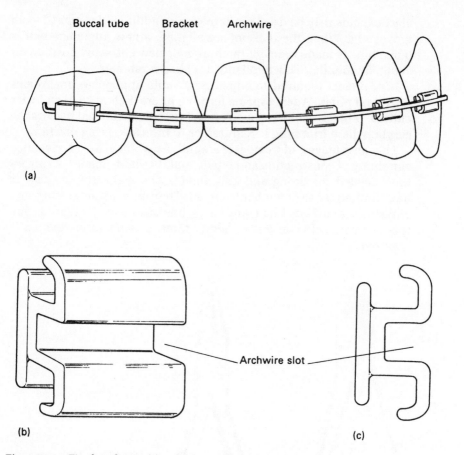

Figure 28.5 *Fixed appliance.* (a) archwire in direct bonded brackets; (b) edgewise orthodontic bracket; (c) side view.

tiny elastic rings or brass pins, depending on the type of bracket and archwire used. The teeth are made to slide along the archwire, or rotate around it, by attaching latex elastics or elastic chains to the brackets.

Instruments used for fixed appliances are: **band drivers** and **pushers** for fitting bands; band **removers** (Figure 28.6); bracket tweezers for direct bonding of brackets; needle holders for placing and tightening ligature wires; **ligature cutters** or serrated scissors for cutting off loose ends, and ligature tuckers for curling the ends away from soft tissues; mosquito forceps for placing elastic rings and chains; **Howe pliers** for fitting bracket pins; and smaller versions of removable appliance pliers for adjusting archwires. A white marking pencil is used to indicate the adjustment or measurement points on archwires.

The advantages of fixed appliances are their precise control over

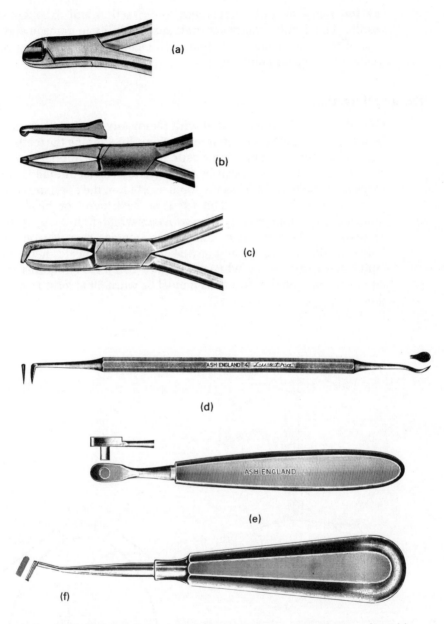

Figure 28.6 *Fixed appliance instruments.* (a) ligature cutters; (b) Howe pliers; (c) molar band remover; (d) Mitchell trimmer; (e) band driver; (f) band pusher.

the full range of tooth movement, rapid action and excellent end results. The disadvantages are their susceptibility to damage and the loss of brackets or bands, difficulty in cleaning, and longer surgery visits for fitting and adjustment.

Extra-oral traction

One of the problems associated with removable and fixed appliances is insufficient space, even after extractions, for aligning the teeth. This can be overcome by applying elastic traction to the appliance from a neck band or headgear worn by the patient. This technique is called **extra-oral traction** (EOT) as the force exerted on the appliance comes from outside the mouth. The external neck band or headgear is attached to the appliance by wire *whiskers* which fit into buccal tubes or hooks on the appliance; and the pull comes from elastic bands between the headgear and whiskers, or an elastic neck band connected direct to the whiskers (Figure 28.7). EOT requires much co-operation from the patient as it must be worn for at least 14 hours a day.

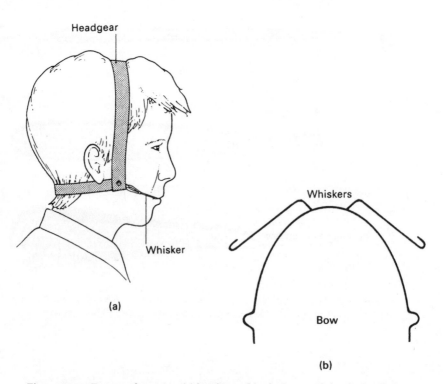

Figure 28.7 *Extra-oral traction.* (a) headgear; (b) whiskers with hooks for elastic traction; bow fits into buccal tubes of appliance.

Functional appliances

These are removable but differ in their mode of action from the type already described. Instead of having springs which engage and move the teeth, functional appliances utilize the forces exerted by muscles. There are two main types: **Andresen** and **Fränkel** appliances.

An Andresen appliance, or monobloc, consists of upper and lower acrylic baseplates which extend over the occlusal surfaces of the back teeth. The two plates are joined together at their occlusal surfaces to form a single unit. They exert their effect by harnessing the pull of the muscles of mastication.

A Fränkel appliance consists of acrylic flanges which fit into the sulcus, labially, buccally and lingually. The flanges are joined together by a wire framework. The effect of the flanges is to influence the forces exerted by the muscles of facial expression and thereby produce the desired tooth movements.

Surgery procedure

Before orthodontic treatment is provided, a thorough assessment is undertaken to check the occlusion and the desire of child and parents for treatment. Unless a child is keen to wear an appliance, the prolonged period of co-operation and strict oral hygiene required are unlikely to be forthcoming. Parents must participate, too, by ensuring that appointments are kept, oral hygiene maintained and instructions for wearing and activating the appliance are followed. These instructions are given orally and in writing. Parents must also realize that time off school for attending appointments may be inevitable.

Orthodontic examination

Apart from a detailed inspection of the teeth, careful observation of the patient is necessary to assess the effects of lip, tongue and swallowing actions; and to detect any deviations or premature tooth contacts during opening and closure of the mouth. A **caliper gauge** is used to measure overjet, overbite, tooth width and spaces. Photographs are often taken at this stage, in addition to X-rays and impressions for models.

X-rays

Children usually attend for orthodontic examination before all their permanent teeth have erupted. X-ray films are necessary at this stage to confirm the presence and position of unerupted permanent teeth; and to detect any supernumerary teeth or other abnormalities.

Cephalometric, OPG, lateral oblique and occlusal films may be taken. These are described in Chapter 29.

Models

Models of upper and lower teeth in occlusion are required before, during and after orthodontic treatment. They are often referred to as study or record models. The first models are studied to decide the treatment plan; subsequent models to record progress; and the final models to monitor stability of the end result.

Impressions for record models and appliances are taken in alginate. A wax squash bite is also necessary to allow the technician to prepare the models in correct occlusion. Disinfection of impressions, appliances and other laboratory work was covered in Chapter 27.

Removable appliances

Patients usually attend monthly on average to check progress. The nurse sets out the patient's records, study models, mouth mirror, caliper gauge, black marking pencil, pliers, wire cutters, straight handpiece and acrylic burs (Figure 27.3) and a large hand mirror.

Appliances often require trimming of the acrylic during tooth movement. This is done with a straight handpiece and acrylic burs. The adjustment of springs and clasps is done with orthodontic pliers.

When a new appliance is fitted the patient and parent are shown how it works and, with the aid of a hand mirror, how to insert, remove and clean it. They are given instructions for it to be worn all day, all night, at meal times, and when swimming or playing contact sports. Contrary to lay belief, appliances can protect and splint the teeth against injury. Removable appliances should be removed after meals for cleaning, and reinserted *immediately.* Instructions are also given where appropriate on the use of a key to activate any screws; or the fitting of elastics and EOT. The importance of keeping all appointments is stressed and information given on how to contact the surgery if any problems arise between appointments. Reassurance is given that any difficulties with eating or speaking will disappear in a few days. The next appointment is then arranged.

Fixed appliances

Patients usually attend monthly to check progress and make any adjustments. The nurse sets out the patient's records and study models, large hand mirror, mouth mirror, caliper gauge, marking pencil, pliers, ligature cutters and tuckers, needle holders and serrated scissors. Mosquito forceps, bracket pins, ligatures or elastic rings and chain may be set out, depending on the type of brackets used.

If bands are to be cemented, the nurse sets out zinc phosphate, polycarboxylate or GIC, band driver and pusher, and a **Mitchell trimmer** (Figure 28.6) for removing excess cement. If brackets are to be bonded, bracket tweezers, acid-etching and composite or GIC bonding materials are needed. In both cases full saliva control is essential, so aspirator tubes, saliva ejectors, cotton wool rolls, absorbent pads and napkins will be required, together with a bib and mouthwash for the patient.

When a fixed appliance is fitted, the patient is given a large hand mirror and the orthodontist explains to patient and parent how it works; how and when to fit and change elastics, and how to wear EOT. They are warned that rapid caries can ensue unless the appliance and teeth are thoroughly cleaned after meals, and instruction is given on how to achieve this by careful, gentle brushing and the use of a water irrigation device. Advice is given to eat a normal diet but to avoid sticky sweets such as toffee or chewing gum as these can get caught up in the appliance. They are told that some toothache may occur at first but should wear off in a day or so. The importance of keeping appointments is emphasized, and so is the need to contact the surgery immediately if any breakages or other problems occur. The patient may be given a supply of elastics; and some soft wax to mould over any parts of the appliance which cause soreness. Finally the nurse arranges the next appointment.

Written examination

(a) What are the causes of malocclusion?
(b) List the aims of orthodontic treatment.
(c) What instructions should be given to the patient after a fixed orthodontic appliance has just been fitted? (May 1994)

What is malocclusion and how may it be classified?
Describe the methods which may be used by the dentist to treat malocclusion. (November 1991)

Summary

Angle's classification of occlusion

- Class 1:   normal jaw relationship
- Class 2 division 1:   protruding upper incisors; overjet increased
- Class 2 division 2:   upper central incisors tilted backwards; overjet decreased; overbite increased
- Class 3:   prominent chin; overjet absent or reversed

Causes of malocclusion

- Abnormal jaw relationship
- Abnormal jaw size
- Supernumerary teeth
- Missing teeth
- Sucking habits

Types of malocclusion

- Crowding – small jaws
- Protruding incisors } Abnormal jaw relationship
- Prominent chin   }

Aims of treatment

- Improve appearance
- Obtain good occlusion
- Reduce plaque retention areas

Treatment

- Extractions – relieve crowding
- Removable appliance } Springs move teeth into correct position
- Fixed appliance   } Extra-oral traction conserves space
- Functional appliance – muscles move the teeth

Care of appliances

- Wear as directed
- Clean after meals – take care with springs
- Avoid sticky sweets ← toffee, chewing gum
- Do not wait for next appointment if difficulties arise

Surgery procedure

- X-rays: show unerupted teeth
- Models: alginate impressions; wax squash bite
- Appliance adjustment: hand mirror, caliper gauge, marking pencil, pliers, wire cutters

Removable appliance instruments

- Adams universal pliers
- Adams spring forming pliers
- Wire cutters
- Straight handpiece and acrylic burs

Fixed appliance instruments

- Cementing bands: zinc phosphate, polycarboxylate or GIC; saliva ejector or aspirator; cotton wool rolls, absorbent pads, napkins; band driver and pusher; Mitchell trimmer
- Bonding brackets: acid etching and composite or GIC materials; saliva ejector or aspirator, cotton wool rolls, absorbent pads, napkins; bracket tweezers
- Adjustments: pliers, ligature cutters and tuckers, needle holders, serrated scissors, mosquito forceps

29 Dental Radiography

Dental radiography is the taking and processing of X-ray films of the teeth and jaws. When an X-ray set is switched on, X-rays are generated and pass out of the set through a plastic cone or metal tube which is pointed towards the required area. To take an X-ray, the tube and film are placed so that the part to be X-rayed lies between them (Figures 29.4 and 29.2). The tube through which the X-ray beam emerges from the set is called a **collimator** and its purpose is to restrict the area of the beam and facilitate aiming the beam.

Although X-rays can travel unimpeded through soft tissues, such as skin and muscle, they are unable to pass through hard tissues so easily and therefore project a shadow of the teeth and bone on to the film. This shadow, which forms the finished X-ray film when it is processed, varies in depth according to the thickness and density of the hard tissues, thus allowing enamel, dentine and bone to be easily recognized. Enamel and metal fillings appear dense white; dentine and bone are less white; while soft tissues such as periodontal membrane and pulp appear black. The finished X-ray film is called a **radiograph**.

Uses of radiography

Some of the commonest uses of X-rays in dentistry are to show the following:

1 Unerupted teeth, impacted teeth and retained roots
2 Shape, size and number of roots of a tooth, and state of the surrounding bone, prior to extraction
3 Presence of chronic alveolar abscesses on dead teeth
4 Progress of endodontic treatment
5 Bone loss in periodontal disease
6 Early detection of caries
7 Development of the teeth in children, for orthodontic purposes
8 Fractures, cysts and bone disease affecting the jaws

Radiographic changes in disease

Chronic alveolar abscesses show up as a dark circular area at the apex of an affected tooth. This is caused by destruction of the apical lamina dura and spongy bone. Figure 12.2 shows the normal appearance of this area.

Periodontal disease shows up as loss of the lamina dura forming the crest of the alveolar bone, loss of height of the alveolar bone, and a widening of the periodontal membrane space.

Caries shows up as a dark area of destruction extending inwards from the enamel surface.

For examination purposes, nurses are not expected to interpret radiographs, but they can take an interest in normal and abnormal radiographic appearances by asking the dentist to explain what is shown on the films they have processed.

X-ray film

X-ray film consists of ordinary black and white photographic film in a light-proof wrapping. There are two types of film: **intra-oral** and **extra-oral**.

Intra-oral film

Intra-oral film is placed inside the mouth and is used to take detailed films of small areas covering a few teeth only. The standard type of film is called **periapical** (Figure 29.1). It measures 3 × 4 cm but there is a smaller size for children.

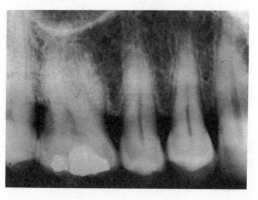

Figure 29.1 *Periapical radiograph.*
Source: *Dental Radiography* (2nd edn.). N.J.D. Smith, Blackwell Science Ltd, Oxford.

A much larger size of intra-oral film is the **occlusal** film (Figure 29.2). This is 6 × 7.5 cm and is used to give a plan view of the mandible or maxilla, usually to show unerupted teeth and cysts.

The contents of an intra-oral film packet are shown in Figure 29.3. When it is unwrapped for developing, the film is seen to be pale green

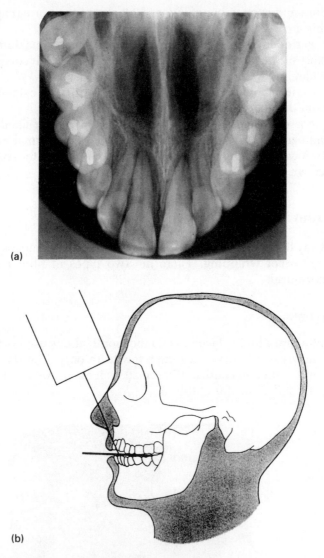

(a)

(b)

Figure 29.2   (a) Occlusal radiograph; (b) Angulation.
Source: Dental Radiography (2nd edn.). N.J.D. Smith, Blackwell Science Ltd, Oxford.

with a mounting pimple on the side which *faces* the X-ray tube. On either side of the film is a piece of black paper to shield it from the light and prevent damage to the film. Behind the black paper, on the side *away* from the X-ray tube, is a piece of lead foil. This absorbs scattered radiation which could spoil the quality of the radiograph. All these layers are enclosed in a light-proof wrapping which has a pimple on the side *facing* the X-ray tube.

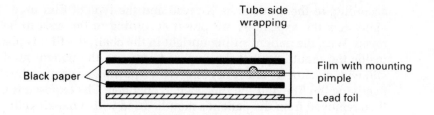

Figure 29.3 *Contents of intra-oral film packet.*

Extra-oral film

Extra-oral film, measuring 13 × 18 cm, is used outside the mouth with ordinary dental X-ray sets. The film is placed against the face over the required area. It covers a large area of the jaws and is used to show unerupted teeth, fractures, cysts and bone diseases. The most commonly taken view is called a **lateral oblique**.

Extra-oral film is packed differently from intra-oral films. The latter are individually packed in light-proof wrappers but extra-oral film is not. Packets of extra-oral film only contain unwrapped film and can only be opened in a darkroom. On removal from the packet in the darkroom, a film is placed immediately in a special light-proof container called a **cassette**, which is then kept closed ready for use.

A cassette opens like a book and the film is placed in the middle. On each inside cover of the cassette there is a white plastic sheet called an **intensifying screen**, and the film is sandwiched between the two screens when the cassette is closed ready for use. The screens fluoresce on exposure to X-rays and allow the exposure time to be reduced to a safe level.

Care of films

If an expiry date is given on a packet of film it should not be used beyond that date. Any remaining films should be discarded, as old film gives poor results.

Films can still deteriorate before their expiry date if stored in hot or damp places, or too near an X-ray set.

Film in poor condition, from any of these causes, will give a radiograph of poor quality which may have to be retaken.

Taking intra-oral radiographs

The X-ray set is plugged into an electricity supply and the time switch is set to the correct exposure. This varies from 0.1 to 0.5 seconds according to the tooth to be X-rayed and the type of film used. On many sets the exposures are preset according to the area to be X-rayed. With the patient sitting upright in the chair, the film is placed inside the mouth against the required area and the patient holds it still with one finger. The X-ray tube is then positioned against the skin overlying the film and the time switch operated. The exposed film is then removed from the patient's mouth, dried with a napkin, clipped on to a film hanger marked with the patient's name, and is now ready for processing.

Cross-infection prevention is facilitated if the film is placed in a clear plastic envelope before insertion in the mouth. The envelope is discarded on removal from the mouth. Some brands of film are supplied with envelopes already fitted.

Angulation

The greatest difficulties in taking intra-oral radiographs are to get the patient to hold the film still in the proper place during exposure, and to angulate the tube correctly. If the tube is tilted too far upwards or downwards the radiograph may be useless as the teeth will appear elongated or foreshortened. However, these difficulties can be easily overcome by using special X-ray beam aiming devices. These consist of a bite-block film holder which enables a film to be held in position in the mouth when the teeth are closed together on the block; and indicate the correct angle and direction for the X-ray beam. Patients do not have to hold the film in place; angulation is simple, irrespective of whether the patient sits upright or in a supine position; and the results are consistently good.

If these devices are not used, the correct way of angulating a tube is to direct it at a right angle to an imaginary line bisecting the angle between the long axis of tooth and film (Figure 29.4 and 29.2). This is called the **bisecting angle technique** and gives correct angulation in the vertical plane. In the horizontal plane the tube must be at a right angle to the film. Wrong angulation in the horizontal plane causes overlapping of teeth on the radiograph.

Even with perfect angulation there is inevitably some distortion in the radiograph. Normally it is insignificant and satisfactory results are produced. However, a different technique using a longer collimator on the X-ray set, and a special aiming device, allows a film to be held parallel to the long axis of a tooth. The collimator fits into a ring on the device, and this eliminates distortion and gives a better quality radiograph. It is particularly useful for showing bone loss in periodontal disease. It is called the *paralleling technique* (Figure 29.5) but has the disadvantage of requiring a longer exposure to compensate for a longer collimator.

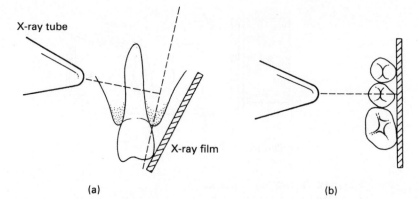

Figure 29.4 *Angulation of the X-ray tube.* (a) bisecting angle technique; (b) horizontal plane; (c) bite-wing.

Bite-wing radiographs

Bite-wing radiographs are X-ray films taken of teeth in occlusion. They show the crowns of opposing upper and lower teeth on the same film and are used to detect caries at the contact points of adjacent teeth, before it can be seen by any other methods (Figure 29.6).

Bite-wing film is periapical intra-oral film with a tab projecting at a right angle from its centre. This tab is bitten between the teeth and holds the film in correct position, covering the crowns of all upper and lower teeth in contact with it. There are no angulation difficulties as the tab can be felt through the cheek, and the tube is simply placed against this point at a 90° angle to teeth and film (Figure 29.4). The aiming devices mentioned earlier are also made for bite-wing film

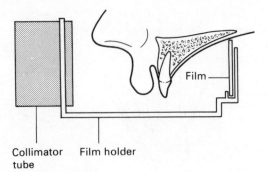

Collimator   Film holder
tube

Figure 29.5 *Paralleling technique.*
Source: Dental Radiography (2nd edn.). N.J.D. Smith, Blackwell Science Ltd, Oxford.

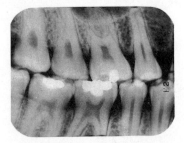

Figure 29.6 *Bite-wing radiograph.*
Source: Dental Radiography (2nd edn.). N.J.D.
Smith, Blackwell Science Ltd, Oxford.

and simplify matters even more; special bite-wing film is unnecessary as the device holds ordinary film without a tab.

Of all the methods of detecting caries at contact points, bite-wing radiographs detect it first and are consequently used widely as part of a general dental examination. In this way small cavities can be discovered and treated early, thus preventing pain and the possible loss of teeth.

Apart from displaying contact points, bite-wing radiographs also show the crest of alveolar bone and any bone loss; restoration overhangs; and occlusal and recurrent caries. This allows them to detect progressive periodontal disease and unsatisfactory fillings, as well as early caries.

Panoramic radiography

A new method of taking radiographs has been introduced into dentistry by a special X-ray set which takes panoramic films of the jaws. The film is called a **dental panoramic tomograph** (DPT) and it shows every single tooth, erupted or unerupted, on each side of both jaws, all on the one film (Figure 29.7). It was originally called an orthopantomograph, and its abbreviation OPG is still in common use.

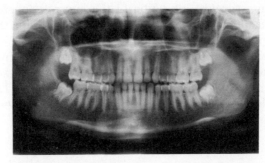

Figure 29.7 *Dental panoramic tomograph.*
Source: Dental Radiography (2nd edn.). N.J.D. Smith, Blackwell Science Ltd, Oxford.

A special DPT machine is used and it takes a panoramic film by having a motor-driven X-ray tube and film cassette holder which circle round the patient's face. The patient stands upright and special supports keep the head still during an exposure time of up to 15 seconds. The cassette holds extra-oral 13 × 31 cm film which is processed in the same way as the smaller size lateral oblique film and intra-oral films.

A DPT is particularly useful for showing teeth which are otherwise difficult to X-ray, such as unerupted third molars and canines. It is also used for screening purposes to show the overall state of development of the dentition and the presence of any abnormalities. However, it is not a substitute for intra-oral films as these are still necessary for giving more detailed views of small areas, particularly the periapical region of incisors.

Cephalometric radiography

Orthodontic diagnosis, treatment planning and recording are greatly facilitated by use of a special X-ray technique which gives standardized views of the whole skull. Side and frontal views are taken with a special machine called a **cephalostat**. The patient's head is positioned in a frame with locating posts which fit into the ear holes; and the most commonly taken films are side views, called lateral skull radiographs (Figure 29.8).

Tracings of these films are used for taking various measurements of the relationships between the skull, jaws and teeth. The cephalostat allows subsequent film tracings to be accurately compared with previous ones, thus enabling the progress and results of treatment to be checked and analysed. The technique is called cephalometric radiography.

Oral surgeons also use frontal and lateral skull films taken in a cephalostat for diagnosis and treatment planning; especially for cases requiring surgical alteration of the jaw relationship. They are also very useful for precise location of the position and angulation of unerupted upper canines.

This technique preceded panoramic radiography and necessitated the use of a cephalostat which could not take any other types of radiographs. However, most DPT machines can be adapted to take cephalometric films as well. Film size for these views is 20 × 25 cm with an exposure time of up to three seconds.

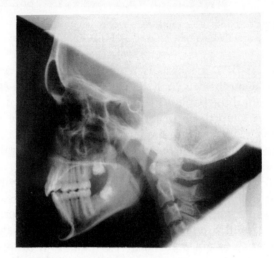

Figure 29.8 *Lateral skull radiograph.*
Source: Dental Radiography (2nd edn.). N.J.D. Smith, Blackwell Science Ltd, Oxford.

Computed radiography

All the radiographic techniques described so far require the use of X-ray film which has to be chemically processed to produce a radiograph. An entirely new technique utilizes computers to produce direct digital intra-oral radiographs which are viewed on a computer monitor screen at the chairside. A normal X-ray set is used but X-ray film and processing are not required. A reusable intra-oral sensor plate is used instead of film and the radiation dose is far less than with ordinary film.

The exposed sensor plate is inserted into a laser scanner which is connected to a compatible personal computer. Less than a minute later the radiograph appears on the monitor screen and can be stored on a hard or floppy disk and retrieved at will.

The scanner may be likened to a CD player and the computer to a word-processor, as the radiograph can be edited to give the effect of different X-ray exposures, and parts magnified or altered, just as words can be altered, moved, erased or otherwise manipulated by a word-processor.

The advantages of this system are the elimination of film-processing; reduced radiation exposure; speed of viewing; reusability of sensor plates; and the ability to retrieve, show and discuss radiographic findings with patients at the chairside.

The disadvantages are the cost of the equipment and a theoretical possibility of legal problems arising from undetectable alterations to the original radiographic image.

Processing

X-ray film is ordinary photographic film and is affected by X-rays in just the same way as film inside a camera is affected by light. The processing procedure for X-ray film is just the same as that for producing an ordinary black and white film negative. After exposure, the film contains the X-ray image but it is not yet visible. The first stage of processing is to *develop* the image so that it can be seen. It cannot be used at this stage, however, as the film is still sensitive to light and would eventually darken all over if viewed in daylight. A second stage of processing is therefore necessary, to *fix* the image, and produce a usable permanent film.

Darkroom procedure

All precautions to prevent unnecessary exposure to radiation are devalued if films are not processed correctly. Such films will be of inadequate diagnostic quality and will have to be retaken. To ensure satisfactory radiographs, processing solutions must be mixed to the correct dilution and replenished as specified by the manufacturer. They must also be replaced at the recommended intervals (at least monthly); and the date when this is due should be prominently displayed in the darkroom. Processing tanks should be made airtight by covering with kitchen clingfilm, as well as with their lids, when not in use. This prevents the premature deterioration of processing solutions. Waterproof gloves should be worn during processing as the chemicals used may irritate sensitive skin.

Under ordinary lighting, the levels of **developer** and **fixer** tank solutions are checked to ensure they are full enough to cover the films. Their temperature is then checked with a thermometer, and raised if necessary with an immersion heater until it reaches the optimum range of 18°–22°C (Figure 29.9). A table giving the correct times for developing and fixing, at various temperatures, is always provided by the manufacturers. It is essential to comply with this as retakes will be necessary if films are over- or under-processed. An

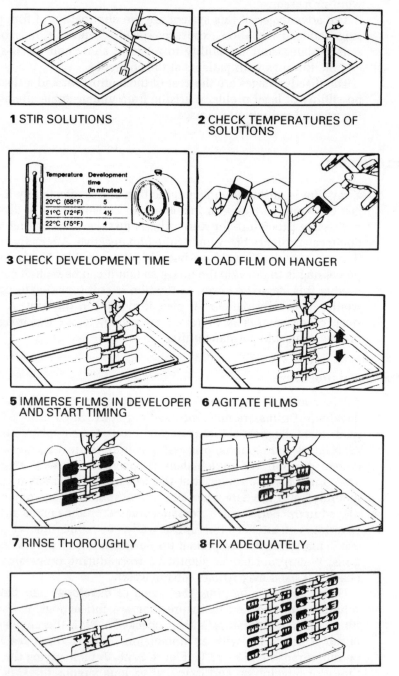

1 STIR SOLUTIONS

2 CHECK TEMPERATURES OF SOLUTIONS

3 CHECK DEVELOPMENT TIME

4 LOAD FILM ON HANGER

5 IMMERSE FILMS IN DEVELOPER AND START TIMING

6 AGITATE FILMS

7 RINSE THOROUGHLY

8 FIX ADEQUATELY

9 WASH THOROUGHLY

10 DRY

Figure 29.9 *Processing.*

accurate alarm-timer and thermometer are necessary as a rise of only 6° halves development time. Before proceeding further, check that all work surfaces are clean and dry. Contamination of films by spilt developer or fixer can ruin a radiograph.

After marking a film hanger with the patient's name, the light is switched off, and the red safelight turned on, giving just sufficient illumination to see without affecting the film. If the safelight seems too dim to see by, wait a few minutes to accustom to it, whereupon you will be surprised how well you can see.

Developing

When you can see well enough under the safelight, remove the film wrapping and clip the film securely to the bottom of the named hanger. The film appears quite blank at this stage. Then set an alarm clock for the required development time and place the film in the developer tank.

When the alarm sounds, remove the hanger with the developed film and hold it over the rinsing tank to prevent any developer dripping on to a work surface. Replace the lid on the developer tank and wash the film in the rinsing tank under clean running water for 30 seconds. This is necessary to prevent the fixer tank being contaminated by developer. After rinsing, let all the drips drain back into the rinsing water. A first trace of the X-ray shadow can now be seen.

Fixing

Dry the work surface and set the alarm for the correct fixing time. Place the developed film in fixer and do not remove it until the alarm sounds. Again allow drips from the hanger to fall back into the rinsing tank and not on a work surface. Then rinse the film in running water as before. The radiograph is now ready for viewing, so switch off the safelight and turn on the ordinary light.

Washing

Although processing is now complete and the radiograph can be viewed, it is necessary to keep it under cold running water for at least ten minutes (only five for extra-oral film) to remove all traces of fixer, before hanging it up to dry. Used film hangers must also be thoroughly washed and dried to prevent the subsequent contamination of solutions and films.

Mounting

Radiographs are mounted on a transparent sheet with the patient's name and date on which they were taken. The purpose of mounting is to ensure that films do not get lost or mixed up with another patient. Retakes are thereby avoided and the dentist has all the radiographs for one patient conveniently arranged for viewing.

In order to mount radiographs correctly, nurses must be able to tell whether a film is upper or lower, left or right. An elementary knowledge of dental anatomy allows a nurse to distinguish between upper and lower teeth. For example most views of upper teeth would show part of the nose or antrum air spaces; and the number of roots may also help (Figures 29.1 and 29.2). To differentiate between left and right there is a small pimple pressed into one corner of every intra-oral film. This indicates the side facing the tube (Figure 29.3); and when held with the top of the convexity of the pimple facing the observer there is no difficulty in deciding which side it belongs to.

Having orientated the radiographs correctly, they are mounted as they would appear on a dental chart. Thus a radiograph of the upper left teeth is mounted at the top right of the mounting sheet, upper right teeth at the top left, lower left teeth at the bottom right, and lower right teeth at the bottom left of the mounting sheet. Radiographs are usually attached to a matt transparent sheet or inserted in a cardboard frame, but whichever method is used the mount must always be clearly marked with the patient's name and date on which the radiograph was taken.

Causes of failure

Although many practices have abandoned manual processing in favour of automatic methods, it is still necessary for *all* nurses to understand what happens to a film during exposure and processing. This will help trace causes of error and prevent any need for retakes.

Any part of a film exposed to X-rays or white light is turned black and opaque by developer. The remaining unexposed part is still sensitive to light and appears green and opaque. Fixer dissolves away the unexposed green part, leaving it completely transparent and no longer sensitive to light. Some common faults are as follows:

Blank film

If the set is not switched on, exposure cannot occur and a blank transparent film will result on processing. It is surprisingly easy to take an X-ray without realizing that the set is not switched on.

Another surprisingly simple error is to forget to reload an extra-oral film cassette in the darkroom immediately after unloading it. Once a cassette is taken out of the darkroom it cannot be opened to check if there is a film inside.

A blank film can also be produced, even when the set is on, if the film is first placed in fixer instead of developer. Tanks should always be clearly labelled to avoid this mistake; but when in doubt, in the dark, a simple way of distinguishing between the two solutions is to sniff them. Fixer smells like vinegar.

Prolonged washing of a processed film, especially in hot water, can dissolve the image and leave a blank film.

Partly blank film

If the edge of the blank area is curved, it is caused by inaccurate aiming or angulation of the pointer cone or circular collimator tube; or using too small an aperture. The X-rays have missed the blank area. If a rectangular collimator is used, the same fault would leave a straight edge.

A more common cause of a straight edge is incomplete immersion in developer when processing. This fault can be avoided by attaching films to the bottom clips of the hanger and ensuring that developer and fixer tanks are full.

Blurred film

This results from movement of the film or tube during exposure. It is usually caused by patients failing to keep their head or the film still. This is one reason for using the fastest (E speed) film as it gives patients (especially children) less time to move.

Distortion or overlapping of teeth

Caused by incorrect angulation of the tube.

Opaque film

The film appears black and almost opaque when held up to the light. This is caused by over-exposure or over-development. The latter is caused by developing for too long, or using developer which is too hot or too strong.

Strict compliance with manufacturers' instructions on film exposure times; and the correct dilution, temperature, immersion time, replenishment and replacement of processing solutions will avoid these faults.

Transparent film

When a film is too transparent to show any detail it is said to be *thin*. This is caused by under-exposure or under-development. The latter may occur if development time is insufficient; or if the developer solution is too old, too weak, or not warm enough.

Under-exposure can occur if the wrong side of the film faces the tube. In such cases it will be seen from Figure 29.3 that the X-rays pass through the lead foil before reaching the film. Some makes of film have a special pattern on the lead foil which shows up on the radiograph if the wrong side is used.

Fogged film

Fogged film is too dark or too grey to show any contrast between hard and soft tissues. There are several possible causes.

It may be due to exposure of the film to light before it is placed in fixer. This can occur if there is a leakage of light into the darkroom. A simple test to confirm darkroom light leakage is to unwrap an unexposed film in the darkroom and place a small coin on it. When it is processed later, it should be completely blank; but if there is light leakage, the part covered by the coin will be blank and the rest black.

It may also occur if films are accidentally exposed to X-rays before or after use. This happens if films are stored too near the X-ray set and are not kept in a lead container. A similar test can also be used to check for storage too near an X-ray set. An unexposed wrapped film is stored with a coin on top. When this is processed it should be completely blank, but if it has been exposed to X-rays it will again show a blank image of the coin with the rest black.

Other causes of fogging are storing film in an excessively hot or humid place; or using film beyond its expiry date.

Discoloured or smudged film

This is caused by carelessness during processing. Blank transparent spots or streaks occur if an undeveloped film is contaminated with fixer spilt over the bench or fingers. To avoid this it is essential to keep hands and bench thoroughly clean and dry during processing.

Diffuse brown or green opaque areas are caused by incomplete fixing. This may occur if the fixer is too old or has been contaminated by developer from an unwashed film or hanger. All processing solutions should be replaced regularly in accordance with manufacturers' instructions.

If an opaque discoloured area has a straight well-defined margin, it is caused by incomplete immersion in fixer. This fault can be avoided by attaching films to the bottom clips of the hanger and ensuring that the processing tanks are full.

White crystalline spots or streaks are residual fixer caused by inadequate washing after fixing.

Some of these faults can be prevented by dividing a darkroom into wet and dry areas. Films are unwrapped, cassettes unloaded and reloaded, and hangers stored in the dry area, with processing confined to the wet area.

When unwrapping intra-oral film, the lead foil should be saved. It can be used in the surgery to absorb spilt mercury; and it also has scrap value.

Dangers of X-rays

X-rays cannot be seen, heard or felt, and therein lies the danger. As they cannot be perceived by any of the senses, it is easily forgotten that they are potentially dangerous to health; and it is just as easy to ignore every safety precaution. An overdose can give rise to serious effects, ranging from a mild burn to leukaemia. Special legal requirements to ensure the health and safety of persons exposed to radiation are now in force for dental practice. They are described later.

In the course of dental radiography the patient never receives an overdose. It is the radiographer, not the patient, who is most at risk, as the former is continually taking X-rays and must therefore take strict precautions to avoid accidental exposure.

The following precautions to protect patients and staff are taken.

1 Radiation safety must be checked at least every three years to ensure that X-ray sets are adequately shielded to prevent stray radiation; and processing procedure is satisfactory. All sets should have regular professional maintenance.
2 Use of the fastest film (E speed) will allow the shortest possible exposure time. Indeed, there is no justification for using anything but the fastest available film. Cassettes should be fitted with the fastest (rare earth) intensifying screens.
3 Sets with adjustable apertures must be correctly set to emit the narrowest beam of X-rays for the size of film used. Plastic aiming cones on X-ray sets should be replaced by rectangular collimator tubes to further reduce beam size to the safest level.

    This combination of fastest film, shortest exposure and narrowest beam will alone reduce the amount of scattered radiation by five times.
4 The special film-holder/beam-aiming devices, already mentioned, should be used for periapical and bite-wing radiographs, and the paralleling technique used in preference to the bisected angle method.
5 The operator must stand well clear of the X-ray beam during exposure, at the full length of the cable on the time switch; this should be not less than two metres. On no account must a nurse hold the film in place for a patient; if a child cannot keep it still, the parent must hold it in place.

6   Exposure of the reproductive organs to X-rays has produced abnormalities in the offspring of experimental animals. Similar exposure may occur from scattered radiation during dental radiography. Although it is insufficient to produce such genetic changes, the possibility can be excluded by strict adherence to all the required safeguards.

7   The amount of stray radiation received by staff should be checked by means of a film badge. This is an intra-oral film which is worn on the chest or waist for up to three months. It is then processed to indicate whether an excessive dosage is being received. If so, expert advice must be sought immediately to trace and eliminate the cause. Staff working in rooms adjacent to the surgery should also wear badges as X-rays can pass through walls.

Film badges are called **personal monitoring dosemeters** and are supplied by the National Radiological Protection Board (NRPB), or a local medical physics department. They process them, notify the dosage received, and can arrange appropriate investigation if it is too high.

8   Every radiograph must not only be necessary but also of diagnostic value. There should be no need for retakes because of faulty technique or processing. Retakes mean unnecessary additional exposure of patients and staff. To ensure perfect results the films must be in good condition, taken correctly, processed carefully and mounted properly.

9   X-ray sets should be disconnected from their electricity supply when not in use.

Legal requirements

All practices with X-ray equipment must comply with the provisions of the *Ionising Radiations Regulations*. The legal requirements are as follows.

Notification

Practices using X-ray sets must notify the local office of the Health and Safety Executive.

Equipment

X-ray sets must be professionally maintained and serviced regularly. No unauthorized persons may interfere with X-ray equipment.

Radiation safety in the practice must be assessed every three years. This is done through the NRPB Dental Monitoring Service. It provides a kit which allows the X-ray set and film-processing technique to be tested. The kit is then returned to the NRPB for assessment of the results.

Radiation protection supervisor

Every practice must appoint a radiation protection supervisor (RPS) to ensure compliance with the regulations. The RPS, who would normally be the dentist, must have a command of the regulations and all the safety measures required.

Staff training

All staff involved in the taking and processing of X-ray films must be adequately trained for their duties.

Staff protection

If more than 150 intra-oral or 50 DPT films a week are taken, staff involved should wear a personal monitoring dosemeter. The RPS will then take appropriate action if excessive radiation is recorded.

Radiation protection adviser

A radiation protection adviser (RPA) must be appointed if a practice uses cephalometric X-ray equipment; or if staff are exposed to a radiation dose equivalent to 360 intra-oral or 40 DPT films a week. An RPA would usually be a radiation physicist who regularly checks, monitors and advises practices on all aspects of radiation hygiene.

Such practices must still comply with all the regulations and appoint their own RPS.

Local rules

Written rules for ensuring radiation protection must be displayed in the practice. They must:

1   Name the RPS and staff qualified to take X-ray films.
2   Designate a **controlled area**. This is an exclusion zone of radius 1.5 metres around the chair where X-ray exposures are made. Nobody but the patient is allowed inside a controlled area during exposure. The operator stands outside the area, out of the direct path of the X-ray beam, at the full length of the cable on the time switch.
3   Describe the safety precautions required in the practice to ensure protection of patients and staff; and to ensure that films are correctly processed. Such details will vary between practices,

according to the type of X-ray set, processing equipment, number of surgeries and workload involved.

4 Provide a contingency plan specifying action to be taken in the event of equipment malfunction. For example, if the exposure warning light or audible signal remains on after the exposure time has elapsed, the mains supply to the set must be switched off *immediately.* The set must not be used again until the cause has been found and rectified.

Role of the dental nurse

In accordance with these legal obligations the GDC requires dentists to ensure that personnel taking X-rays have received adequate training. This means that dental nurses are not allowed to place X-ray films in the mouth or to position the X-ray tube, unless they have been properly trained to the legally specified standards.

Although this training may be given by the dentist, nurses can prove their legal competence to take X-rays by attending and passing a course for the Certificate in Dental Radiography mentioned in Chapter 2. Nurses must possess the National Certificate, and be registered, for entry to such courses.

Nurses without a radiography certificate are allowed to process X-ray films but must be fully trained for this work by their dentist. Furthermore, they are obliged to comply fully with the local rules for correct processing procedure.

Written examination

How should patients and staff be protected when dental radiographs are being taken?

Describe five faults which may occur during the processing of radiographs and how they may be caused. (November 1994)

For what reasons may a dentist take the following radiographic views?

(a)   periapical
(b)   bite-wing
(c)   occlusal
(d)   panoral (OPG)

How may exposure to X-radiation be controlled in the dental surgery? (May 1992)

Summary

X-ray film

Periapical

Contents:

- Tube side wrapping – has *pimple*
- Black paper
- Film (green)
- Black paper
- Lead foil
- Reverse side wrapping

Angulation:

(a) Bisected angle technique: direct tube at a right angle to line bisecting angle between long axis of tooth and film
(b) Paralleling (long cone) technique: film parallel to long axis of tooth → more accurate radiograph
Requires special film holder/beam-aiming device

Uses:

- Unerupted teeth and retained roots
- Prior to difficult extraction
- Chronic alveolar abscesses
- Root treatment
- Periodontal disease
- Orthodontics

Bite-wings

Angulation:

- Tube against tab 90° to teeth and film

Uses:

- Early detection of interproximal caries.

Also shows:

- Occlusal and recurrent caries
- Crest of alveolar bone ⎫ diagnosis of periodontal disease
- Restoration overhangs ⎭

Occlusal

- Plan view of either jaw
- Unerupted teeth
- Cysts

Extra-oral

- Large areas of jaw
- Unerupted teeth
- Cysts
- Fractures
- Bone disease
- Orthodontics

Panoramic

- One film shows both sides of both jaws and every tooth
- Requires special DPT set

Cephalometric

- Lateral or frontal views of skull
- Requires special equipment called a cephalostat
- Used for orthodontic and jaw surgery measurements

Computerized

- Special reusable sensor instead of film
- No processing required
- Radiographic image appears on computer monitor screen
- Exposure faults easily rectified
- Magnification and alterations possible
- Allows immediate chairside viewing

Taking X-ray films

1 Connect X-ray set to electricity supply
2 Set time switch to correct exposure
3 Patient sitting upright in chair
4 Place film in patient's mouth
5 Angulate tube
6 Stand clear and switch on
7 Remove film and dry with napkin
8 Clip on to hanger marked with patient's name
9 Disconnect X-ray set

Processing

1 Wear waterproof gloves
2 Check temperature of solutions and raise if necessary to 18°–22°C with immersion heater
3 Switch off darkroom light and switch on safelight
4 Unwrap film and set alarm clock for developing time
5 Start clock and place film in developer
6 When alarm goes, remove film and wash in water. Replace lid on developer
7 Reset alarm and place film in fixer
8 When alarm goes, remove from fixer and wash in water
9 Switch on light and inspect film
10 Leave film under cold running water for ten minutes (five for extra-oral film)
11 Leave to dry

Causes of failure

- Blank film – set not switched on; *developed* in fixer; cassette not loaded
- Partly blank – curved edge: incorrect angulation or aim; aperture too small
                 – straight edge: incomplete immersion in developer
- Blurred film – patient, film or tube moved during exposure
- Distortion or overlapping of teeth – incorrect angulation
- Opaque film – over-exposed or over-developed; developer too strong or too hot
- *Thin* film – under-exposed or under-developed; (c)old developer; wrong side of film
- Fogged film – exposed to light before fixing; storage too near X-ray set; too hot or too humid; old film
- Discoloured film – blank spots: film contaminated with fixer before developing
                    – brown or green opaque area: incomplete fixing
                    – white crystalline spots: inadequate wash after fixing

Mounting

- Arrange films as on dental chart
- Mount with top of pimple facing observer
- Write name of patient and date taken

Precautions with X-rays

- Check machine for leakage
- Use fastest (E speed) film and rare earth intensifying screens
- Use smallest aperture for film size
- Replace plastic aiming cone with square collimator tube
- Use film holders and paralleling technique.
- Only the patient or parent may hold the film in place
- Stand well clear of X-ray beam, at full length of cable, during exposure
- Personal monitoring dosemeters for surgery staff

Ionising Radiations Regulations

- Notify use of X-ray set to Health and Safety Executive
- Regular maintenance and servicing of set
- Check radiation safety every three years with NRPB monitoring kit
- Appoint RPS to ensure compliance with regulations
- Adequate training for all practice staff
- Wear personal monitoring dosemeter if 150 intra-oral or 50 DPT films a week are taken
- Appoint RPA if cephalometric set used; or if 360 intra-oral or 40 DPT films a week are taken
- Produce and display written *Local Rules* for radiation safety:
  - (a) Designate controlled area – exclusion zone, radius 1.5 m round X-ray chair. Only the patient allowed inside area during exposure
  - (b) Describe safety precautions for patients and staff; and correct processing procedure
  - (c) Contingency plan for equipment malfunction

30 Records

The purpose of dental records is to provide an up-to-date case history of each patient's condition, and includes the examination findings and treatment given on each attendance at the surgery. By referring back to previous visits the dentist can assess the results of earlier courses of treatment and thereby decide the best line of treatment on future occasions. Adequate records also facilitate the transfer of patients between dentists in the practice when absence or staff changes occur. Another dentist can then continue any previous treatment with all the required information already available.

Recording methods, and the amount of detail recorded, vary considerably from practice to practice, but patients' records consist basically of personal and clinical information. They include radiographs, clinical photos, study models, medical history, consent forms, correspondence and accounts, as well as treatment charts.

For new patients the personal details, medical and dental history are recorded, and clinical details are entered on a new chart. At subsequent visits the date and treatment given are entered on the patient's chart and in a day book. The day book is a daily record of work done for each patient attending the surgery and forms a valuable cross-reference system with the charts.

Apart from clinical records, those relating to practice administration are just as important. Such records concern the supply and purchase of equipment, materials and drugs used for treatment, details of despatch and receipt of work done by dental laboratories; and staff personnel records.

Many practices use computers and word-processors for dealing with records, recall systems, correspondence, accounts and stock control. They permit rapid access to information, save much storage space and secretarial time, and can greatly enhance the efficiency of practice administration.

Importance of records

Under NHS regulations, dentists are expected to keep adequate records. In all branches of dentistry, within or without the NHS, records taken at the time are legally valid documents and serious legal difficulties may arise if they are inadequate or inaccurate. Errors or omissions in recording information may result in incorrect treatment or failure to provide necessary treatment.

Dental records are also extremely valuable as a means of establishing identity. In fatal accidents where facial features are destroyed, the teeth are usually unaffected and can be compared with dentists' records to identify a victim.

Proper records allow correct treatment planning and provide a check on details of past treatment. They form the basis on which fees are calculated and accounts rendered to patients. Failed appointments and refusals of treatment are noted and the patient's attitude to dental health assessed. Appropriate recall arrangements can then be made for each patient.

The nurse must accurately record information given by the patient or dictated by the dentist. She must ensure that records are filed properly, made available at each appointment, and signed as necessary by patient and dentist.

Adequate records allow the practice to run with the greatest efficiency for all concerned; and should be retained for at least 11 years after completion of treatment. Many difficulties concerning individual patients can be prevented altogether if complete records are available of all attendances at the practice, while no time is wasted in putting such information at the dentist's disposal. Recording and filing systems may vary considerably in different practices but whichever method is used, records must always be accurate, legible, comprehensive and easily accessible.

Confidentiality

Nurses must clearly understand that unauthorized disclosure of any sort of information concerning patients is absolutely forbidden. This is of such fundamental importance that breach of confidentiality constitutes grounds for dismissal. The duty of confidentiality applies not only to history and treatment details, but even to the fact that a patient attends the practice.

Personal records

Personal records include the patient's name, address, telephone number, age and occupation. The address will indicate any travelling difficulties or problems regarding appointment times. It may also be important to note the fluoride content of the water supply for that address.

Age

A carious deciduous molar in a child under seven may be conserved with a permanent filling; but in a child of ten a temporary filling will usually suffice until the tooth is shed naturally. NHS patients over 60 are entitled to free prescriptions.

Occupation

A missing upper incisor may be replaced with a bridge or partial denture. A wind instrumentalist obviously requires a fixed form of restoration and would probably prefer a bridge; whereas a professional player of contact sports might be better off with a partial denture as it can be removed when exposed to occupational hazards.

Clinical records

Clinical records consist of the past and present appointment and day books, as well as records of each patient attending the practice. Individual patient records include the medical history, dental history, present condition, charting and treatment; consent forms, estimates, accounts and correspondence.

Medical history and present condition

Full details of patients' past and present illnesses and drugs taken must be obtained. All relevant information is recorded and must be regularly updated. Taking, assessing and updating a medical history is the sole responsibility of a dentist and is not part of a nurse's duty.

In order to ensure complete confidentiality, a medical history must be taken in private where it cannot be overheard. Patients cannot be expected to provide full details unless they are satisfied of privacy.

Many conditions or drugs may influence the dental treatment plan. For example:

1 The choice between LA or GA (Chapter 14) may depend on the condition of the patient's heart and chest; and whether drugs are being taken for medical treatment.
2 If a patient has suffered from any heart conditions or rheumatic fever it may be necessary to give antibiotic cover (Chapter 11) before extractions, scaling, surgery and root filling, as a precautionary measure against infective endocarditis.
3 Extractions may be inadvisable whilst a patient is being treated with certain drugs such as anticoagulants and corticosteroids; or after irradiation treatment of the jaws. Special care is needed for patients with bleeding disorders.
4 Allergy to certain drugs may cause a severe anaphylactic reaction (Chapter 15). Patients are asked if any untoward reactions have

occurred before. Penicillin and its derivatives, such as amoxycillin, are the drugs most likely to be involved in dental practice.

5   Adverse reactions can occur because of an interaction between drugs being taken for medical treatment and drugs administered during dental treatment (Chapters 11 and 15).

6   Special care is necessary during pregnancy.

   (a)   There must be no contact with staff or other patients who are rubella (German measles) contacts.

   (b)   LA is safe but GA and drugs of any other kind should be avoided (Chapter 11).

   (c)   In the late stages of pregnancy, patients should not be treated in the supine position.

7   Patients who have been in contact with infectious diseases such as mumps and German measles should not attend the surgery while these illness are still active (Chapter 10).

8   Careful observation of patients will detect signs which may affect treatment: breathlessness and pallor are suggestive of anaemia; while cyanosis (blue complexion) and jaundice are indicative of heart and liver disease respectively.

9   Special precautions may be necessary for treatment of known HBV and HIV carriers (Chapter 10); and immunocompromised patients (Chapter 9).

The name of the patients' doctor should always be included in the records. Then, if any doubts arise, the doctor can be consulted before treatment is undertaken.

Dental history

Diagnosis of the present condition and determination of the treatment plan may depend on details of earlier dental disorders and their treatment. Knowledge of previous difficulties such as excessive bleeding, poor response to anaesthetics, difficult extractions; allergy to dental materials, latex gloves or rubber dam; or any other complications, will help the dentist to avoid their recurrence.

Present condition

The present condition of the teeth is recorded on the dental chart as shown in Figure 12.8; and any other conditions such as the state of existing restorations and dentures, poor oral hygiene, periodontal disease, malocclusion, close bite, discoloured teeth, etc., which may affect treatment are also noted. The dentist can then assess the patient's general attitude towards dental health and accordingly advise the most appropriate treatment.

Treatment

Full details of treatment and the date on which it is given are recorded on the dental chart. This will include special examinations such as X-rays, vitality tests, study models, etc., together with the type of filling and lining, any retained roots after extraction, drugs and dosage administered or prescribed, shade of artificial teeth, crown or filling, broken appointments, and any other information considered necessary by the dentist.

The charts (Figures 12.8 and 25.3) and treatment notes folder will also include the radiographs, clinical photos, consent forms, referral letters and reports, treatment plans and estimates, and any other relevant documents or correspondence.

As in the case of a medical history, the dentist, not the nurse, is responsible for obtaining consent to treatment. Such consent is not legally valid unless the necessity, nature, complications, alternative options and costs are personally explained by the dentist and understood by the patient.

National Health Service records

The NHS provides a standard chart (Form FP25) for recording the treatment required and provided (Figure 12.8) and patient visits. Although practitioners are not obliged to use these particular charts, they are expected to keep adequate records.

Form FP17DC/GP17DC is given to the patient. It outlines treatment required and the NHS charges; as well as the details and cost of any agreed private treatment.

The Dental Estimates Form (Form FP17) is used by practitioners to record details of treatment required, and subsequently given, and provides a form of account on which payment can be claimed.

The law

Legal requirements for practice records include those relating to patients, practice equipment and materials, and health and safety matters. The latter are covered in Chapter 31 and the remainder in the following paragraphs.

Patients have a legal right of access to their records, whether they are filed manually or held in computer storage. Under consumer protection law, dentists must keep records of all equipment and materials used for treatment and/or supplied to patients.

The *Data Protection Act* obliges dentists to register under the Act if they keep patients' records on a computer. The purpose of the Act is to protect patients' privacy by ensuring that computer records are accurate, relevant, kept securely and are not disclosed to unauthorized persons. Patients have a right of access to such records and for the correction of any inaccuracies therein.

The *Access to Health Records Act* gives patients a right of access to their manually held records. They can also request correction of any entries or, in the event of refusal, to have their request noted in the records.

These Acts require dentists to ensure that:

1 Recorded information is accurate and up to date
2 Records are securely filed to prevent unauthorized disclosure of information

In view of these rights of access to records, great care must be taken to ensure that no derogatory comments are included.

The *Consumer Protection Act* requires dentists to keep records for at least 11 years; or until the age of 25, whichever is the longer. Beyond these limits records may be destroyed, but this must be done by incineration or shredding so that their information is irretrievable. This Act also applies to records of all supplies of equipment, materials, drugs and laboratory work; as any harm suffered by a patient which is attributable to such products can render the supplier or dentist liable to legal action for damages.

Written examination

What precautions need to be taken when treating a dental patient who:

(a)   is pregnant
(b)   is a known hepatitis B carrier
(c)   has suffered from rheumatic fever? (November 1994)

(a)   Why is accurate dental record keeping important and what information should be included on patients' record cards?
(b)   What instructions should be given to the patient when making an appointment for a general anaesthetic? (May 1994)

What information does a dental record card give and why is it important?

List the additional information which should be recorded about a patient. (May 1991)

Summary

Personal records

- Name, address (? fluoridated area), telephone number
- Age
- Occupation
- Travelling time to practice
- Convenient appointment times

Clinical records

1 Past and present medical history

- Illnesses
- Drugs and dosage prescribed or administered
- Drug reactions
- Allergy
- Pregnancy
- Contact with infectious diseases
- HBV and HIV carriers, contacts and groups at risk
- Name and address of doctor

2 Dental history:

- Bleeding
- Difficult extractions
- Anaesthetics
- Allergy
- Attendance record

3 Present condition:

- Chart, radiographs, models, photos
- State of restorations and dentures
- Discoloured teeth
- Occlusion
- Oral hygiene
- Periodontal condition

4 Diagnosis and treatment
5 Referral letters and reports
6 Consent forms
7 Treatment plans and estimates
8 Payments and receipts
9 Appointment and day books
10 Keep records for 11 years or until age 25, whichever is longer

11 Patients have right of access to their records
12 Confidentiality

Administrative records

- Correspondence
- Accounts
- Stock control
- Equipment, supplies, materials and drugs purchased
- Laboratory work
- Practice personnel files

31 Health and Safety at Work

All dental premises, their staff and patients are covered by the provisions of the **Health and Safety at Work Act**. This legislation seeks to protect staff and patients by making the staff aware of hazards at work, and encouraging them to find the best ways of making their particular premises safer for all concerned.

Dentists are required under this law to ensure, so far as is reasonably practicable, the health, safety and welfare at work of all their employees. Every dental practice is required to:

1   Provide a working environment for employees that is safe, without risks to health, and adequate as regards facilities and arrangements for their welfare at work.
2   Maintain the place of work, including the means of access and egress, in a safe condition
3   Provide and maintain safe equipment, appliances and systems of work. This includes proper seating and eye protection for staff using computer keyboards and monitors
4   Ensure safe handling and storage of any dangerous or potentially harmful articles or substances
5   Provide such instruction, training and supervision as is necessary to ensure health and safety

To comply with these statutory obligations dentists must keep their staff informed of the safety measures adopted. Practices with five or more employees must produce a safety policy and provide all staff with a copy. It classifies the practice health and safety procedures and names the person responsible for them.

Role of the dental nurse

All nurses have a legal obligation to co-operate with their employers in carrying out the practice requirements in respect of these safety measures. They are designed to protect not only the staff and patients, but anybody else using or visiting the premises. In a large practice or clinic, a nurse may be appointed as *safety representative* under the Act for the purpose of improving liaison within the practice about health and safety matters.

Inspection of premises

The Act empowers inspectors to visit dental practices, examine equipment and question staff in order to ascertain whether a reasonable standard of safety and welfare prevails.

Staff welfare

Legal requirements for the welfare of staff include: regular maintenance of equipment; provision of adequate and suitable washing and toilet facilities, cloakroom space, heating, ventilation and lighting, seating, rest room facilities; no-smoking areas and general cleanliness.

General safety measures

These relate to any premises where people are employed to provide a service to the public. They are all common-sense precautions for preventing injury to anybody using or visiting the premises. For example:

1 Safe means of access and egress, adequately lit and unobstructed. Stairs should have firm secure handrails.
2 Floor coverings should be non-slip and secure at the edges to prevent tripping.
3 Walls and ceilings should be washable and free of any dust traps.
4 Furniture and fittings should not have sharp edges.
5 All fires and heaters must be adequately guarded, and electrical appliances should be so positioned as to avoid trailing leads and be out of reach of children.
6 All fixed and movable electrical equipment and appliances, and their supply lines, must be correctly installed, fused, regularly checked by approved persons, and records kept.
7 Gas and electricity should be turned off at source before leaving the premises at the end of the day.
8 A first-aid kit must be provided in a special marked container or cupboard. It should be easily accessible and contain, with relevant instructions: sterile eye dressings and eye bath; an assortment of bandages and disinfectants for the treatment of burns, cuts, lacerations, fractures and sprains; and 4% sodium bicarbonate solution for treatment of acid burns. At least one member of the staff should be specially trained in the provision of first aid.

Notification of accidents

All employers are legally required to notify the **Health and Safety Executive** of serious accidents and dangerous occurrences at work. Notifiable incidents are those involving staff and members of the public; but patients undergoing treatment are specifically excluded. Thus an injury to a patient in the surgery is not notifiable, whereas a major injury occurring elsewhere in the practice is notifiable.

The definition of major injury includes such things as any injury resulting in death; most fractures; the loss of a hand, foot or sight of an eye; or any other injury resulting in hospital in-patient treatment for more than one day. Dangerous occurrences in a dental practice include: compressor or autoclave explosion; a serious mercury spillage; a serious spillage or leakage of any other substance which could affect a person's health; hepatitis B resulting from cross-infection in the surgery; a dangerous fire resulting in closure of the premises for more than one day.

Serious accidents and dangerous occurrences must be recorded in a special accident book and notified without delay to the local office of the Health and Safety Executive. It is a wise precaution in practice to record all accidents and potentially dangerous incidents in an accident book even though they may, at the time, appear to be trivial and not serious enough to be notifiable. Needlestick and similar injuries with a risk of cross-infection should always be entered in an accident book.

Fire precautions

These will vary according to the size and nature of each practice but should be checked by seeking the advice and approval of the local fire prevention officer. Fire precautions in a dental practice are, in general, the same as those applying to any other place of work. However, certain materials and drugs used in dentistry are flammable and special care must be taken with them, for example, acrylic monomer, alcoholic disinfectants and methylated spirit. Again, the precautions to be taken are all common-sense measures.

1 Smoke detectors should be installed.
2 There should be an alarm system and a planned means of escape from any part of the premises. Doorways must be unobstructed and fire exit doors clearly marked.
3 Fire-fighting equipment must be easily accessible and properly maintained. Depending on the particular practice, fire extinguishers, fire blankets and hoses should be provided, as advised by the local fire prevention officer.

4   Flammable substances should be stored in non-spill containers in locked cabinets in a no-smoking area, again as advised by the fire prevention officer.

5   Instructions for the procedure to be adopted in case of fire should be prominently displayed and understood by all the staff. A person designated as Fire Officer for the premises should provide training in use of fire extinguishers and arrange for fire drill to be practised periodically.

In the event of a fire, the first and foremost consideration is the safety of everybody on the premises. On discovery of an outbreak of fire:

1   Raise the alarm.

2   Unless the fire can be contained immediately with the equipment available, make an emergency call (999) to the local fire brigade.

3   Evacuate the premises.

4   Every room must be checked to see that nobody is left inside; gas and electricity must be turned off; and windows and doors closed.

5   Do not use lifts for evacuation.

6   All persons evacuated from the premises should assemble, as instructed, in a safe area and a check made to ensure that everybody is accounted for. The appointment or day book may be very useful in this respect.

7   No risks should be taken in misguided attempts to salvage property or equipment. Safety of life is the prime consideration.

Substances hazardous to health

Under the *Control of Substances Hazardous to Health Regulations* (COSHH), dentists are required to make an assessment of hazardous substances in their practice This must be followed by the issue of written instructions on accident procedure and staff training to reduce any risks as much as possible. The regulations cover laboratory chemicals, disinfectants, mercury, biological hazards, clinical waste disposal and staff protection. Records of the practice COSHH assessment must be kept and updated regularly. Failure to comply with these regulations is an offence under the Health and Safety at Work Act.

Storage

All chemicals should be stored in cupboards with separate storage for inflammable substances and poisons. Mercury must be stored in a cool cupboard in properly sealed containers. Glutaraldehyde should be stored away from heat and direct sunlight.

Ventilation

Adequate ventilation is essential to minimize any risk of dangerous or irritant vapours from mercury, disinfectants, anaesthetic gases and laboratory chemicals.

Disinfectants

Some disinfectants used in dental practice can irritate skin, airway and eyes. Gloves, mask and glasses should be worn when handling them and working areas must be well ventilated to avoid irritation of the airway.

Glutaraldehyde is the most irritant disinfectant and its use should accordingly be confined to applications unsuitable for hypochlorite.

Waste disposal

Surgery (clinical) waste must not be included or collected with normal domestic waste. It should be separately packaged in hazard-labelled, yellow plastic sacks, together with chemical waste. Sharps and glass (ampoules and cartridges) must be sealed in special rigid, puncture-proof containers complying with the British Standard; and to avoid injury to refuse handlers, they must not be overfilled. All clinical waste must be collected for incineration by authorized and registered operatives and records of these arrangements should be kept.

Non-clinical (office and domestic) waste is stored in black plastic sacks to distinguish it from clinical waste; and the normal domestic waste-collection service should be used for its disposal.

Staff protection

Staff should be provided with waterproof aprons, gloves, masks and glasses for handling irritant chemicals, disinfectants and X-ray processing solutions. Biological hazards such as exposure to blood-borne infection are covered by the practice cross-infection procedure.

Laboratory hazards

Dentists and dental staff are legally required to practise and maintain rigorous standards of safety within their own laboratory.

1 Laboratory compressors, like surgery compressors, present an explosion risk and must be regularly inspected, tested and serviced in accordance with manufacturers' instructions. They

should be covered with a protective shield and sited safely. Records of inspection and maintenance must be kept.

2 Grinding and polishing dentures, especially chrome-cobalt ones, produces a great deal of dust. Masks and goggles must be worn to prevent the inhalation of dust or injury to eyes from flying debris.

3 Staff working in the vicinity of lathes should not have long hair, ties or loose clothing which could get caught in rotating machinery. All such equipment should have guards fitted.

4 Heat-treatment and casting equipment must be housed so as to avoid fire risks and injury to the user. Protective clothing and special handling instruments must be provided for carrying heated casting rings.

5 Acid and electro-plating baths must be properly housed as they may emit toxic fumes or cause burns if splashed on the skin. A 4% sodium bicarbonate solution is used for treatment of acid burns and all dental first aid kits should contain a bottle.

6 Efficient ventilation equipment must be installed to extract dust, toxic fumes and irritant vapours. The inhalation of vapour from acrylic monomer, acid and electro-plating baths can be very dangerous.

7 Flammable substances must be kept well away from sources of fire.

Surgery hazards

The most important hazards facing dental staff arise from cross-infection, use of mercury and taking X-ray films. General anaesthesia and sedation are potentially hazardous procedures for patients and they, too, must be protected under the Health and Safety at Work Act. These hazards are covered in the chapters on infection control, general anaesthesia, amalgam and radiography; but the precautions to be taken are summarized in this chapter for the sake of completeness.

Other risks in dental practice include:

1 Use of toxic or corrosive materials
2 Inhalation of waste anaesthetic gases
3 Injury from faulty or improper use of sterilizers and air compressors

These particular risks are also covered in other chapters, but in general they may be guarded against as follows:

1 Correct storage, handling and use of drugs. They must be kept in a separate locked cabinet
2 Good ventilation. A scavenging system for waste anaesthetic gases should be used during GA and RA

3 Meticulously following manufacturers' instructions on the use and maintenance of all equipment and materials
4 Wearing protective clothing

Protective clothing

Gowns, masks and gloves minimize the transmission of infection from patient or instruments to staff. Surgical gloves prevent absorption of mercury when handling amalgam, and will also prevent irritation of sensitive skin by X-ray processing solutions. Heavy-duty gloves protect against injury when scrubbing instruments prior to sterilization.

Protective glasses with full lenses and side-shields can prevent eye damage from infected material or amalgam particles when a water spray is used. They should also be worn by patients undergoing treatment in a supine position, where they are at risk of injury from dropped instruments, acid etching liquids and other materials. Dark glasses or shields are necessary when using light-cured filling materials.

Jewellery, wrist watch and open-toed shoes should not be worn in the surgery.

Cross-infection

Dental staff are at constant risk of infection from patients and used instruments. The sources of infection are:

1 Direct contact with a patient's blood or saliva
2 Droplet infection from a patient's exhaled air
3 The aerosol cloud produced by a water spray when using a high-speed handpiece or ultrasonic scaler
4 Instruments awaiting sterilization
5 Inoculation injury such as needlestick

Pathways by which infection is transmitted to staff are skin cuts or abrasions, the airway and eyes.

Ways of avoiding these risks would be outlined in the practice infection control policy (Chapter 10), issued to all members of staff to clarify their duties and indicate who is responsible for dealing with them. The following precautions are taken to prevent cross-infection of staff and patients:

1 Wear protective clothing at all times in the surgery:
   (a) uniform coat or gown
   (b) new mask and gloves for each patient
   (c) protective glasses for staff and patients

2   If any blood splashes on to an exposed part of the body, wash it off with water immediately

3   Use an efficient aspirator whenever water spraying equipment is used

4   Use rubber dam whenever possible to minimize the infected aerosol effect of water spray and compressed air

5   Keep the surgery well ventilated

6   Use as much disposable material as possible

7   All clinical waste must be packed in heavy-duty yellow plastic sacks and approved sharps containers ready for incineration

8   Wear heavy-duty waterproof gloves when cleaning instruments prior to sterilization

9   Sterilize instruments for the correct time at the correct temperature

10   Work surfaces should be cleaned and disinfected or covered with a waterproof disposable sheet between patients

11   Great care must be taken to ensure that sterile instruments are not contaminated before use on another patient

12   Hands must be washed and new gloves worn before laying up for the next patient or handling clean instruments

13   Laboratory work should be disinfected with hypochlorite

Special care must be taken if child patients have been in contact with virus infections such as mumps and German measles (*rubella*). The virus is present in saliva before any signs of illness are apparent, and surgery staff may become infected in this way from an apparently fit child.

1   Rubella in the first three months of pregnancy can cause serious physical defects in the unborn child; and there are strong medical grounds for advising the termination of pregnancy in such cases.

2   Mumps can cause sterility in mature males.

If there is any evidence of contact with these diseases, treatment of the children concerned should be postponed. This will protect staff, and adult patients in the waiting room, from any risk of infection.

Staff should be immunized against hepatitis B, rubella, poliomyelitis, and bacterial infections such as pertussis (whooping cough), diphtheria, tetanus and tuberculosis.

Hepatitis B and AIDS

These diseases can be fatal and are transmitted by contact with the blood of a sufferer or carrier. Special care must accordingly be taken when known sufferers or carriers are being treated. The basic safety principle involved is the avoidance of any contact with the patient's blood or blood-stained saliva. The hepatitis B virus (HBV) or AIDS virus (HIV) can infect via the skin, mucous membrane, eyes or airway.

The precautions already given for prevention of cross-infection must be followed for *every* patient seen in a dental practice because the majority of carriers are either unaware of their condition or unwilling to disclose it. However, for known carriers or sufferers some extra precautions are recommended.

1 Reserve the last appointment of the day for their treatment. This allows ample time after completion of treatment for sterilization of instruments and disinfection of the surgery
2 Move all unnecessary equipment and furniture away from the working area
3 Regard steel burs and matrix bands as disposable
4 Items which cannot be sterilized by heat, or disinfected with hypochlorite, should be immersed in glutaraldehyde for three hours
5 If any blood splashes on to an exposed part of the body, wash it off with water immediately
6 All staff must be vaccinated against HBV
7 Patients with the active disease, or carriers requiring procedures involving much loss of blood, should be referred to a specialist unit

Surgery water supply

Dental equipment must be prevented from contaminating the public water supply. It should accordingly be modified if necessary to incorporate an air gap for the prevention of backflow into the mains supply.

Mercury

Mercury is poisonous. It is used in dentistry solely for amalgam fillings; but as these are the commonest fillings used, mercury is a continual hazard in dental practice and constant vigilance is necessary. It can enter the body from mercury itself, from mixed amalgam or during the removal of old amalgam fillings. Absorption is by inhalation of mercury vapour and amalgam particles; or through bare skin by contact with amalgam or mercury.

Mercury vapour is invisible and odourless. It is released from mercury or waste amalgam which is exposed to the air; and the higher the temperature, the greater the amount of vapour released.

Early symptoms of mercury poisoning are vague and usually unrecognizable as such. Later, however, serious effects can occur and the vision and kidneys may be affected. Mercury has been used for so long in dentistry, with so little obvious harm, that its dangers should be kept in proper perspective. It is perfectly safe to use, provided that appropriate precautions are taken to prevent the release of mercury vapour into the surgery and to avoid all contact with the skin. To avoid unnecessary exposure to mercury, staff should not use the surgery as a changing room, rest room or dining room.

Precautions

To avoid absorption of mercury through the skin:

1   Wear gloves when using mercury, handling amalgam and cleaning amalgam instruments
2   Do not wear open-toed shoes as floors could be contaminated by dropped amalgam

To avoid pollution of the air by mercury vapour:

1   Containers of mercury must be tightly sealed and stored in a cool place
2   Great care must be taken not to spill mercury or drop any amalgam. Use funnels or squeeze bottles when transferring mercury from a stock container to a smaller bottle or an amalgamator
3   Store amalgam and mercury waste in a sealed, labelled container of old X-ray fixer solution
4   Do not re-use disposable amalgamator capsules
5   When removing old amalgam fillings, wear a mask, gloves and glasses; use an efficient aspirator, rubber dam, and keep the surgery well ventilated
6   All traces of amalgam must be removed from instruments before sterilization.

Surgery hygiene

1   Storage and handling of mercury can be avoided altogether by the use of prepacked capsules of mercury and alloy.
2   Dispensing of mercury and preparation of amalgam must be done over a drip tray (lined with kitchen foil) on a special work surface. A drip tray prevents loss of spilled mercury and facilitates recovery. The work surface must not have a slope which allows spilled mercury to fall on the floor; and must not have any joints, cracks or crevices which could prevent the recovery of spilled mercury or amalgam.
3   Floor coverings, too, must not have any joint, cracks, gaps or other

places which are inaccessible for the recovery of spillages. Carpets should never be used.

4 Efficient ventilation is essential at all times of the year and high surgery temperatures should be avoided.

5 Waste amalgam has recycling value and recorded arrangements should be made for its collection by authorized scrap-dealers. It must not be sent by post.

Mercury spillage

Accidental spillage of mercury or waste amalgam must always be reported to the dentist. *Never be afraid to do this.* If a spillage occurs, globules of mercury can be sucked up with a disposable syringe or bulb aspirator and transferred to a mercury container. Lead foil from intra-oral X-ray film packets can be used to absorb small spillages. Waste amalgam can be gathered with a damp paper towel.

Globules of mercury or particles of amalgam which are too small or too numerous to be recovered in this way can be rendered safe by smearing the contaminated area with a mercury absorbent paste. Special mercury spillage kits are available commercially.

Always wear disposable gloves for the recovery of mercury or amalgam. Never use a vacuum cleaner as this will vaporize the mercury and discharge it back into the surgery.

Detection of mercury vapour

If a serious spillage occurs, or there are other reasons for suspecting mercury contamination in the surgery, tests are available for determining the amount of mercury vapour in the air.

If such tests show an excessive concentration of mercury vapour, expert advice should be sought to trace and eradicate the cause. Hospital tests can also be arranged to check whether staff have absorbed dangerous amounts of mercury.

Radiation

X-rays are dangerous. An overdose can give rise to serious effects ranging from a mild burn to leukaemia. As X-rays cannot be perceived by any of the senses, and any harmful effects may take years to develop, it is only too easy to forget their dangers and ignore safety precautions. Dental X-ray dosage is too low to adversely affect patients; the most vulnerable persons are those actually taking the radiographs.

Under the Health and Safety at Work Act, dentists are legally obliged to protect their staff and patients against the harmful effects of radiation. All practices using X-ray sets must notify the local office of the Health and Safety Executive; and must comply with the *Ionizing Radiations Regulations*. The legal requirements are as follows:

1   X-ray sets must be professionally maintained and serviced regularly. No unauthorized persons may interfere with X-ray equipment. Radiation safety in the practice must be assessed every three years by the National Radiological Protection Board (NRPB).
2   Every practice must appoint a radiation protection supervisor (RPS) to ensure compliance with the regulations. This would normally be the dentist.
3   Written local rules for ensuring radiation protection must be displayed in the practice. They must:

   (a)   Designate a *controlled area*. This is an exclusion zone of radius 1.5 m around the chair where X-ray exposures are made. Nobody but the patient is allowed inside a controlled area during exposure. The operator stands outside the area, out of the direct path of the X-ray beam, at the full length of the cable on the time switch.
   (b)   Describe the safety precautions required in the practice to ensure protection of patients and staff; and to ensure that films are correctly processed.
   (c)   Provide a contingency plan specifying action to be taken in the event of equipment malfunction. For example, if the exposure warning light or audible signal remains on after the exposure time has elapsed, the mains supply to the set must be switched off *immediately*. The set must not be used again until the cause has been found and rectified

4   All staff involved in the taking and processing of X-ray films must be adequately trained for their duties.
5   If more than 150 intra-oral or 50 DPT films a week are taken, staff involved should wear a personal monitoring dosemeter. The RPS will take appropriate action if excessive radiation is recorded.
6   Practices using cephalometric equipment, or taking more than 40 DPT or 360 intra-oral films a week, must have a radiation protection advisor (RPA). An RPA would usually be a radiation physicist who regularly checks, monitors and advises practices on all aspects of radiation hygiene.

Precautions

The basic principles of radiation protection are to take the minimum number of films, with the shortest possible exposure times, confining the X-ray beam to no more than the film area; and for the operator to keep out of the direct beam, as far away as possible. Correct procedure is as follows.

1 Do not take unnecessary films
2 Use the fastest possible film (E speed) and rare earth intensifying screens to give the shortest exposure time
3 For sets with adjustable apertures, always use the minimum size aperture for the film area used
4 Replace plastic director cone with rectangular collimator tube
5 Use film holder/beam-aiming devices and the paralleling technique whenever possible
6 Operators must stand at the full length of the cable (at least 2 metres) and out of the direct beam of X-rays
7 The operator must *never* hold a film in place for a patient
8 No unnecessary personnel should be in the surgery when an X-ray set is used
9 There must be no need for retakes due to faulty technique. To ensure perfect results, films must be in good condition, taken correctly, processed carefully and mounted properly

General anaesthesia and sedation

GDC requirements for the safety of patients undergoing these procedures are as follows.

1 Before GA or sedation procedures a full medical history must be taken; precise written pre- and post-operative instructions given; and adequate records of the procedure kept
2 For GA, an anaesthetist and a dentist must be present
3 For GA, three fully trained dental nurses must be present throughout: one to assist the anaesthetist with monitoring the patient's condition and any resuscitation measures; the second to assist the dentist with the operative procedure; and a third must be in constant attendance in the recovery room
4 A dentist may use sedation techniques and act as operator, provided that a nurse, fully trained and experienced in sedation, monitoring and resuscitation procedures, is present throughout
5 Whenever GA or sedation is used, proper facilities and equipment must be available for their administration; monitoring of patients' condition; resuscitation; and recovery. All staff taking part must be fully trained for these procedures
6 Patients must not be left unattended in the recovery room, or allowed to return home without an escort. Only the anaesthetist or dentist may specify the patient as fit for discharge

Apart from GA and sedation, patients may require resuscitation for reasons other than dental treatment. All practice staff are therefore required to be fully trained and practised in basic life support (Chapter 15).

Written examination

Write short notes on:

(a) protection of the eyes
(b) protection of the hands
(c) needlestick injuries (May 1996)

How should a dental establishment ensure the health and safety of staff and patients in relation to:

(a) premises
(b) fire (November 1995)

What should a dental nurse do in the event of these mishaps occurring?

(a) pricking a finger with a needle which has just been used for a dental injection
(b) a spillage of mercury in the surgery
(c) a patient slipping on a wet floor on the dental premises (November 1990)

Summary

Health and Safety at Work Act

Requires:

- Provision and maintenance of safe equipment, appliances and systems of work
- Safe handling and storage of dangerous substances
- Safe premises, access and egress
- Safe working environment
- Adequate and suitable staff welfare facilities
- Staff training to ensure health and safety

- Provision of first-aid facilities
- Co-operation between employer and staff on safety measures adopted
- Notification of accidents – major injury and dangerous occurrences

Fire precautions

- Consult fire brigade for advice
- Alarm system and escape routes
- Extinguishers, fire blankets and hoses
- Evacuation procedure
- Regular fire drill
- Safe storage of flammable material

Outbreak of fire

1 Raise alarm
2 Close doors and windows
3 Attempt to extinguish fire
4 Call fire brigade if unsuccessful
5 Switch off gas and electricity
6 Evacuate premises
7 Roll call

Control of Substances Hazardous to Health (COSHH)

- Staff training obligatory
- Written instructions for staff protection and accident procedure involving:

  o mercury
  o disinfectants
  o X-ray processing solutions
  o waste anaesthetic gases
  o laboratory chemicals
  o disposal of clinical waste

Laboratory hazards

1 Compressors → explosion risk
   Regular inspection, testing and maintenance required
2 Grinding and polishing → inhalation of dust, eye injuries
   Wear mask and goggles; good ventilation; guards on lathes → no long hair, ties or loose clothing

3 Heat treatment and casting equipment → fire risk, burns
   Wear protective clothing; correct handling
4 Acid and electro-plating baths → burns, toxic fumes
   Protective clothing; good ventilation

Surgery hazards

1 Cross-infection
2 Mercury poisoning
3 Radiation
4 Toxic or corrosive materials
5 Inhalation of waste anaesthetic gases
6 Faulty equipment → compressors, autoclaves → explosion risk

General precautions

Protective clothing:

(a) Operating gown or uniform coat
(b) Glasses → water spray, curing light, supine patient
(c) Mask → droplet infection ← colds, coughs, sore throat, water spray
(d) Operating gloves → cuts, abrasions, handling mercury and disinfectants, processing radiographs
(e) Heavy-duty gloves → cleaning instruments

• Efficient suction
• Good ventilation
• Correct storage, handling and use of drugs
• Prevent contamination of main water supply:
  ○ Surgery equipment water lines must have air gap to prevent backflow into mains supply

Follow manufacturers' instructions on use, care and maintenance of equipment.

Cross-infection

• From patient's blood, saliva, droplet infection, water spray
• Enters airway, eyes, skin cuts and abrasions

1 Protective clothing
2 Efficient suction
3 Good ventilation
4 Disposable equipment
5 Safe waste disposal

6 Correct sterilization procedure
7 Clean and disinfect work surfaces or use sterile disposable covers
8 Wash hands and fit new gloves and mask between patients and before handling clean instruments
9 Postpone treatment of mumps and rubella contacts
10 Vaccination: HBV, rubella, poliomyelitis, tetanus, pertussis, diphtheria, tuberculosis

Hepatitis B and AIDS

Extra precautions for known carriers:

1 Refer to hospital for:

  (a) patients with active disease
  (b) multiple extractions and minor oral surgery

2 Last appointment
3 Move unnecessary equipment and furniture out of way
4 Use glutaraldehyde to sterilize items unsuitable for heat or other disinfectants
5 Contact public health authority if accidental infection suspected
6 HBV vaccination for all staff

Mercury poisoning

- Absorbed through skin or inhaled
- Wear gloves
- Prepare amalgam over drip tray on special work surface
- Use prepacked capsules of alloy and mercury
- Keep waste mercury and amalgam in sealed, labelled container of old X-ray fixer solution
- Remove all traces of amalgam from instruments prior to sterilization
- Do not flush waste amalgam particles down surgery spittoons or sinks
- Arrange collection of waste amalgam for recycling. Do not send by post
- No carpets or open-toed shoes
- Keep surgery well ventilated

Mercury spillage

- Must be reported
- Collect mercury with disposable syringe, bulb aspirator or lead foil

- Gather amalgam with damp paper towel
- Remove remainder with mercury absorbent paste

Radiation

- Staff training
- Comply with practice local rules for radiation safety
- Regular professional maintenance of X-ray set
- Use fastest (E speed) film and rare earth intensifying screens
- Use rectangular collimator tube, film holder/beam-aiming devices and paralleling technique.
- Only the patient or parent must hold the film in place
- Stand well clear of X-ray beam, at full length of cable, during exposure
- Wear personal monitoring dosemeter

General anaesthesia and sedation

For protection of patient:

1 Full medical history and written pre- and post-operative instructions required before GA or sedation given. Records of procedure must be kept
2 GA must not be given single-handed by an operator/anaesthetist
3 GA may only be given by a second dentist or doctor who is properly trained and experienced and remains with the patient throughout the procedure
4 At least three fully trained nurses for GA:

- assist dentist
- assist anaesthetist
- recovery room

5 Sedation can be given by a dentist single-handed if a properly trained and experienced dental nurse is present throughout
6 Adequate equipment, facilities and training for all concerned with GA, sedation, monitoring and resuscitation

Collapse

Collapse may occur for many reasons, other than GA or sedation, in a dental practice. All practice staff are required to be fully trained, equipped and practised in basic life support.

Index

The most important references are printed in **bold** type.